Review Questions for
HUMAN PATHOLOGY

A Review for the USMLE
Step 1, 2 and 3 Examinations

Review Questions for HUMAN PATHOLOGY

A Review for the USMLE
Step 1, 2 and 3 Examinations

by

Robin R. Jones, MD, PhD

Professor, Department of Pathology
University of Arkansas for Medical Sciences

Review Questions Series
Series Editor: Thomas R. Gest, PhD
University of Arkansas for Medical Sciences

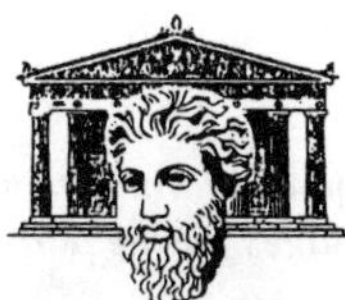

The Parthenon Publishing Group
International Publishers in Medicine, Science & Technology

NEW YORK   LONDON

Published in the USA by
The Parthenon Publishing Group Inc.
One Blue Hill Plaza,
PO Box 1564, Pearl River,
New York 10965, USA

Published in Europe by
The Parthenon Publishing Group Limited
Casterton Hall, Carnforth,
Lancs., LA6 2LA, UK

Library of Congress Cataloging-in-Publication Data

Jones, Robin, R.
    Review questions for human pathology / by Robin R. Jones.
       p.   cm. -- (Review questions series)
    ISBN: 1-85070-599-2
    1. Human pathology -- Examinations, questions, etc. I. Title.
II. Series.
    [DNLM: 1. Pathology -- examination questions. QZ 18.2 J78r 1998]
RB119.J66 1998
616.07'076 -- dc21
DNLM/DLC
for Library of Congress   97-47206
                                                   CIP

British Library Cataloguing in Publication Data

Jones, Robin R.
    Review questions for human pathology. – (Review questions series)
    1. Human pathology – Examinations, questions, etc.
    I. Title
    616'.07'076

    ISBN 1-85070-599-2

Printed in the USA

Acknowledgements

I would like to acknowledge the Department of Pathology faculty at the University of Arkansas for Medical Sciences (UAMS) who wrote the questions used in this review text. The questions in this text were chosen from pathology examinations administered at UAMS over the past 5 years. I especially want to thank the following colleagues at UAMS who wrote the feedback responses for various parts of the section on hematopathology: Tom Rozenzweig, MD and Carla Wilson, MD, for their work on lymphomas and leukemias, myelomas, and related disorders; Darrell W. Swank, MD, for his work on anemias; and Bruce Marshall, MD, for his work on coagulation and transfusion therapy.

In addition, I wish to thank my colleagues Harry Brown, MD, for writing the feedback responses for the sections on pediatric diseases and diseases of the eye, and Tony Butch, PhD, for his contributions to the feedback responses in the section on immune disorders.

Finally, I owe a great deal of thanks to a friend, Mr Jaime Hurtado, who spent many hours editing and formatting the manuscript of this book.

Reference resources for this book include:

Cotran RS, Kumar V, Robbins SL. *Robbins Pathologic Basis of Disease*, 5th edn. Philadelphia: WB Saunders, 1994

Harmening DM, ed. *Modern Blood Banking and Transfusion Practices,* 3rd edn. Philadelphia: FA Davis, 1994

Hathaway WE, Goodnight SH, eds. *Disorders of Hemostasis and Thrombosis: A Clinical Guide*. New York: McGraw–Hill, 1993

Hull R, Pino GF, eds. *Disorders of Thrombosis*, 1st edn. Philadelphia: WB Saunders, 1996

Ratnoff OD, Forbes CD, eds. *Disorders of Hemostasis*, 3rd edn. Philadelphia: WB Saunders, 1996

Rubin E, Farber JL. *Pathology*, 2nd edn. Philadelphia: JB Lippincott, 1994

Sandstad JS, McKenna RW, Keffer JH. *Handbook of Clinical Pathology*. Chicago: American Society of Clinical Pathology Press, 1992

Robin R. Jones, MD, PhD

Preface

This book is designed to be a review guide in preparation for examinations in pathology. I would like to stress the word "review", as this book can only be helpful after a student has thoroughly learned the subject by reading traditional textbooks on the subject and participating in formal educational courses in pathology. After a student has mastered a certain topic, this book will be helpful as a means of self-assessment as well as a source of information in the form of feedback reinforcement of the correct answers. After using this book as a self-assessment tool, defined areas of weakness should be corrected by returning to traditional textbooks for further study.

The questions in this book are all taken from pathology examinations administered at the University of Arkansas for Medical Sciences (UAMS) over the past 5 years. The information presented in courses in pathology does not vary greatly from school to school and, therefore, the questions in this book will, for the most part, reflect the core information presented at most medical schools.

Most of the questions in this book are standard National Board format four- or five-choice questions, requiring a single best answer. Some of the questions are similar to the National Board extended format, and include more than five choices.

Throughout the book, you may find several questions that appear to be similar. This is because testing on an important concept with questions that use slightly different approaches often proves to be particularly helpful.

My recommendation to users of this book is to take one page at a time, covering the right-hand side of the page with a sheet of paper so that the answers and feedback responses cannot be seen. Answer each question by writing your response on the sheet of paper. After you have finished a page, check your answers, read the feedback responses, and continue on to the next page. After completing a section, identify areas of weakness and consult a textbook of pathology to strengthen those areas. After some time has elapsed, you may wish to return to the same questions in this book to determine if you have improved your knowledge of the subject.

GOOD LUCK!!

Contents

The number in parentheses indicates the number of questions available.

SECTION 1: CELLULAR REACTION TO INJURY

1.001   The increased level of the serum enzyme aspartate aminotransferase following a myocardial infarction is due to:
    A. mitochondrial swelling
    B. nuclear lysis
    C. increased permeability of plasma membranes
    D. increased endoplasmic reticulum
    E. increased Golgi activity

C is correct.
After ischemic cell injury, there is membrane injury which results in the leaking out of cytoplasmic contents such as enzymes. This is reflected by an elevation of the serum concentration of those enzymes.

1.002   Which one of the following is the earliest morphologic sign of hypoxic cell injury?
    A. karyorrhexis
    B. pyknosis
    C. cell swelling
    D. rupture of cell membranes
    E. glycogen accumulation

C is correct.
In hypoxic injury, there is decreased ATP and ATP-ase, resulting in failure of the cell membrane sodium pump. This allows sodium and water to enter the cell, causing cell swelling.

1.003   The pathogenesis of reversible fatty change in the liver is BEST described by which one of the following general mechanisms?
    A. lack of a degradative enzyme normally present in lysosomes
    B. accumulation of indigestible materials
    C. inability to degrade phagocytosed particles
    D. autophagy of abnormal cell organelles
    E. abnormal metabolism of normal lipid constituents

E is correct.
Lipid may abnormally accumulate in hepatocytes due to excessive entry of free fatty acids, enhanced fatty acid synthesis, decreased fatty acid oxidation, increased esterification of fatty acids, decreased apoprotein synthesis, or impaired lipoprotein secretion. The lipid constituents, however, are normal.

1.004 Which one of the following is LEAST likely to be associated with an organ of abnormal size?
    A. hypoplasia
    B. metaplasia
    C. congestion
    D. atrophy
    E. hyperplasia

B is correct.
Hypoplasia and atrophy both cause decreased size of an organ. Congestion, due to the increased amount of blood, and hyperplasia (due to increased numbers of cells), cause organ enlargement. Metaplasia in itself only involves an alteration in cell type, such as ciliated respiratory epithelium changing to squamous.

1.005   The MOST likely 'final common pathway' of cell injury in such varied processes as reperfusion injury, chemical and radiation injury, oxygen toxicity, cellular aging, and inflammatory damage involves:
    A. activation of proteases
    B. free radical generation
    C. increased phospholipid degradation
    D. polyribosome detachment
    E. decreased DNA synthesis

B is correct.
Free radicals have a single unpaired electron in the outer orbital. As a result, they are highly reactive and enter into reactions with cell membrane components. Many processes may initiate free radical generation within cells.

1.006 Which of the following is MOST likely to occur in cells injured by hypoxia?
   A. decreased intracellular sodium
   B. increased intracellular potassium
   C. decreased cell membrane surface area
   D. increased intracellular pH
   E. decreased intracellular proteins

E is correct.
In hypoxic injury, cells accumulate sodium and water, lose potassium, and have a decreased pH due to anaerobic metabolism. The cell membrane surface area is increased due to the swelling. Proteins (including enzymes) leak out of the cell due to the damaged, leaky, membrane.

1.007 Which one of the following is LEAST likely to be seen in cell injury?
   A. lipid accumulation
   B. cell swelling
   C. alterations in nuclear chromatin
   D. increase in intracellular glycogen
   E. mitochondrial dilation

D is correct.
All occur in cell injury except glycogen accumulation. Glycogen in fact decreases in cells injured by hypoxia due to the conversion to anaerobic metabolism and activation of glycolysis.

1.008 Which one of the following is the BEST indicator of necrosis?
   A. karyolysis
   B. cessation of mitosis
   C. accumulation of polymorphonuclear
      leukocytes
   D. cellular and interstitial edema
   E. decrease in membrane-bound ATP

A is correct.
Good indicators of necrosis are found in the nucleus. Karyolysis, or nuclear fading, is one of the classic nuclear changes seen in necrosis.

1.009 Irreversible ischemic damage in the nervous system typically presents morphologically as:
   A. coagulation
   B. liquefaction
   C. caseation
   D. neurofibrillary tangles
   E. neuronal lipid accumulation

B is correct.
Irreversible ischemic damage in the nervous system characteristically presents as liquefaction necrosis. Due to the high lipid content of neural tissue, there is rapid dissolution of the tissue with no cell outlines visible.

1.010 The nature of the cell response to viral replication may take any of the following forms EXCEPT:
   A. cell lysis
   B. cytoskeletal alterations
   C. coagulation necrosis
   D. formation of syncytial giant cells
   E. development of inclusion bodies

C is correct.
Coagulation necrosis is typically seen in infarcts, and is not associated with viral injury.

1.011 Which one of the following morphologic features is LEAST helpful in distinguishing post-mortem autolysis from coagulation necrosis?
   A. polymorphonuclear leukocyte infiltrate
   B. a zone of active hyperemia
   C. karyolysis, pyknosis, and karyorrhexis
   D. wedge-shaped zone of dead cells surrounded
      by normal-looking cells

C is correct.
Karyolysis, pyknosis, and karyorrhexis are nuclear changes which are seen in both coagulation necrosis and post-mortem autolysis. Leukocyte infiltration and active hyperemia are vascular responses which cannot occur after death. A focal zone of dead cells surrounded by normal cells is not seen in post-mortem autolysis.

1.012   Each of the following changes occur in a cell damaged by hypoxia EXCEPT:
   A. decreased pH
   B. alteration in intracellular osmotic load
   C. dissociation of polysomes into monosomes
   D. decreased rate of anaerobic glycolysis
   E. decreased membrane ATP-ase activity

D is correct.
Due to the hypoxia, energy production becomes more dependent on anaerobic glycolysis. Therefore, the rate of anaerobic glycolysis increases rather than decreases in hypoxia. All of the other changes listed characteristically occur in hypoxia.

1.013   Which one of the following morphologic changes is irreversible?
   A. swelling of the endoplasmic reticulum
   B. mitochondrial swelling
   C. karyolysis
   D. surface-membrane blebs
   E. clumping of nuclear chromatin

C is correct.
All of the morphologic changes listed in this question are reversible except for karyolysis. Karyolysis is nuclear fading due to breakdown of DNA by enzymatic action.

1.014   Which one of the following elements is believed to be an important mediator of the biochemical alterations leading to cell death?
   A. sodium
   B. potassium
   C. calcium
   D. magnesium
   E. copper

C is correct.
Although the exact event responsible for cell death has not been identified, influx of calcium into the injured cell plays a significant role in cell death.

1.015   The BEST example of adaptive hypertrophy is:
   A. endometrium during the menstrual cycle
   B. adrenal glands after excess ACTH secretion
   C. prostate gland in aging
   D. myocardium in systemic hypertension
   E. thyroid gland in iodine-deficient goiter

D is correct.
In systemic hypertension, the heart must work against increased pressure to pump blood. To meet this increased demand for work, the myocardial cells adapt by undergoing hypertrophy. The other examples given are various types of hyperplasia.

1.016   Hyperplasia is LEAST likely to be associated with:
   A. ischemia
   B. DNA synthesis
   C. partial hepatectomy
   D. pregnancy
   E. prostatic enlargement

A is correct.
Ischemia, or inadequate oxygen delivery to tissues, is likely to be associated with atrophy, or decreases in organ size in an attempt to adapt to the environmental stress by decreasing the metabolic needs of the tissue. All of the other choices are associated with hyperplasia.

1.017   A final common pathway of cell injury in such varied processes as chemical and radiation injury, cellular aging, and microbial killing by phagocytic cells is closely linked to:
   A. free radicals
   B. phosphorylase
   C. opsonins
   D. fatty acids
   E. carbon dioxide

A is correct.
Free radicals are chemical forms which have a single unpaired electron in an outer orbital. They are extremely unstable and enter reactions with cell constituents. Free radicals may be formed within cells in a wide variety of injuries.

1.018 When phenobarbital is given to an experimental animal over a period of time, there is a marked increase in the smooth endoplasmic reticulum of hepatocytes. This is an example of:

A. neoplasia
B. hyperplasia
C. hypertrophy
D. metaplasia
E. hydropic change

C is correct.
The increased demand for metabolism of phenobarbital by the hepatocytes is met by the cells increasing their endoplasmic reticulum. These ER-filled cells become larger. There is no cell division involved; therefore, this represents hypertrophy.

1.019 In enzymatic fat necrosis, there is a deposit formed from the chemical combination of free fatty acids and:

A. calcium
B. magnesium
C. sodium
D. potassium
E. glycerol

A is correct.
Pancreatic lipase cleaves triglycerides into glycerol and free fatty acids. The free fatty acids combine with ionized calcium and precipitate as calcium soaps.

1.020 Occlusion of one of the arcuate arteries of the right kidney is MOST likely result in which one of the following types of necrosis?

A. gangrenous
B. caseous
C. liquefaction
D. enzymatic fat
E. coagulation

E is correct.
Sudden occlusion of a renal end-artery will result in sudden tissue hypoxia, which results in necrosis of the coagulation type. The necrotic zone is an infarct.

1.021 Which one of the following types of necrosis is associated with granulomatous inflammation?

A. gangrenous
B. caseous
C. liquefaction
D. enzymatic fat
E. coagulation

B is correct.
Granulomatous inflammation is seen in a variety of situations, one of which is tuberculosis. In this disease, the granulomas characteristically undergo a central necrosis which is called 'caseous' or 'cheese-like' because it grossly resembles white, crumbly cheese.

1.022 Cerebral abscess is MOST likely to contain which one of the following types of necrosis?

A. gangrenous
B. caseous
C. liquefaction
D. enzymatic fat
E. coagulation

C is correct.
Liquefaction, or complete dissolution of cells, typically occurs in infarcts of the central nervous system and in suppurative or purulent necrosis in any organ. Since abscesses are localized areas of suppuration, there is prominent liquefaction necrosis.

1.023 When denaturation is the primary feature in necrosis, the necrotic tissue has which one of the following morphologic patterns?

A. caseous
B. coagulation
C. fatty
D. gangrenous
E. liquefaction

B is correct.
Coagulation necrosis is characterized by cell swelling, breakdown of intracellular organelles, and denaturation of cytoplasmic proteins. There is preservation of the cell outlines presumably because protein denaturation also affects intracellular hydrolases, thus preventing proteolytic degradation of the cell membranes.

1.024   Exposure of cells to anoxia may result in all of the following EXCEPT:
   A. impaired oxidative phosphorylation
   B. decreased ATP reserve
   C. release of enzymes into blood
   D. induction of smooth endoplasmic reticulum
   E. anaerobic glycolysis

D is correct.
Induction of smooth endoplasmic reticulum is an adaptive response which follows the administration of phenobarbital. This is an example of hypertrophy. Such a change would not be expected to occur under conditions of anoxia.

1.025   Of the following, which MOST characteristically causes coagulation necrosis?
   A. bacterial infection
   B. obstruction of blood flow
   C. decrease in hormones
   D. genetic enzyme abnormality
   E. chemical toxins

B is correct.
Coagulation necrosis is a pattern of necrosis where there is conversion of the cell to an opaque acidophilic structure with preservation of cell outlines. This is almost always secondary to sudden loss of blood supply.

1.026   Metaplasia is thought to be caused in MOST cases by:
   A. genetic mutation
   B. oncogenic virus
   C. chronic irritation
   D. immunologic reaction
   E. congenital defect

C is correct.
Metaplasia is commonly seen in the epithelial surfaces of the bronchial tree secondary to chronic irritation of cigarette smoke. Metaplasia may also be seen in areas of long-standing, chronic infections.

1.027   The BEST explanation for the change in cytoplasmic glycogen content in a cell injured by hypoxia is:
   A. active secretion of glycogen by the cell membrane
   B. increased anaerobic glycolysis
   C. sequestration of glycogen inside the mitochondria
   D. increased glycogen synthesis
   E. increased gluconeogenesis

B is correct.
In hypoxic situations, the metabolism of the cell shifts to anaerobic glycolysis so that ATP may be synthesized under conditions of low oxygen. This results in a decrease in glycogen concentration in the hypoxic cell.

1.028   Which one of the following plays the MOST significant role in the pathophysiology of irreversible cell injury?
   A. intracellular changes in potassium concentration
   B. intracellular changes in sodium concentration
   C. mitochondrial swelling
   D. membrane interaction with free radicals
   E. loss of ribosomes

D is correct.
Many varied processes may cause cell injury by a final common pathway which involves generation of chemical species with a single unpaired electron in the outer orbital. These species are termed 'free radicals'.

1.029   Which of the following pairs of terms is MOST appropriately matched?
A. renal infarct / liquefaction necrosis
B. lung infarct / caseous necrosis
C. brain infarct / coagulation necrosis
D. pancreatic abscess / enzymatic fat necrosis
E. hepatic abscess / liquefaction necrosis

E is correct.
An abscess is a focal collection of suppurative inflammation, or pus, within a solid organ. Due to the large accumulation of polys releasing their hydrolytic enzymes, there is liquefactive necrosis of the tissue.

1.030   Each of the following is associated with an increase in cell size EXCEPT:
A. hypoxia to renal tubular epithelial cells
B. alcohol injury to hepatocytes
C. hepatic amyloidosis
D. viral hepatitis
E. Gaucher's disease

C is correct.
In hepatic amyloidosis, the intercellular amyloid accumulation causes pressure atrophy of the hepatocytes. This is probably secondary to interference with the delivery of oxygen and nutrients to the hepatocytes.

1.031   All of the following are potentially reversible EXCEPT:
A. squamous metaplasia
B. adrenal cortical hyperplasia
C. early necrosis
D. skeletal muscle atrophy

C is correct.
Any kind of necrosis at any stage is an irreversible situation. Hyperplasia, atrophy and metaplasia are all potentially reversible, depending on the environmental conditions.

1.032   A rise in serum enzymes after ischemic injury is MOST closely related to:
A. alterations in cell membranes
B. dissociation of polysomes into monosomes
C. clumping of nuclear chromatin
D. swelling of the endoplasmic reticulum
E. terminal 'burst' of synthesis

A is correct.
Ischemic injury leads to cell membrane damage, which results in an increased permeability of the cell. Intracellular enzymes begin to leak from the cell through the damaged cell membranes.

1.033   All of the following occur in cellular hypertrophy EXCEPT:
A. increase in the number of mitochondria
B. increase in functional capacity
C. ability to revert to normal size
D. increase in nuclear-to-cytoplasmic ratio
E. increase in cell size

D is correct.
There is no increase in nuclear-to-cytoplasmic ratio in cell hypertrophy. Increased nuclear-to-cytoplasmic ratio is a feature which may be seen in certain malignant neoplasms.

1.034   The major difference between metastatic and dystrophic calcification is the:
A. rate of deposition
B. metabolic activity of the tissue
C. serum calcium level
D. age of the patient
E. serum phosphorus level

C is correct.
Dystrophic calcification occurs in damaged or necrotic tissues with normal serum calcium levels. Metastatic calcification occurs in normal tissues due to an elevation of the serum calcium level. Favored sites for metastatic calcification are lung, gastric mucosa and kidney.

1.035   Which one of the following diseases is caused by α-L-iduronidase deficiency?
  A. McArdle's disease
  B. Tay–Sachs disease
  C. Hurler's disease
  D. von Gierke's disease
  E. Gaucher's disease

C is correct.
Hurler's disease or mucopolysaccharidosis-I (MPS-I) results from a deficiency of α-L-iduronidase. Patients with this disease may present with dwarfism, corneal clouding, hepatosplenomegaly, coronary artery and heart valve lesions and skeletal deformities.

1.036   Which one of the following diseases is caused by muscle phosphorylase deficiency?
  A. McArdle's disease
  B. Tay–Sachs disease
  C. Hurler's disease
  D. von Gierke's disease
  E. Gaucher's disease

A is correct.
McArdle's disease results from a deficiency of muscle phosphorylase. This leads to glycogen storage in skeletal muscles, muscle weakness, muscle cramps after exercise, and failure of exercise-induced rise in blood lactate.

1.037   Which one of the following diseases is caused by glucocerebrosidase deficiency?
  A. McArdle's disease
  B. Tay–Sachs disease
  C. Hurler's disease
  D. von Gierke's disease
  E. Gaucher's disease

E is correct.
This disease results in the accumulation of cerebrosides in the mononuclear phagocytic system and, in some forms, in the central nervous system. Patients may present with splenomegaly and bone marrow involvement. Some patients may have central nervous system disorders.

1.038   Massive cardiomegaly and cardiac failure by 2 years of age are findings MOST consistent with which one of the following diseases?
  A. Niemann–Pick disease
  B. von Gierke's disease
  C. Pompe's disease
  D. Hurler's disease
  E. Gaucher's disease

C is correct.
In this disease, there is a deficiency of the lysosomal enzyme acid maltase (α-glucosidase). Glycogen storage is prominent in the heart, resulting in cardiomegaly and cardiac failure usually by 2 years of age.

1.039   Coarse facial features, hepatosplenomegaly, narrowing of coronary arteries are findings MOST consistent with which one of the following diseases?
  A. Niemann–Pick disease
  B. von Gierke's disease
  C. Pompe's disease
  D. Hurler's disease
  E. Gaucher's disease

D is correct.
This is one of the mucopolysaccharidoses in which there is a deficiency of α-L-iduronidase.

1.040   Hepatomegaly, growth retardation, and severe hypoglycemia are features MOST consistent with which one of the following diseases?
  A. Niemann–Pick disease
  B. von Gierke's disease
  C. Pompe's disease
  D. Hurler's disease
  E. Gaucher's disease

B is correct.
This is a glycogen storage disease caused by a deficiency of the enzyme glucose-6-phosphate phosphatase which is essential for the conversion of glucose-6-phosphate to glucose. There is prominent hepatic glycogen accumulation.

1.041 Which one of the following diseases is NOT a lysosomal storage disease?
   A. Gaucher's (glucocerebrosidase deficiency)
   B. von Gierke's (glucose-6-phosphatase deficiency)
   C. Tay–Sachs (hexosaminidase A deficiency)
   D. Pompe's (α-glucosidase deficiency)
   E. Hurler's (α-L-iduronidase deficiency)

B is correct.
von Gierke's disease involves the deficiency of an enzyme which is normally present in the cytosol. This disease results in the accumulation of intracytoplasmic glycogen principally in the liver and kidney.

1.042 All of the following would be expected to occur in widespread, extensive enzymatic fat necrosis EXCEPT:
   A. hypercalcemia
   B. activation of pancreatic lipases
   C. destruction of adipose cell membranes
   D. increased breakdown of triglycerides into fatty acids
   E. focal chalky white deposits in adipose tissue

A is correct.
In fat necrosis, pancreatic enzymes escape, causing hydrolysis of triglcerides. The fatty acids which are released combine with calcium to produce calcium soaps which precipitate in the necrotic tissue. Widespread extensive fat necrosis may deplete serum calcium levels, resulting in hypocalcemia.

1.043 Which one of the following occurs within cells injured by hypoxia?
   A. increased glycogen accumulation
   B. decreased anaerobic glycolysis
   C. increased sodium ion concentration
   D. decreased membrane permeability
   E. increase in pH

C is correct.
In the early stages of hypoxic injury to cells, there is increased anaerobic glycolysis with decreased glycogen concentration within cells and decreased intracellular pH, increased membrane permeability with loss of potassium and an increase in intracellular water and sodium.

1.044 The MOST common etiology of squamous metaplasia involving respiratory epithelium is:
   A. bacterial pneumonia
   B. herpes simplex virus
   C. alcoholism
   D. cigarette-smoking
   E. chronic inhalation of carbon monoxide

D is correct.
The chronic irritation of the respiratory mucosa by cigarette smoke is a stimulus for metaplasia of the respiratory epithelium. It is the most common cause of this change in the respiratory tract.

1.045 Skeletal muscle enlarged by exercise and skeletal muscle decreased in size due to immobilization have which one of the following features in common?
   A. increased glycogen in myocytes
   B. increased numbers of myocyte subcellular organelles
   C. decreased size of individual myocytes
   D. fibrosis
   E. ability to revert to normal size

E is correct.
Atrophy and hypertrophy are both potentially reversible changes.

1.046   Serum elevation of which one of the following substances gives the MOST useful clinical information regarding cell injury?
A. enzymes
B. steroids
C. carbohydrates
D. lipids
E. sodium

A is correct.
Measurement of serum enzymes provides valuable information regarding cell injury. The increased cell permeability of injured cells allows intracellular enzymes, among other cell components, to leak out into the serum. The finding of elevation of certain enzyme concentrations in the serum indicates injury to cells. Some enzymes may be relatively organ-specific, thus indicating which cells are injured.

1.047   The major difference between heterolysis and autolysis is:
A. degree of preservation of cell outlines
B. organ involved
C. reversibility
D. oxygen saturation of the tissue
E. source of the catalytic enzymes

E is correct.
In heterolysis, many of the enzymes responsible for the cell digestion come from inflammatory cells, such as polymorphonuclear leukocytes. In autolysis, the enzymes which cause cell digestion arise from within the lysosomes of the dead cells.

1.048   Each of the following are characteristic morphologic features of apoptosis EXCEPT:
A. cell swelling
B. chromatin condensation
C. cytoplasmic blebs
D. membrane-bound bodies

A is correct.
Apoptosis is a process which is important in programmed cell death. The cells shrink in this process.

1.049   Tay–Sachs disease is a genetic disease due to a deficiency in which one of the following enzymes?
A. hepatic phosphorylase
B. lysosomal glucosidase (acid maltase)
C. hexosaminidase
D. α-L-iduronidase
E. glucocerebrosidase

C is correct.
In this disease, there is a deficiency of hexosaminidase resulting in the lysosomal accumulation of gangliosides, mainly in the brain.

1.050   Pompe's disease is associated with a deficiency of:
A. hepatic phosphorylase
B. lysosomal glucosidase (acid maltase)
C. hexosaminidase
D. α-L-iduronidase
E. glucocerebrosidase

B is correct.
Pompe's disease is a lysosomal storage disease involving glycogen metabolism. A deficiency of lysosomal glucosidase results in the accumulation of glycogen in organs. The heart is especially affected, resulting in cardiomegaly and congestive failure.

1.051   Hypoxia to renal tubular epithelial cells and alcohol injury to hepatocytes have which one of the following findings in common?
A. alteration in cell size
B. metaplastic alteration
C. induction of smooth endoplasmic reticulum
D. increased intracellular glycogen concentration
E. increased lipoprotein synthesis

A is correct.
Hypoxia results in cell swelling in the early stages. There is an influx of water and sodium, causing enlargement of the cell. Alcohol injury to hepatocytes results in the intracellular accumulation of fats, causing enlargement of the cells.

1.052   Increased intracellular concentrations of which one of the following ions has been implicated in the activation of phospolipases, resulting in degradation of membrane phospholipids in cell injury?
    A. magnesium
    B. copper
    C. potassium
    D. sodium
    E. calcium

E is correct.
A prominent decrease in membrane phospholipids occurs in irreversible ischemic injury. It is suggested that the phospholipids are degraded because of activation of endogenous phospholipases by increases in intracellular calcium ion concentrations.

1.053   Tay–Sachs disease and Pompe's disease have which one of the following features in common?
    A. predominant clinical feature is congestive heart failure
    B. accumulation of cytosolic and lysosomal glycogen
    C. deficiency of gangliosidase
    D. accumulation of substance within lysosomes
    E. predominant central nervous system involvement

D is correct.
Tay–Sachs disease is associated with lysosomal accumulation of gangliosides. Pompe's disease is associated with lysosomal accumulation of glycogen.

1.054   The finding of an area of coagulation necrosis in the kidney is MOST likely to be associated with which one of the following conditions?
    A. renal amyloidosis
    B. nephrotic syndrome
    C. aortic atherosclerosis
    D. pulmonary embolism
    E. sepsis

C is correct.
Coagulation necrosis is typically a result of vascular occlusion resulting in an infarct. Atherosclerosis of the aorta could cause renal infarcts due to embolism of atherosclerotic material to the renal arteries, or from embolization of thrombi forming over aortic atherosclerotic plaques.

1.055   A 43-year-old woman presents with systemic amyloidosis. It is confirmed that the amyloid consists predominantly of AL-type amyloid protein. Which one of the following clinical tests is MOST likely give definitive information regarding the underlying disease process in this patient?
    A. serum electrophoresis
    B. hemoglobin electrophoresis
    C. blood culture
    D. lung biopsy
    E. renal biopsy

A is correct.
AL (amyloid light chain)-type amyloid protein is composed of immunoglobulin light chains. This type of amyloid is found in B-cell dyscrasias such as multiple myeloma. Serum electrophoresis detects an abnormal immunoglobulin spike due to the monoclonal proliferation of plasma cells.

1.056   A 3-year-old child has hepatosplenomegaly, skeletal deformities, valvular heart lesions, and brain lesions. Which one of the following substances would you expect to find in abnormal amounts?
    A. glycogen
    B. GM_2 gangliosides
    C. galactocerebrosides
    D. glycosaminoglycans
    E. sphingomyelin

D is correct.
The clinical findings suggest one of the mucopolysaccharidoses. In this group of diseases, enzyme deficiencies lead to lysosomal accumulations of mucopolysaccharides (glycosaminoglycans).

1.057 The focal yellowish-white lesions of enzymatic fat necrosis are a result of:
   A. metastatic calcification
   B. pancreatic lipase activity on adipose cells
   C. excess accumulation of triglycerides
   D. pancreatic amylase activity on lipoproteins
   E. caseous necrosis

B is correct.
In enzymatic fat necrosis, release of pancreatic enzymes causes hydrolysis of triglycerides. The free fatty acids combine with calcium ions to form soaps. These soaps precipitate in the adipose tissue and appear as yellowish-white areas.

1.058 In ischemic cell injury, there is an:
   A. efflux of K^+ and Na^+
   B. influx of K^+ and Ca^{++}
   C. influx of K^+ and H_2O
   D. influx of Na^+ and Ca^{++}
   E. influx of Na^+ and K^+

D is correct.
In ischemic injury to cells, there is an influx of water, sodium and calcium ions, and an efflux of potassium ions and other intracellular molecules, such as enzymes.

1.059 Squamous metaplasia of the bronchial epithelium and adrenal cortical hyperplasia have which one of the following features in common?
   A. accumulation of amyloid protein
   B. fibrosis
   C. etiology
   D. premalignant
   E. reversible

E is correct.
Both squamous metaplasia and adrenal cortical hyperplasia have the potential to revert to normal tissue when the cause of these alterations is removed.

1.060 Hypertrophy is MOST likely to be the result of which one of the following conditions?
   A. chronic increased pulmonary vascular pressure
   B. pregnancy
   C. partial hepatectomy
   D. residence at high altitude
   E. estrogen-producing ovarian tumor

A is correct.
Chronic increased pulmonary vascular pressure causes an increased work load on the right ventricle of the heart. Heart muscle responds by undergoing hypertrophy. All of the other conditions listed may cause hyperplasia.

1.061 A 42-year-old man with a long history of chronic bronchiectasis presents with proteinuria. A thorough work-up is done and a renal biopsy is performed. Routine H & E sections of the kidney show a hyaline substance in most of his glomeruli. Which one of the following would you expect to be present in this hyaline material?
   A. granulomatous inflammation
   B. lipoproteins
   C. AA protein
   D. AL protein
   E. plasma cells

C is correct.
AA (amyloid-associated) protein accumulates in association with long-standing chronic inflammatory conditions. It is derived from a serum precursor protein which is synthesized in the liver and found in increased concentrations in the serum in chronic inflammatory conditions.

1.062 A 24-year-old man is found to have an increased total body iron concentration. Biopsy of his liver shows large amounts of granular golden-brown pigment which stains blue with Prussian blue stain. The presence of which one of the following diseases BEST explains these findings?

    A. iron-deficiency anemia
    B. systemic amyloidosis
    C. chronic congestive heart failure
    D. advanced atrophy
    E. hemophilia

E is correct.

The studies indicated that this patient has an accumulation of iron-containing pigment in his liver. One of the causes of this is multiple transfusions which increases the total iron load on the body. A patient with hemophilia typically requires multiple blood transfusions over the years.

1.063 A 54-year-old man is admitted to the hospital with an acute occlusion of the left anterior descending coronary artery. Which one of the following findings is MOST likely to occur in the myocardium supplied by this artery?

    A. decreased intracellular sodium
    B. increased ATP reserves
    C. induction of smooth endoplasmic reticulum
    D. cell-volume regulation impairment
    E. increased oxidative phosphorylation

D is correct.

The tissue supplied by the occluded artery undergoes ischemic damage. One of the classic early changes of ischemic cell injury is failure of the membrane sodium pump with influx of sodium and water, causing cell swelling.

1.064 The BEST explanation for the reduction of intracellular pH after hypoxic cell injury is:

    A. influx of hydrogen ions
    B. efflux of hydroxyl ions
    C. sequestration of hydrogen ions inside
       mitochondria
    D. increased rate of anaerobic glycolysis
    E. increased gluconeogenesis

D is correct.

In hypoxic cell injury, there is an increase in anaerobic glycolysis which results in increased lactic acid production. This causes a decrease in intracellular pH.

1.065 The increased damage which may occur to ischemic tissue on reperfusion of the area (reperfusion injury) is believed to be primarily due to:

    A. free radicals
    B. ATP depletion
    C. cytosolic calcium
    D. hydrostatic pressure
    E. cellular phosphatases

A is correct.

An important mechanism of cell membrane damage in reperfusion injury is induced by the presence of free radicals, especially activated oxygen species.

1.066 Hyperplasia is LEAST likely to be the result of:

    A. ACTH-producing pituitary tumor
    B. partial hepatectomy
    C. wound-healing
    D. puberty
    E. systemic hypertension

E is correct.

Systemic hypertension creates an increased work load on the left ventricle of the heart. Heart muscle adapts to such conditions by undergoing hypertrophy, not hyperplasia.

1.067   The pathogenesis of the hypoglycemia in patients with von Gierke's disease is:
   A. insulin hypersensitivity
   B. hepatocyte synthesis of protein with insulin-like activity
   C. inability to convert glucose into glycogen
   D. failure of conversion of glucose-6-phosphate to glucose
   E. a deficiency of the enzyme hexosaminidase

D is correct.
von Gierke's disease is a genetic disease resulting in a deficiency of the enzyme glucose-6-phosphatase. The inability to rapidly convert glucose-6-phosphate to glucose results in hypoglycemia.

1.068   A 45-year-old man has been diagnosed with a plasma cell neoplasm (multiple myeloma). Several years later, he develops cardiomegaly, atrophy of myocardial fibers, and abnormalities in the conduction system. Which one of the following substances is MOST likely to have accumulated in this patient's myocardium?
   A. glycogen
   B. immunoglobulin light chains (AL)
   C. amyloid-associated (AA) protein
   D. plasma cells
   E. GM_2 ganglioside

B is correct.
Amyloidosis consisting of AL amyloid is associated with plasma cell dyscrasias, such as multiple myeloma. The amyloid collects in an extracellular location in various organs, including the heart, where it may cause atrophy of adjacent parenchymal cells and interference with the conduction system. Overall, there is cardiomegaly due to the accumulation of amyloid in the heart.

1.069   Each of the following situations is associated with enlargement of an organ or tissue. In which one of the following situations is hyperplasia MOST likely to be responsible for the enlargement?
   A. stenosis of the ascending aorta
   B. pulmonary hypertension
   C. Gaucher's disease
   D. chronic blood loss
   E. venous obstruction

D is correct.
In chronic blood loss, there is a reactive hyperplasia of the bone marrow in an attempt to replenish blood cells. Stenosis of the ascending aorta and pulmonary hypertension cause organ enlargement primarily by hypertrophy. Gaucher's disease causes organ enlargement due to the accumulation of a substance within cells, and venous obstruction results in enlargement due to edema.

1.070   You would expect to find increased size and numbers of subcellular organelles within cells in:
   A. hyperplasia
   B. hypertrophy
   C. cellular edema
   D. ischemia
   E. amyloidosis

B is correct.
In hypertrophy, there is cellular enlargement associated with an increase in the size and numbers of subcellular organelles.

1.071   Injury to hepatocytes by chlorinated hydrocarbons typically results in the accumulation of intracellular:
   A. potassium
   B. protein
   C. glycogen
   D. lipid
   E. chloride

D is correct.
Injury to hepatocytes by toxins is reflected by the accumulation of lipids within the hepatic cells. This occurs because of the central role of the liver in lipid metabolism. Damage to lipid metabolic pathways results in the inability of the hepatocyte to properly secrete intracellular lipids.

1.072   A 54-year-old woman has a long history of chronic rheumatoid arthritis. She develops renal disease. A biopsy of the kidney is MOST likely to show an accumulation of which one of the following substances?

    A. amyloid protein AA

    B. amyloid protein AL

    C. transthyretin

    D. glycogen

    E. mucopolysaccharides

A is correct.

AA (amyloid-associated) protein accumulates in association with long-standing chronic inflammatory conditions. It is derived from a serum precursor protein which is synthesized in the liver and found in increased concentrations in the serum in chronic inflammatory conditions. The amyloid may accumulate in various organs, including the kidney.

1.073   A liver biopsy shows the accumulation of a yellowish-brown granular pigmented substance within the Kupffer's cells. Special stains are performed which indicate that the source of this pigment is from the red blood cell. The special stain was positive for:

    A. hemoglobin

    B. globin

    C. iron

    D. heme

    E. red cell membrane component

C is correct.

The yellow-brown pigment is hemosiderin derived from red blood cells. To identify this pigment, a special stain (Prussian blue) is used which stains iron deep blue.

1.074   Cellular edema following hypoxic injury can be MOST directly linked to:

    A. increased ATP levels

    B. failure of the sodium pump

    C. break-up of polysomes

    D. increased posterior pituitary ADH secretion

B is correct.

Hypoxic injury to cells results in decreased membrane-bound ATP with failure of the ATP-dependent membrane sodium pump. This results in the influx of sodium and water into the cell.

1.075 Metaplasia is thought to arise from which one of the following mechanisms?

    A. interaction of free radicals

    B. aging

    C. action of polypeptide growth factors

    D. genetic reprogramming of stem cells

D is correct.

Metaplasia is a reversible alteration where one adult cell type is replaced by another adult cell type. It is believed to occur by the genetic reprogramming of stem cells. These reprogrammed cells then develop into the new adult cell type.

1.076   In reperfusion injury, one important mechanism of membrane damage is injury induced by chemical species that have:

    A. one more proton than electrons

    B. one more electron than protons

    C. ferric iron present

    D. a single unpaired electron in an outer orbital

    E. a single proton with no electron

D is correct.

Free radicals have a single unpaired electron in the outer orbital. As a result, they are highly reactive and enter into reactions with cell membrane components. Many processes may initiate free radical generation within cells.

SECTION 2: ACUTE AND CHRONIC INFLAMMATION AND WOUND-HEALING

2.001 Multinucleated inflammatory giant cells originate from:
    A. endothelial cells
    B. fibroblasts
    C. granulocytes
    D. epithelioid cells

D is correct.
Inflammatory giant cells form from the coalescence and fusion of epithelioid cells. Epithelioid cells are modified macrophages.

2.002 Focal inflammatory lesions include each of the following EXCEPT:
    A. abscess
    B. cellulitis
    C. granuloma
    D. ulcer

B is correct.
Cellulitis is a diffuse, spreading infection caused by certain organisms which have the ability to break down intercellular components. One example is group A streptococci, which produce the enzyme hyaluronidase that breaks down hyaluronic acid, allowing the infection to spread through tissue planes. All of the other processes listed in the question are focal lesions.

2.003 The suppurative response of inflammation is the result of:
    A. hydrolases released from neutrophils
    B. action of mast cells
    C. bacterial toxins
    D. extrusion of enzymes from macrophages
    E. activity of eosinophils

A is correct.
Suppuration only occurs under conditions where huge numbers of polymorphonuclear leukocytes collect at the site of certain bacterial infections. Suppuration or liquefaction necrosis of the tissue occurs due to the release of hydrolases from the polys. Polys live only a short time in tissues and, as they die, they release their enzymes in the area.

2.004 The primary vascular mechanism for the edema in acute inflammation is:
    A. venous congestion
    B. lymphatic obstruction
    C. increased arterial flow
    D. increased arterial pressure
    E. increased vascular permeability

E is correct.
In acute inflammation, there is loss of intravascular fluid primarily due to a leaky endothelium. The immediate–transient phase of increased vascular permeability is due to the action of histamine as well as other chemical mediators of inflammation.

2.005 The specific site of the microcirculation exclusively involved in the immediate–transient leakage induced by histamine is:
    A. veins
    B. venules
    C. arteries
    D. arterioles
    E. capillaries

B is correct.
Histamine and most other chemical mediators induce leakage from small- and medium-sized venules exclusively. This occurs through gaps between endothelial cells which are created by the contraction of the endothelial cells.

2.006   Children with chronic granulomatous disease (CGD) of childhood have a defect in:
   A. neutrophil membrane receptors for C3
   B. neutrophil hydrogen-peroxide production
   C. neutrophil membrane receptors for the Fc fragment
   D. complement activation via the classical pathway
   E. macrophage activation

B is correct.
Hydrogen-peroxide production by neutrophils is deficient, leading to failure of the myeloperoxidase/hydrogen-peroxide killing system. CGD is most commonly an X-linked disease of male children characterized by recurrent infections.

2.007   Granulation tissue contains each of the following EXCEPT:
   A. abundant cross-linking of collagen
   B. macrophages
   C. numerous branching capillaries
   D. phagocytic cells
   E. proliferating fibroblasts

A is correct.
All are typical features of granulation tissue except abundant cross-linking of collagen. Granulation tissue is the early phase of repair whereas cross-linking of collagen occurs later and does not normally become prominent until after the disappearance of the granulation tissue.

2.008   Chronic granulomatous disease of childhood is an inherited enzymatic defect that primarily affects the:
   A. extracellular release of leukocyte products
   B. myeloperoxidase-dependent killing of bacteria
   C. migration and chemotaxis of leukocytes
   D. activity of lysozyme within neutrophils
   E. Fc and C3b receptors on the leukocyte membrane

B is correct.
In this disease, there is a failure of production of hydrogen peroxide in sufficient quantities for effective killing of bacteria after phagocytosis. This makes the patients susceptible to recurrent infections.

2.009   Which one of the following characteristically occurs in acute inflammation?
   A. increased osmotic pressure of interstitial fluid
   B. fibroblastic proliferation
   C. increased intravascular osmotic pressure
   D. increased return of fluid to the blood on the venous end of the capillary
   E. infiltration of macrophages

A is correct.
In acute inflammation, there is an outpouring of protein-rich fluid into the interstitial space. This high protein concentration increases the osmotic load in the interstitium.

2.010   Following emigration, motile white cells migrate into sites of inflammation by:
   A. margination
   B. degranulation
   C. cytokinesis
   D. chemotaxis

D is correct.
Chemotaxis is the term used for the unidirectional migration of cells towards an attractant.

2.011   Which one of the following biosubstances is MOST closely involved with vasoconstriction and platelet aggregation?
    A. endothelial leukocyte adhesion molecules (ELAM-1)
    B. histamine
    C. leukotriene B_4
    D. thromboxane A_2
    E. colony-stimulating factor

D is correct.
Thromboxane A_2, derived from cyclooxygenase activity on arachidonic acid, is a powerful vasoconstrictor and has prominent platelet-aggregation activity.

2.012   Which one of the following biosubstances is the MOST chemotactic?
    A. endothelial leukocyte adhesion molecules (ELAM-1)
    B. histamine
    C. leukotriene B_4
    D. thromboxane A_2
    E. colony-stimulating factor

C is correct.
Of the substances listed, leukotriene B_4 has potent chemotactic properties. It is derived from the action of lipoxygenase on arachidonic acid.

2.013   Which one of the following biosubstances is MOST closely associated with vascular leakage?
    A. endothelial leukocyte adhesion molecules (ELAM-1)
    B. histamine
    C. leukotriene B_4
    D. thromboxane A_2
    E. colony-stimulating factor

B is correct.
Histamine which is released from mast cells has potent effects on increasing vascular permeability. The other substances listed do not significantly increase vascular leakage.

2.014   Most chemical mediators of inflammation cause increased vascular permeability by:
    A. increasing the intravascular hydrostatic pressure
    B. decreasing tissue oncotic pressure
    C. causing microscopic ruptures in the wall of the microcirculation
    D. opening gaps in intercellular junctions
    E. altering the chemical composition of the vascular basement membrane

D is correct.
Using carbon-labeling techniques, it has been determined that the immediate–transient leakage induced by most chemical mediators is through interendothelial gaps which form by contraction of endothelial cells, widening their junctions.

2.015   The MOST likely mechanism for the increased permeability in immediate–sustained reactions of acute inflammation such as is seen in burns is:
    A. increased transendothelial transport
    B. increased intravascular hydrostatic pressure
    C. decreased tissue oncotic pressure
    D. widening interendothelial gaps
    E. direct damage to endothelial cells

E is correct.
Immediate–sustained reactions occur in severe injuries and are associated with necrosis on lining endothelium. All levels of the microcirculation are affected.

2.016   Defects in Fc and C3b receptors on phago-
cyte membranes MOST directly affect:
   A. oxygen-dependent bactericidal mechanisms
   B. extracellular release of leukocyte products
   C. myeloperoxidase-independent killing of
      bacteria
   D. adhesion to endothelium
   E. engulfment

E is correct.
In phagocytosis, engulfment involves the attachment
and binding of Fc and C3b receptors on the leukocyte membrane.

2.017   Aspirin, indomethacin and corticosteroids
have anti-inflammatory properties because they
inhibit the biosynthesis of:
   A. prostaglandins
   B. complement
   C. interleukin-1
   D. bradykinin
   E. histamine

A is correct.
Corticosteroids interfere with arachidonic acid production from cell membrane phospholipids. Aspirin
and indomethacin interfere with cyclooxygenase
activity on arachidonic acid. Since prostaglandins
are synthesized from cyclooxygenase activity on
arachidonic acid, these compounds inhibit prostaglandin synthesis.

2.018   Macrophages in an inflammatory site are
derived from:
   A. plasma cells
   B. lymphocytes
   C. monocytes
   D. neutrophils
   E. basophils

C is correct.
The majority of macrophages at the site of inflammation are derived from blood monocytes which are
chemotactically attracted to the inflammatory focus.

2.019   The LEAST likely finding in early acute
inflammation is / are:
   A. polymorphonuclear leukocytes
   B. hyperemia
   C. tissue exudate
   D. fibroblasts
   E. pain

D is correct.
Fibroblast activity appears later during the healing
process with the appearance of granulation tissue.
Fibroblasts are prominent in long-standing or
chronic inflammation.

2.020   The characteristic cell common to every
chronic infectious granulomatous lesion is:
   A. Langhans' giant cell
   B. plasma cell
   C. mast cell
   D. fibrocyte
   E. epithelioid macrophage

E is correct.
The definition of a granuloma is the collection of
epithelioid macrophages.

2.021   Features common to chronic non-specific
inflammation include:
   A. lymphocytes, epithelioid cells, and necrosis
   B. macrophages, neutrophils, and fibrosis
   C. lymphocytes, plasma cells, and fibrosis
   D. eosinophils, neutrophils, and osseous
      metaplasia
   E. neutrophils, Langhan's giant cells, and
      necrosis

C is correct.
Foci of chronic non-specific inflammation typically
contain mononuclear cell infiltrates such as lymphocytes, plasma cells and macrophages, along with
fibroblasts and collagen deposition.

2.022 In foci of chronic inflammation, you are likely to find more __________ than you would find in foci of acute inflammation.

    A. edema
    B. polymorphonuclear leukocytes
    C. hemorrhage
    D. hyperemia
    E. fibrosis

E is correct.
All of the other features listed are typical of acute inflammation. Fibrosis is associated with long-standing or chronic inflammatory processes.

2.023 Granulation tissue contains each of the following EXCEPT:

    A. abundant cross-linked collagen
    B. macrophages
    C. numerous branching capillaries
    D. phagocytic cells
    E. active fibroblasts

A is correct.
Granulation tissue is a young, soft, edematous tissue which forms during the healing phase. As the granulation tissue is replaced with scar tissue, there is prominent collagen deposition; a late feature is cross-linking of collagen.

2.024 Which of the following is MOST characteristic of repair?

    A. exudate
    B. fibrin
    C. giant cells
    D. granulation tissue
    E. granuloma

D is correct.
Repair is a healing process involving regeneration of parenchymal cells and replacement by connective tissue. The first step in connective-tissue replacement of damaged tissue is the formation of granulation tissue, which is a soft edematous tissue composed of fibroblasts, phagocytic cells and branching capillaries.

2.025 Because of the great number of biologically active products it can produce, which cell type is the central figure in chronic inflammation?

    A. plasma cell
    B. macrophage
    C. neutrophil
    D. mast cell

B is correct.
Activated macrophages may produce a wide variety of products including proteases, chemotactic factors, arachidonic acid metabolites, reactive oxygen metabolites, complement components, coagulation factors, growth-promoting factors, and cytokines.

2.026 Local proliferation by mitotic division at inflammatory foci occurs in:

    A. neutrophils
    B. macrophages
    C. both
    D. neither

B is correct.
Macrophages may undergo mitotic division in tissue. Neutrophils do not undergo mitosis. The neutrophil has a lifespan of only a few days; therefore, without continued chemotactic attraction, neutrophils decrease in number fairly rapidly in acute inflammation.

2.027 Which one of the following responds to chemotactic stimuli?

    A. neutrophils
    B. monocytes
    C. both
    D. neither

C is correct.
Both neutrophils and monocytes respond to a variety of chemotactic stimuli.

2.028 The local warmth in areas of acute inflammation is primarily due to:
    A. release of platelet factor 3
    B. action of tumor necrosis factor
    C. vasodilatation
    D. action of interleukin-1
    E. metabolic 'burst' in polymorphonuclear leukocytes

C is correct.
In acute inflammation, there is vasodilatation of the vessels which results in increased blood flow. This is responsible for the local warmth and redness in acute inflammation.

2.029 Chronic granulomatous inflammation differs from non-specific chronic inflammation in which one of the following ways?
    A. presence of cross-linked collagen
    B. absence of lymphocytes
    C. presence of tissue destruction
    D. potential for resolution
    E. presence of epithelioid macrophages

E is correct.
The presence of modified macrophages called epithelioid cells by definition is a component of granulomatous inflammation.

2.030 Suppurative inflammation is LEAST likely to be associated with:
    A. abscesses
    B. staphylococcal pneumonia
    C. liquefaction necrosis
    D. gastric ulcers
    E. acute appendicitis

D is correct.
Gastric ulcers are localized defects in the gastric mucosa secondary to acid-peptic digestion of the stomach surface. The base of the ulcer may contain fibrin and necrotic debris, but suppuration is not a feature.

2.031 The main determining factor for the formation of an exudate instead of a transudate is:
    A. endothelial injury
    B. hydrostatic pressure
    C. serum osmotic pressure
    D. tissue osmotic pressure
    E. serum ratio of albumin to globulin

A is correct.
Increased hydrostatic pressure and decreased serum osmotic pressures predispose to transudate formation. An exudate containing higher protein concentrations occurs when there is sufficient damage to the endothelium to allow large amounts of large protein molecules to escape into the tissues.

2.032 Of the following, the MOST potent mediator of chemotaxis is:
    A. leukotriene B_4
    B. histamine
    C. leukotriene E_4
    D. bradykinin
    E. C3a

A is correct.
Leukotriene B_4, which is derived from leukocytes, is a very potent mediator of chemotaxis. Leukotriene E_4, histamine, and bradykinin and C3a are active in producing vascular leakage.

2.033 Which one of the following statements is TRUE of a patient who has had a previous Cesarean delivery?
    A. the patient is less likely to rupture her uterus than she was before her operation
    B. if a rupture occurs, it will most likely be in the old scar
    C. if a rupture occurs, it will most likely be in normal uterine wall of the anterior fundus
    D. if a rupture occurs, it will most likely be in normal uterine wall of the posterior fundus

B is correct.
A scar never regains the tensile strength of normal tissue.

2.034 Theoretically, chemotaxis could be blocked by preventing the cytosolic accumulation of which one of the following substances?
    A. sodium
    B. potassium
    C. calcium
    D. magnesium
    E. hydrogen ion

C is correct.
Increased cytosolic calcium triggers the formation and arrangement of contractile elements which are responsible for cellular motion in chemotaxis.

2.035 Two factors determine the formation of tuberculous granulomas. These factors are the presence of poorly digestible irritants and:
    A. T cell-mediated immunity
    B. B-cell activation
    C. fibroblastic proliferation
    D. neovascularization
    E. squamous epithelial cell migration

A is correct.
Products of activated T lymphocytes are associated with the transformation of macrophages into epithelioid cells and multinucleate giant cells in granulomas.

2.036 The MOST common mechanism of the immediate–transient response of vascular leakage in acute inflammation is:
    A. leukocyte-mediated endothelial injury
    B. leakage from regenerating capillaries
    C. endothelial cell contraction
    D. cytoskeletal and junctional reorganization
    E. direct endothelial injury

C is correct.
Contraction of endothelial cells with widening of the interendothelial junctions is the most common mechanism of increased vascular permeability. This type of increased permeability is rapid and short-lived.

2.037 The richest source for the principal mediator of the immediate phase of increased vascular permeability in acute inflammation is:
    A. plasma cells
    B. mast cells
    C. lymphocytes
    D. polymorphonuclear leukocytes
    E. capillary endothelium

B is correct.
The principal mediator of the immediate phase of increased vascular permeability in acute inflammation is histamine. The richest source of histamine is in the granules of mast cells.

2.038 A major component of granulation tissue is:
    A. fibroblasts
    B. polymorphonuclear leukocytes
    C. plasma cells
    D. epithelioid cells
    E. remodeled collagen

A is correct.
Granulation tissue primarily consists of proliferating fibroblasts and vascular endothelial cells. Granulation tissue is part of the repair process.

2.039 One of the hallmarks of chronic inflammation is:
    A. reactive parenchymal hyperplasia
    B. tissue destruction
    C. prolonged hyperemia
    D. prolonged increased vascular permeability
    E. prolonged polymorphonuclear mitotic activity at the inflammatory site

B is correct.
Chronic inflammation takes place over a duration of weeks, months, or even years. The continual inflammatory process leads to tissue destruction and fibrosis.

2.040   Which one of the following statements BEST describes the nature of E-selectin (ELAM-1)?
   A. induced in endothelium after stimulation by inflammatory mediators
   B. normally present on the surface of endothelial cells
   C. stored in granules within platelets and released in platelet activation
   D. synthesized by leukocytes at sites of endothelial injury

A is correct.
The selectin group of molecules is responsible for the loose transient adhesion of leukocytes to endothelium that results in the rolling phase in early inflammation. ELAM-1 is not present in normal endothelium, but is induced after stimulation by specific mediators such as IL-1 and TNF. ELAM-1 binds to sialated oligosaccharides of leukocyte surface glycoproteins.

2.041   During an acute inflammatory response, the initial attachment of a circulating neutrophil to the endothelial cell surface is mediated by:
   A. basement membranes
   B. platelets bound to endothelial cells
   C. selectins
   D. kinins
   E. interleukins

C is correct.
Selectins consist of E-selectin (ELAM-1), which is present only in endothelium, P-selectin (GMP140) present in endothelium and platelets, and L-selectin (LAM-1), present in most leukocytes. The selectins are involved in the initial, loose adhesion of neutrophils to the endothelial surface in acute inflammation.

2.042   The MOST consistent finding associated with chronic inflammation is:
   A. amyloid deposition
   B. tissue destruction
   C. epithelioid cells
   D. inflammatory giant cells
   E. neovascularization

B is correct.
Whereas epithelioid cells and inflammatory giant cells may occur in a specific type of chronic inflammation (granulomas), they are not consistent in all forms of chronic inflammation. Tissue destruction and fibrosis are consistent in all types of chronic inflammation.

2.043 Epithelioid cells are associated with:
   A. granulomas
   B. granulation tissue
   C. squamous metaplasia
   D. squamous neoplasia

A is correct.
Epithelioid cells are modified macrophages. Accumulations of these cells define a granuloma.

2.044   The MOST common mechanism of the immediate–transient response of vascular leakage in acute inflammation involves:
   A. leakage from regenerating capillaries
   B. leukocyte-mediated endothelial injury
   C. direct endothelial injury
   D. endothelial cell swelling
   E. formation of widened intercellular junctions

E is correct.
Contraction of endothelial cells with widening of the interendothelial junctions is the most common mechanism of increased vascular permeability. This type of increased permeability is rapid and short-lived.

2.045   Which one of the following plays a prominent role in leukocyte adhesion to the endothelium in areas of acute inflammation?
   A. histamine
   B. ELAM-1
   C. thromboxane A_2
   D. leukotriene B_4
   E. 5-HETE

B is correct.
ELAM-1 (E-selectin) is found in endothelial cells. It is involved in the initial adhesion of neutrophils to the endothelial surface in acute inflammation.

2.046   Which of the following is activated by the binding of chemotactic agents to leukocyte membrane receptors?

    A. leukotriene B_4
    B. histamine
    C. phospholipase C
    D. tumor necrosis factor
    E. serotonin

C is correct.

The binding of chemotactic agents to receptors on leukocyte cell membranes causes activation of phospholipase C. A hydrolysis reaction ensues resulting in the release of calcium from intracellular stores. The increased cytosolic calcium is important in the movement of the cells in chemotaxis.

2.047   After phagocytosis, bacterial killing is accomplished largely by:

    A. oxygen-dependent mechanisms
    B. bactericidal permeability-increasing protein
    C. lysozyme
    D. lactoferrin
    E. defensins

A is correct.

The major pathway for bacterial killing after phagocytosis is by oxygen-dependent mechanisms. Substances in leukocyte granules can also kill bacteria by mechanisms not related to the oxidative burst which occurs after phagocytosis.

2.048   One of the major differences between the exudates of fibrinous and suppurative inflammation is the quantity of:

    A. epithelioid cells
    B. fibroblasts
    C. plasma cells
    D. polymorphonuclear leukocytes
    E. macrophages

D is correct.

Fibrinous exudates contain large amounts of fibrin, but few leukocytes. By definition, suppurative exudates contain huge numbers of polymorphonuclear leukocytes.

2.049   A chemical mediator which interacts with vascular receptors in the thermoregulatory center of the hypothalamus, thereby producing fever, is:

    A. colony-stimulating factor
    B. interleukin-1
    C. bradykinin
    D. nitric oxide
    E. C3a

B is correct.

Interleukin-1 along with interleukin-6 produce fever by interacting with vascular receptors in the hypothalamic thermoregulatory center. This interaction involves the induction of prostaglandin (PGE) production.

2.050   Children who have a defect in their neutrophil myeloperoxidase/hydrogen-peroxide system typically present clinically with:

    A. severe acute viral illness
    B. leukemoid reactions
    C. bone marrow atrophy
    D. hepatomegaly
    E. recurrent bacterial infections

E is correct.

A defect in oxygen-dependent bacterial killing mechanisms is present in a congenital disorder called chronic granulomatous disease. Due to the defect in bacterial killing after phagocytosis, these children suffer repeated bacterial infections.

2.051   Abscesses, caseating granulomas, and infarcts all have which one of the following features in common?

    A. prominent infiltrate of polymorphonuclear
       leukocytes
    B. epithelioid cells
    C. etiology
    D. method of healing
    E. pathogenesis

D is correct.

Abscesses, caseating granulomas, and infarcts all have in common the destruction of an entire zone of parenchymal and stromal elements. Under such circumstances, healing can only occur by repair or fibrosis.

2.052 The usual fate of apoptotic cells is:
   A. metaplastic transformation
   B. neoplastic transformation
   C. phagocytosis
   D. calcification
   E. hypertrophy

C is correct.
After the cell undergoes shrinkage and chromatin condensation, the apoptotic cell is phagocytized by adjacent healthy parenchymal cells or macrophages.

2.053 Epithelioid cells in granulomatous inflammation are derived from:
   A. lymphocytes
   B. plasma cells
   C. endothelial cells
   D. squamous cells
   E. macrophages

E is correct.
Products of activated T lymphocytes help transform macrophages into epithelioid cells.

2.054 All of the following mechanisms contribute to the edema of acute inflammation EXCEPT:
   A. reduced intravascular osmotic pressure
   B. increased interstitial osmotic pressure
   C. increased hydrostatic pressure
   D. increased lymphatic flow

D is correct.
Increased lymphatic flow would in fact decrease the edema by carrying the fluid away from the tissue into the vascular system.

2.055 Most scars ultimately attain tensile strength of approximately what percent of normal tissue?
   A. 10–20%
   B. 40–50%
   C. 70–80%
   D. 100%

C is correct.
Scars never attain the strength of uninjured tissue. After about 3 months of injury, wound strength reaches about 70–80% of the tensile strength of unwounded skin and plateaus.

2.056 Which one of the following is activated by the binding of chemotactic agents to leukocyte membrane receptors?
   A. histamine
   B. integrin
   C. prostacyclin PGI_2
   D. thromboxane A_2
   E. colony-stimulating factor
   F. ICAM-1
   G. leukotriene B_4
   H. phospholipase C

H is correct.
The binding of chemotactic agents to receptors on leukocyte cell membranes causes activation of phospholipase C. A hydrolysis reaction ensues, resulting in the release of calcium from intracellular stores. The increased cytosolic calcium is important in the movement of the cells in chemotaxis

2.057 Which molecule found on leukocytes binds to endothelial receptors in leukocyte adhesion?
   A. histamine
   B. integrin
   C. prostacyclin PGI_2
   D. thromboxane A_2
   E. colony-stimulating factor
   F. ICAM-1
   G. leukotriene B_4
   H. phospholipase C

B is correct.
Integrins are transmembrane glycoproteins which may be found on leukocyte cell membranes. These integrins bind to endothelial receptor adhesion molecules (ICAM-1 and VCAM-1) during leukocyte adhesion in acute inflammation.

2.058   Which one of the following stimulates platelet aggregation and vasoconstriction?
   A. histamine
   B. integrin
   C. prostacyclin PGI$_2$
   D. thromboxane A$_2$
   E. colony-stimulating factor
   F. ICAM-1
   G. leukotriene B$_4$
   H. phospholipase C

D is correct.

Thromboxane A$_2$ is a major product of platelets. It is a very powerful platelet-aggregating substance as well as a vasoconstrictor. Thromboxane A$_2$ is unstable and is quickly converted to an inactive form (thromboxane B$_2$)

2.059   Which one of the following is an adhesion receptor found on endothelial cell membranes?
   A. histamine
   B. integrin
   C. prostacyclin PGI$_2$
   D. thromboxane A$_2$
   E. colony-stimulating factor
   F. ICAM-1
   G. leukotriene B$_4$
   H. phospholipase C

F is correct.

ICAM-1 (intercellular adhesion molecule 1) belongs to the immunoglobulin family of molecules. This molecule, along with VCAM-1 (vascular cell adhesion molecule 1), interacts with integrins located on leukocyte cell membranes to bind leukocytes to endothelium during the early phases of acute inflammation.

SECTION 3: HEMODYNAMIC DISORDERS

3.001 An infarct of the kidney heals by:
   A. resolution
   B. regeneration
   C. organization
   D. calcification

C is correct.
In an infarct, there is necrosis of both the parenchymal and stromal elements. The necrotic zone is filled with granulation tissue, followed by fibrosis. This is the process of organization.

3.002 One of the earliest events in thrombosis is:
   A. platelet activation
   B. thromboxane A_2 secretion
   C. platelet adhesion to vascular wall
   D. platelet factor 3 release
   E. activation of the extrinsic coagulation system

C is correct.
Whereas all of the other events occur in thrombosis, the earliest is platelet adhesion to exposed subendothelial collagen at sites of endothelial injury.

3.003 Pulmonary emboli may originate from any of the following sites EXCEPT:
   A. pulmonary veins
   B. prostatic veins
   C. mural thrombus in right atrium
   D. hepatic veins
   E. superior vena cava

A is correct.
This is really an anatomy question. All sites listed other than the pulmonary veins drain into the right ventricle of the heart and then into the lungs. Pulmonary veins drain into the left side of the heart, and could give rise to systemic emboli.

3.004 Hemorrhagic infarcts are MOST likely to occur in the:
   A. kidney
   B. spleen
   C. liver
   D. lung
   E. heart

D is correct.
The dual blood supply as well as the loose spongy texture of the lung sets the stage for hemorrhagic infarcts. The only other organ listed with dual blood supply is the liver, but it is quite compact and does not predispose to the spread of blood through the tissue.

3.005 Twenty-four to seventy-two hours following traumatic injury involving broken bones, a patient develops progressive pulmonary insufficiency, mental deterioration, and thrombocytopenia. The BEST explanation is:
   A. systemic thromboemboli
   B. septic shock
   C. hypovolemic shock
   D. fat-embolism syndrome
   E. paradoxical embolus

D is correct.
Fat-embolism syndrome is attributed to the release of fat microglobules into sinusoids and venules following severe trauma, especially involving bone fractures. Many microglobules are trapped in the lungs, but some squeeze through to the systemic circulation to cause occlusion of small vessels in other organs, notably the brain. Several complex injury mechanisms are invoked.

3.006 Left ventricular failure is MOST likely to be a cause of which one of the following?
   A. sinusoidal dilation in the liver
   B. pulmonary alveolar transudate
   C. hypovolemia
   D. decreased pulmonary venous pressure
   E. congestive splenomegaly

B is correct.
Left ventricular failure results in increased hydrostatic pressure in the left side of the heart which is transmitted to the pulmonary veins and then to the pulmonary vascular bed. According to Starling's law, this creates a loss of low-protein fluid into the alveolar spaces.

3.007 MOST pulmonary emboli arise from thrombi originating in the:
- A. deep veins of the legs
- B. inferior vena cava
- C. pulmonary artery
- D. hepatic veins
- E. periprostatic veins

A is correct.
Although all of the other sites listed may be a source of pulmonary emboli, over 95% arise in thrombi in the deep veins of the legs.

3.008 The MOST common outcome of pulmonary embolism is:
- A. death during the acute stages
- B. pulmonary infarction
- C. chronic pulmonary hypertension
- D. shock
- E. resolution

E is correct.
From 60–80% of all pulmonary emboli are so small that they are clinically silent. These small emboli are rapidly removed by fibrinolysis.

3.009 Virchow's triad consists of:
- A. endothelial injury, right heart failure, and hypercalcemia
- B. right heart failure, hypercoagulability of blood, and endothelial injury
- C. hypercoagulability of blood, alteration in normal blood flow, and platelet-release reaction
- D. alteration in normal blood flow, endothelial injury, and hypercoagulability of blood
- E. platelet activation, platelet adhesion, and platelet aggregation

D is correct.
The major changes which predispose to thrombosis are alteration in blood flow, endothelial injury, and alteration (hypercoagulability) of blood. These three factors are known as Virchow's triad.

3.010 All of the following play a pathogenic role in the edema of heart failure EXCEPT:
- A. decreased glomerular filtration rate
- B. increased central venous pressure
- C. decreased renal tubular sodium resorption
- D. increased transudation
- E. increased aldosterone production

C is correct.
In congestive heart failure, there is decreased effective blood volume, sensed by the juxtaglomerular apparatus; a compensatory mechanism is activated which results in an increased tubular resorption of sodium.

3.011 The primary pathogenic mechanism in the development of edema secondary to venous thrombosis is:
- A. increased hydrostatic pressure
- B. endothelial damage
- C. decreased plasma osmotic pressure
- D. decreased tissue osmotic pressure
- E. reflex arterial vasodilatation

A is correct.
In venous thrombosis, there is increased hydrostatic pressure proximal to the occlusion. In accordance with Starling's law, fluid leaves the intravascular compartment, leading to local tissue edema.

3.012 The MOST accurate name for a blood clot in the pericardial sac is:
- A. mural thrombus
- B. pericardial thrombus
- C. antemortem thrombus
- D. hemopericardium
- E. pericardial petechiae

D is correct.
One of the issues in this question is the definition of a thrombus. For a blood clot to be correctly called a thrombus, it must have formed during life within the vascular system. The pericardial sac is not intravascular; therefore, any blood in this location is referred to as hemopericardium.

3.013   An important pathogenic feature in the initiation of thrombosis is:
   A. decreased serum calcium
   B. exposure of subendothelial fibrillar collagen
   C. fibrinolysis
   D. clearance of clotting factors
   E. binding of thrombin

B is correct.
The exposure of subendothelial fibrillar collagen, allowing contact with blood elements, is a powerful stimulus to platelet adhesion and, hence, the initiation of thrombosis.

3.014   The earliest step in thrombogenesis is:
   A. platelet adhesion to sites of endothelial injury
   B. platelet secretion of alpha granules and dense bodies
   C. platelet activation
   D. thromboxane formation
   E. platelet factor 3 activation

A is correct.
The first step in thrombus formation is the adhesion of platelets at the site of endothelial injury. All of the other items listed occur after platelet adhesion.

3.015   The MOST likely site for the formation of a mural thrombus is:
   A. aorta
   B. renal arcuate arteries
   C. saphenous vein
   D. hepatic sinusoids
   E. pericardium

A is correct.
A mural thrombus is one which forms on the wall of a large chamber or large-caliber vessel without occluding the lumen. The aorta is the only large vessel listed. A blood clot in the pericardium cannot be called a thrombus because it is not within the vascular system.

3.016   MOST pulmonary emboli behave clinically in which one of the following ways?
   A. result in sudden death
   B. are clinically silent
   C. cause pulmonary infarction
   D. precipitate respiratory failure
   E. lead to shock

B is correct.
Most pulmonary emboli are small and go unnoticed. They are usually removed by fibrinolysis.

3.017   The MOST fundamental definition of shock is:
   A. hypotension
   B. widespread hypoperfusion
   C. decreased blood volume
   D. increased heart rate
   E. generalized arteriolar dilation

B is correct.
Although all of the other findings may occur in the shock syndrome, at the most fundamental level, hypoperfusion of tissues is the common denominator of all forms of shock.

3.018   Chronic right ventricular cardiac failure is MOST likely to present with:
   A. pulmonary edema
   B. centrilobular hepatic hypoxia
   C. splenic infarcts
   D. cerebral atrophy
   E. systemic active hyperemia

B is correct.
Right ventricular failure causes increased venous pressure in the superior and inferior vena cavae and their tributaries. This increased venous pressure is transmitted through the hepatic veins into the hepatic sinusoids, slowing normal sinusoidal blood flow. Oxygenated blood enters at the portal triad and flows toward the central vein. With decreased flow, by the time sinusoidal blood reaches the centrilobular zone, it is low in oxygen saturation.

3.019 The fate of a thrombus is LEAST likely to include:
  A. embolization
  B. organization
  C. propagation
  D. fibrinolysis
  E. suppuration

E is correct.
Suppuration is the term to describe the formation of pus in pyogenic bacterial infections. Thrombi may commonly undergo any of the other changes listed.

3.020 A potent mediator of platelet aggregation is:
  A. sodium
  B. plasmin
  C. adenosine diphosphate (ADP)
  D. phosphorylase
  E. heparin

C is correct.
ADP is released from platelets and initiates platelet aggregation, forming a temporary hemostatic plug. ADP, thrombin, and thromboxane then interact to convert the temporary platelet plug into a larger secondary plug.

3.021 The MOST frequent source of pulmonary emboli is from thrombi in the:
  A. superficial varicose veins of the legs
  B. hepatic veins
  C. right cardiac atrium
  D. popliteal, femoral and iliac veins
  E. superior and inferior vena cavae

D is correct.
Over 95% of pulmonary emboli arise in the large veins of the leg (popliteal, femoral and iliac veins).

3.022 Disseminated intravascular coagulation (DIC) is LEAST likely to be associated with:
  A. bleeding diathesis
  B. multiple thrombi in the microcirculation
  C. consumption of platelets and clotting factors
  D. left ventricular mural thrombus
  E. fibrinolysis

D is correct.
DIC is a coagulopathy resulting in multiple thrombi in the microcirculation which consumes platelets and clotting factors, resulting in a bleeding diathesis. Fibrinolytic activity results in the finding of fibrin split products in the blood. Large thrombi are not a usual component of this syndrome.

3.023 MOST infarcts are caused by:
  A. thrombosis or embolism
  B. shock
  C. disseminated intravascular coagulation
  D. atherosclerotic narrowing of arteries
  E. compression of vessels by expansile tumor
    masses

A is correct.
Infarcts are focal areas of necrosis caused by sudden loss of blood supply. The two most frequent causes of sudden loss of blood supply are thrombosis or embolism.

3.024 Migratory thrombosis (Trousseau's syndrome) is caused by:
  A. abnormal platelets
  B. disseminated intravascular coagulation
  C. embolization
  D. tumor-associated procoagulant release
  E. widespread endothelial injury

D is correct.
Tumor-associated procoagulant release plays a prominent role in the thromboses which may occur in disseminated cancers.

3.025   Factors which increase the probability of infarction after vascular occlusion include all of the following EXCEPT:
- A. hypoxemia
- B. anemia
- C. rapid development of the occlusion
- D. increased vulnerability of a tissue to hypoxia
- E. prominent anastomotic channels

E is correct.
Prominent anastomotic channels in an organ serve as a protective mechanism against infarction by allowing oxygenated blood to reach the tissue around the point of occlusion. All of the other features listed render infarction more probable after vascular occlusion.

3.026   Each of the following commonly occurs in shock EXCEPT:
- A. reduction in urinary output
- B. hypotension
- C. generalized tissue ischemia
- D. metabolic alkalosis
- E. decreased glomerular filtration rate (GFR)

D is correct.
In shock, due to the hypoperfusion and tissue hypoxia, there is an increase in anaerobic metabolism and lactic acid production which results in a metabolic acidosis.

3.027   The edema of congestive heart failure can be attributed in part to renal hypoperfusion. The pathogenic mechanism underlying this effect involves an increase in:
- A. aldosterone production
- B. cardiac output
- C. plasma osmotic pressure
- D. sodium excretion
- E. vascular permeability

A is correct.
Hypoperfusion of the kidneys stimulates the release of renin from the renal tissue. This, in turn, stimulates alsosterone production, which results in increased sodium reabsorption. The effect is retention of sodium and water.

3.028   Small renal infarcts undergo:
- A. caseation
- B. fibrosis
- C. gangrenous change
- D. regeneration
- E. resolution

B is correct.
In an infarct, there is loss of both parenchyma and stroma. Healing occurs by fibrosis or scarring.

3.029   Mural thrombi are LEAST likely to occur in the:
- A. aorta
- B. left atrium
- C. left ventricle
- D. pulmonary capillaries
- E. right ventricle

D is correct.
Mural thrombi form on the wall of a large vascular channel. They are not occlusive due to the large size of the chamber in which they form. Any thrombi forming in pulmonary capillaries would be occlusive because of the very small lumen of these structures.

3.030   Which one of the following organs is the LEAST susceptible to damage by pure hypovolemic shock?
- A. brain
- B. heart
- C. kidneys
- D. lungs

D is correct.
The lungs are usually not affected in pure hypovolemic shock. When shock is secondary to bacterial sepsis or trauma, lung injury may occur in the form of diffuse alveolar damage.

3.031 All of the following phenomena may produce edema EXCEPT:
- A. depletion of sodium
- B. increased vascular permeability
- C. decrease in plasma protein
- D. increased hydrostatic blood pressure
- E. lymphatic obstruction

A is correct.
Increased sodium retention will cause water retention and contribute to edema, not a depletion of sodium.

3.032 The fate of a thrombus may include all of the following EXCEPT:
- A. propagation
- B. metaplastic transformation
- C. embolization
- D. lysis
- E. organization

B is correct.
A thrombus may continue to grow or propagate; it may break loose and form an embolus, or it may slowly be removed by fibrinolysis. In some thrombi, there is ingrowth of granulation tissue or organization. Metaplastic transformation is not a likely event in a thrombus.

3.033 All of the following disorders predispose to thrombosis EXCEPT:
- A. pancreatic carcinoma
- B. obesity
- C. diabetes mellitus
- D. vitamin K deficiency
- E. myocardial infarction

D is correct.
Vitamin K deficiency may in fact contribute to a defect in coagulation with a resulting bleeding tendency. Many adenocarcinomas cause hypercoagulability of the blood. Obesity increases the predisposition to thrombosis in an undefined way. In diabetics, there is likely to be advanced atherosclerosis and, in myocardial infarcts, there is a likelihood of endothelial damage overlying the infarct.

3.034 A postoperative patient develops a swollen, painful right leg with a positive Homans' sign. The next day, the patient develops chest pain followed by hemoptysis. The earliest stage in the pathologic process leading to these symptoms is:
- A. trapping of embolic material in the lung
- B. aggregation and cross-linking of fibrin
- C. trapping of erythrocytes
- D. adhesion of platelets to intima
- E. invasion by leukocytes and fibroblasts

D is correct.
This patient has probably developed a venous thrombus in his right leg which has broken loose, forming an embolus which has lodged in the lung. The first step in thrombogenesis is platelet adhesion to the vascular endothelium.

3.035 A patient is admitted to the hospital with crushing substernal chest pain, and electrocardiographic abnormalities consistent with acute myocardial necrosis. Five days later, the patient develops left flank pain and hematuria. The process causing the renal pathology in this patient MOST likely began in the:
- A. left ventricle
- B. femoral vein
- C. pulmonary veins
- D. abdominal aorta
- E. renal artery

A is correct.
This patient most likely has developed a mural thrombus on the damaged endothelium overlying the infarct. Pieces of this thrombus may break loose, forming systemic emboli that may become lodged in various locations. One has probably lodged in a small renal artery, causing a renal infarct which has resulted in the flank pain and hematuria.

3.036   An obese pregnant woman suffers acute shortness of breath and chest pain. Physical examination reveals bulging neck veins. The MOST likely pathophysiologic mechanism operating in this patient is:
    A. hypovolemic shock
    B. left ventricular failure
    C. systemic arterial embolization
    D. acute pulmonary hypertension
    E. paradoxical embolism

D is correct.
Obesity increases the predisposition to thrombosis. The enlarged uterus of pregnancy causes lower abdominal pressure, which may slow venous return from the lower extremities. This is a second factor in increasing the predisposition to thrombosis. She has probably had a pulmonary embolus which has caused a sudden increase in pulmonary resistance, increasing pulmonary pressure, and causing right heart failure. The bulging neck veins are secondary to right heart failure.

3.037   The edema which occurs in patients with congestive heart failure is primarily due to:
    A. increased hydrostatic pressure
    B. decreased plasma osmotic pressure
    C. lymphatic obstruction
    D. increased endothelial permeability

A is correct.
In congestive failure, blood pools in the venous system, resulting in an increased venous hydrostatic pressure. According to Starling's law, this results in fluid moving from the vascular system into the interstitial spaces. This low-protein fluid is called a transudate.

3.038   The edema which occurs in patients with the nephrotic syndrome is primarily due to:
    A. increased hydrostatic pressure
    B. decreased plasma osmotic pressure
    C. lymphatic obstruction
    D. increased endothelial permeability

B is correct.
In the nephrotic syndrome, large amounts of protein are lost in the urine. This results in a decreased serum osmotic pressure which, according to Starling's law, results in loss of intravascular fluid into the interstitial tissues.

3.039   All of the following contribute to the edema of heart failure EXCEPT:
    A. decreased aldosterone
    B. increased renal sodium resorption
    C. increased renin
    D. increased ADH (antidiuretic hormone)

A is correct.
Decreased effective blood volume results in increased renin production, increased renal sodium resorption, increased ADH, and INCREASED aldosterone. All of these changes produce water retention, contributing to edema.

3.040   A thrombus is undergoing organization when you can detect:
    A. lines of Zahn
    B. fibrinolysis
    C. granulation tissue
    D. propagation

D is correct.
Organization is the process of ingrowth of fibroblasts. Granulation tissue consists of young fibroblasts and new capillaries.

3.041   Mural thrombi are LEAST likely to occur in which one of the following locations?
    A. left atrium
    B. left ventricle
    C. thoracic aorta
    D. abdominal aorta
    E. right coronary artery

E is correct.
Mural thrombi are thrombi which form on one wall of a structure, thus occurring in large-caliber vascular spaces such as the cardiac chambers or the aorta. Thrombi which occur in smaller-caliber vessels, such as coronary arteries, are usually occlusive thrombi.

3.042 A 72-year-old woman had a partial colectomy for carcinoma of the colon. Three days postoperative, she developed a painful swollen left leg. The pathologic process in her leg was initiated by:
    A. pavementing of leukocytes
    B. fibrin aggregation
    C. trapping of erythrocytes
    D. platelet adhesion to intima
    E. fibroblastic attachment to endothelium

D is correct.
The finding of swelling in only one leg suggests a local event, such as venous thrombosis. This patient has at least two risk factors for thrombosis, carcinoma and postoperative state. Thrombosis is initiated by the adhesion of platelets to intimal surfaces at points of endothelial injury.

3.043 The increased total body fluid load in patients with congestive heart failure is largely due to:
    A. renal retention of sodium and water
    B. antidiuretic medication
    C. decreased plasma osmotic pressure
    D. widespread hypoxic endothelial damage
    E. decreased venous hydrostatic pressure

A is correct.
In congestive heart failure, there is a decreased effective arterial blood volume. This stimulates increased renin and aldosterone secretion, resulting in increased renal sodium resorption, and retention of sodium and water.

3.044 A 34-year-old woman with known renal disease presents with generalized edema. She is diagnosed as having the nephrotic syndrome, a condition characterized by a leaky glomerular basement membrane. The mechanism MOST likely to be responsible for her edema is:
    A. renal sodium and water retention
    B. decreased plasma osmotic pressure
    C. widespread lymphatic obstruction
    D. increased vascular hydrostatic pressure
    E. increased permeability of endothelial cells

B is correct.
Many diseases which affect the glomeruli result in damage to the selective filtration barrier, allowing larger protein molecules such as albumin to be lost in the urine. The urinary loss of albumin results in hypoalbuminemia and decreased plasma osmotic pressure. According to Starling's law, decreased plasma osmotic pressure moves fluid from the intravascular compartment to the extravascular compartment.

3.045 Each of the following clinical features is characteristic of shock EXCEPT:
    A. hypotension
    B. renal insufficiency
    C. rapid cardiac rate
    D. metabolic alkalosis

D is correct.
In shock, there is hypoperfusion of tissues resulting in cellular hypoxia. This causes a shift to anaerobic metabolism with increased lactate production. This leads to a lactic (metabolic) acidosis.

3.046 Each of the following situations may result in edema EXCEPT:
    A. hypoalbuminemia
    B. increased renal tubular excretion of sodium
    C. increased vascular permeability
    D. increased vascular hydrostatic pressure
    E. lymphatic obstruction

B is correct.
Retention of sodium will contribute to edema by causing an associated retention of water. However, loss of sodium, as in increased renal tubular excretion, would not contribute to edema.

3.047 All of the following characteristically occur in chronic failure of the left ventricle EXCEPT:
    A. pulmonary edema
    B. accumulation of hemosiderin in pulmonary macrophages
    C. interference with gas exchange in the lung
    D. microhemorrhages in alveolar spaces
    E. decreased pulmonary capillary pressure

E is correct.
With left ventricular heart failure, there is increased venous pressure in the pulmonary veins and in the pulmonary capillary bed. This is the mechanism of the pulmonary edema that occurs in left heart failure.

3.048   In septic shock, tumor necrosis factor (TNF) is produced by mononuclear phagocytes in response to:
A. bacterial wall lipopolysaccharides (LPS)
B. complement
C. interleukin-1 (IL-1)
D. nitric oxide
E. tissue necrosis

A is correct.
Septic shock is usually caused by endotoxin-producing Gram-negative bacilli. The endotoxins are bacterial wall lipopolysaccharides (LPS), which induce mononuclear phagocytes to produce TNF which, in turn, causes the production of IL-1. Both TNF and IL-1 induce endothelial cells to produce additional cytokines.

3.049   A patient with which one of the following conditions is LEAST predisposed to thrombosis?
A. leukopenia
B. pregnancy
C. pancreatic carcinoma
D. chronic right-sided congestive heart failure
E. acute myocardial infarction

A is correct.
Leukopenia or decreased white blood cell count in the peripheral blood does not predispose to thrombosis.

3.050   The processes of organization and recanalization of a venous thrombus would primarily involve which pair of the following components?
A. mast cells and fibroblasts
B. endothelial cells and plasma cells
C. platelets and fibroblasts
D. epithelioid cells and endothelial cells
E. fibroblasts and endothelial cells

E is correct.
Organization of a thrombus is defined as the ingrowth and proliferation of fibroblasts and endothelial cells from the attachment site of the thrombus to the vessel wall.

3.051   Disseminated intravascular coagulation is referred to as a consumptive coagulopathy because:
A. there is an underlying platelet disorder
B. platelets and coagulation factors are depleted
C. hypothrombocytemia is the underlying cause
D. it occurs predominantly in disseminated tuberculosis
E. there is an associated profound anemia

B is correct.
In disseminated intravascular coagulation, there is widespread development of fibrin thrombi in the microcirculation. The formation of the numerous small microthrombi causes consumption of platelets, prothrombin, fibrinogen, and factors V, VII, and X.

3.052   A 52-year-old woman is admitted to the hospital with a swollen left leg. Several hours later, she is found in acute respiratory distress. It is noted that her neck veins are bulging. Which one of the following conditions do you expect to find in this patient?
A. septic shock
B. infarcts of multiple organs
C. paradoxical embolism
D. increased right ventricular pressure
E. aortic stenosis

D is correct.
Unilateral swelling of a leg suggests a local phenomenon such as venous thrombosis. This woman has apparently experienced a pulmonary embolus from a femoral vein thrombus. Occlusion of pulmonary arteries creates increased resistance to blood flow and increased right ventricular pressure.

3.053   The MOST likely site for an occlusive thrombus is in the:
- A. aorta
- B. left atrium
- C. left ventricle
- D. right ventricle
- E. coronary artery

E is correct.

Occlusive thrombi occur in vessels of small- to medium-caliber such as coronary arteries. Thrombi occurring in large-caliber vascular spaces are usually attached to one wall (mural thrombi) and do not totally occlude the lumen.

3.054   Endotoxin-mediated activation of the mononuclear phagocyte system and the consequent release of which pair of the following mediators is believed to be a key event in the pathogenesis of septic shock?
- A. histamine and serotonin
- B. interleukin-1 and tumor necrosis factor-α
- C. leukotrienes B_4 and E_4
- D. prostaglandins and immunoglobulins
- E. integrins and selectins

B is correct.

Release of IL-1 and TNF-α as a result of activation of the mononuclear phagocyte system is a key event in septic shock.

3.055   Bilateral pitting edema of the lower extremities is MOST often secondary to:
- A. lymphatic obstruction
- B. bilateral venous thromboses
- C. arterial embolization
- D. cardiac failure
- E. renal failure

D is correct.

Bilateral edema of the lower extremities suggests a systemic rather than a local problem. So-called 'pitting' edema of the lower extremities is a common manifestation of right-sided cardiac failure.

3.056   A 64-year-old woman develops a mural thrombus in the left ventricle over an area of recent myocardial infarction. Her vital signs are stable and her temperature is normal. She develops sudden left costovertebral angle pain and blood in her urine. The BEST explanation for this is:
- A. renal infarct
- B. bilateral renal cortical necrosis
- C. acute bacterial infection of the kidney
- D. septic shock

A is correct.

A mural thrombus in the left ventricle may give rise to systemic thromboemboli. If one of these emboli lodge in an end-artery such as in the kidney, infarction of the tissue usually occurs. Renal infarct may present clinically with pain and hematuria.

3.057   In congestive heart failure, a significant etiologic factor in the edema which occurs is:
- A. increased hydrostatic pressure
- B. hypoalbuminemia
- C. increased vascular permeability
- D. increased renal tubular excretion of sodium

A is correct.

In heart failure, there is decreased venous return to the heart, resulting in increased venous hydrostatic pressure. According to Starling's law, this increased hydrostatic pressure moves fluid from within to outside of the vascular spaces.

SECTION 4: IMMUNE DISORDERS

4.001 Which one of the following is derived from a serum precursor synthesized in the liver?
- A. amyloid light chain protein (AL)
- B. amyloid-associated protein (AA)
- C. both of the above
- D. neither of the above

B is correct.

AA or amyloid-associated protein is a non-immunoglobulin protein derived from a serum precursor known as SAA (serum amyloid-associated) protein, which is synthesized in the liver and elevated in chronic inflammatory states.

4.002 Which one of the following is associated with chronic inflammatory states?
- A. amyloid light chain protein (AL)
- B. amyloid-associated protein (AA)
- C. both of the above
- D. neither of the above

B is correct.

AA or amyloid-associated protein is a non-immunoglobulin protein derived from a serum precursor known as SAA (serum amyloid-associated) protein, which is synthesized in the liver and elevated in chronic inflammatory states.

4.003 Which one of the following may occur in an intracellular location?
- A. amyloid light chain protein (AL)
- B. amyloid-associated protein (AA)
- C. both of the above
- D. neither of the above

D is correct.

Amyloid is deposited between cells in an extracellular location. It is not found intracellularly.

4.004 Electron microscopy reveals which one of the following as non-branching fibrils of indeterminate length associated with pentagonal subunits?
- A. amyloid light chain protein (AL)
- B. amyloid-associated protein (AA)
- C. both of the above
- D. neither of the above

C is correct.

The morphology of all types of amyloid, as determined by electron microscopy, is in groups of non-branching fibrils 7.5–10 nm in diameter and of indeterminate length. These fibrils are associated with a minor ('P') component, consisting of stacks of pentagonal structures composed of five glycoprotein subunits.

4.005 Amyloid deposits associated with chronic inflammatory states have which one of the following characteristics?
- A. intracellular accumulations of amyloid derived from amyloid-associated protein
- B. intracellular accumulations of amyloid derived from immunoglobulin light chains
- C. extracellular accumulations of amyloid derived from immunoglobulin light chains
- D. extracellular accumulations of amyloid derived from a serum precursor protein synthesized in the liver
- E. intracellular and extracellular accumulations of amyloid derived from amyloid-associated protein

D is correct.

The amyloid that accumulates in chronic inflammatory conditions such as rheumatoid arthritis is of the AA (amyloid-associated) type of protein. This is a non-immunoglobulin protein derived from a serum precursor protein which is synthesized in the liver.

4.006   All of the following are possible mechanisms by which T-helper cell tolerance can be bypassed, resulting in autoimmunity, EXCEPT:
  A. complexing of self-antigens with certain drugs
  B. antibodies to bacterial determinants that cross-react with receptors on B cells.
  C. enhanced T-suppressor cell activity
  D. emergence of sequestered antigens
  E. development of anti-idiotypic antibodies

C is correct.
Suppressor cells prevent autoimmune reactions by controlling the magnitude and duration of immune responses. A loss of suppressor cells, but not enhanced activity, may lead to immune reactions against self.

4.007   Tissue damage in autoimmune diseases is commonly mediated by all of the following EXCEPT:
  A. deposition of circulating immune complexes
  B. cell-mediated hypersensitivity resulting in lymphokine production by sensitized T cells
  C. formation of IgG antibodies that bind antigen, resulting in phagocytosis by the reticuloendothelial system
  D. binding of antibody and complement to various tissues
  E. development of antibodies that mimic the action of biologically active molecules

B is correct.
Cell-mediated hypersensitivity reactions (type IV) can be mediated by cytotoxic T lymphocytes or activated macrophages at sites of inflammation. Tissue damage in autoimmune diseases is mediated by antibody (type II) and immune complex-mediated (type III) hypersensitivity reactions.

4.008   All of the following autoantibodies are highly associated with the accompanying autoimmune disease EXCEPT:
  A. antibodies to ribonucleoproteins designated SS-A and SS-B, Sjögren's syndrome
  B. antibodies to DNA topoisomerase I, diffuse-type systemic sclerosis
  C. antibodies to histones, drug-induced systemic lupus erythematosus (SLE)
  D. antibodies to double-stranded DNA, SLE
  E. antibodies to the ribonucleoprotein designated U1RNP, CREST syndrome (systemic sclerosis)

E is correct.
Antibodies against ribonucleoproteins, such as U1RNP and Smith (Sm) antigen, are associated with systemic lupus erythematosus (SLE). Anticentromere antibodies are highly associated with CREST syndrome (systemic sclerosis).

4.009 All of the following are associated with the accompanying autoimmune disease EXCEPT:
- A. in Hashimoto's thyroiditis, the cardinal feature is enlargement of the thyroid gland and increased thyroid hormone levels
- B. in Hashimoto's thyroiditis, destruction of the thyroid gland can be mediated by direct T-cell killing and immune-complex deposition
- C. although the majority of patients with SLE have antinuclear antibodies, this finding is not specific for the disease
- D. clinical manifestations commonly associated with SLE include lesions involving blood vessels, kidneys, and skin
- E. in SLE, polyclonal activation of B cells results in increased production of antibodies to both self and non-self antigens

A is correct.

Cardinal features of Hashimoto's thyroiditis are an enlarged thyroid gland and hypothyroidism. Early in the disease, patients can have normal thyroid hormone levels with an elevation of serum TSH levels.

4.010 Each of the following statements is matched with the appropriate autoimmune disorder EXCEPT:
- A. CREST syndrome is a relatively benign form of scleroderma associated with limited skin involvement, often confined to fingers, forearms, and face.
- B. in Sjögren's syndrome, numerous autoantibodies are often present which are directed against salivary duct cells, smooth muscle mitochondria and thyroid antigens
- C. mixed connective tissue disease is characterized by high titers of antibodies against ribonucleoproteins which often appear 'speckled' by indirect immunofluorescence staining
- D. it has been postulated that the immunologic abnormalities in systemic sclerosis (scleroderma) are due to immune complex-mediated tissue injury
- E. skeletal muscle weakness in dermatomyositis may be mediated by CD4-positive cells which are present within areas of myofiber injury

D is correct.

In systemic sclerosis (scleroderma), fibroblast activation and collagen deposition are believed to contribute to the pathogenesis of the disease.

4.011 Each of the following is a true statement for SLE (systemic lupus erythematosus) EXCEPT:
   A. predominately a disease of women occurring in the second and third decades of life
   B. skin, joints and kidneys are commonly affected
   C. incidence is higher among those with certain class II histocompatibility complex antigens
   D. polyclonal activation of B cells results in antibodies against both self and non-self
   E. the finding of antinuclear antibodies is diagnostic of SLE

E is correct.
Antinuclear antibodies can be found in many autoimmune disorders. Antibodies against double-stranded DNA are highly specific for SLE.

4.012 Each of the following is true regarding inflammatory myopathy EXCEPT:
   A. myocyte necrosis in polymyositis is primarily mediated by B cell production of antibodies
   B. patients often produce antibodies against transfer RNA (tRNA) synthetase
   C. they are a heterogeneous group of disorders characterized by inflammation of skeletal muscles
   D. skin involvement in childhood dermatomyositis is associated with immune complex-mediated tissue injury
   E. in polymyositis, there is a lack of cutaneous involvement

A is correct.
Myocyte damage in polymyositis is caused by cell-mediated injury. CD8-positive cytotoxic T cells and macrophages can be found near damaged muscle fibers. In dermatomyositis, antibodies and complement produce foci of myocyte necrosis.

4.013 Which one of the following antibodies is highly associated with the accompanying autoimmune disease?
   A. tRNA synthetase, polymyositis
   B. DNA topoisomerase I, SLE
   C. double-stranded DNA, CREST syndrome (systemic sclerosis)
   D. ribonucleoprotein U1RNP, drug-induced SLE
   E. histones, diffuse-type systemic sclerosis

A is correct.
Antibodies against double-stranded DNA and Sm antigen are associated with SLE, anticentromere antibodies with CREST syndrome (systemic sclerosis); antihistone antibodies with drug-induced SLE; and anti-DNA topoisomerase I antibodies (Scl-70) with diffuse-type systemic sclerosis.

4.014 Which one of the following is NOT a postulated mechanism resulting in loss of self-tolerance and development of autoimmunity?
   A. complexing of self-antigens with certain drugs
   B. direct activation of B cells by bacterial components
   C. thymic and/or macrophage defects
   D. loss of T-helper cell function
   E. emergence of sequestered antigens

D is correct.
Increased T-helper cell function contributes to the development of autoimmunity by driving B cells to produce extremely high levels of autoantibody.

4.015   Tissue injury in autoimmune diseases is NOT mediated by which of the following?
   A. deposition of immune complexes
   B. cytokine release by T-suppressor cells
   C. antibody and complement
   D. antibodies that mimic biologically active molecules
   E. cytotoxic T cell-mediated reactions

B is correct.
T-suppressor cells normally down-regulate immune responses and do not mediate tissue damage by producing cytokines.

4.016   Which one of the following statements is TRUE of Hashimoto's thyroiditis?
   A. the defect is a deficiency of T-helper cell activity
   B. the classic presentation is an enlarged thyroid gland and increased thyroid hormone levels
   C. autoantibodies are formed against thyroglobulin and TSH receptors
   D. extensive destruction of thyroid parenchyma results in release of thyroid hormones and hyperthyroidism
   E. an association with major histocompatibility complex (MHC) genes has not been shown

C is correct.
The defect in Hashimoto's thyroiditis is thought to be a deficiency in antigen-specific suppressor T cells. Patients normally present with decreased T3 and T4 hormone levels. Extensive destruction of the thyroid parenchyma results in hypothyroidism and there is a well-defined association with HLA-DR5.

4.017   The diffuse form of scleroderma (systemic sclerosis):
   A. is associated with antibodies to histones
   B. is associated with vascular abnormalities and activation of fibroblasts
   C. involves only the skin and mucous membranes
   D. is characterized by excessive deposition of amyloid throughout the body
   E. is not associated with antinuclear antibodies in the majority of cases

B is correct.
The diffuse form of scleroderma is associated with antibodies against DNA topoisomerase I (Scl-70), widespread skin and visceral involvement, excessive deposition of collagen, and antibodies against many nuclear antigens.

4.018   All of the following are possible mechanisms by which T-helper cell tolerance can be bypassed, resulting in autoimmunity, EXCEPT:
   A. complexing of self-antigens with drugs or microorganisms
   B. direct stimulation of T-suppressor cells
   C. partial degradation of autoantigen
   D. direct activation of autoreactive B cells
   E. infectious agents bearing haptenic determinants that cross-react with human tissues

B is correct.
Suppressor cells prevent autoimmune reactions by controlling the magnitude and duration of immune responses. A loss of suppressor cells, but not direct stimulation, may lead to immune reactions against self.

4.019   All of the following autoantibodies are highly associated with the accompanying autoimmune disease EXCEPT:
  A. antibodies to double-stranded DNA, SLE
  B. antibodies to centromeric proteins, CREST syndrome (systemic sclerosis)
  C. antibodies to ribonucleoproteins designated SS-A and SS-B, Sjögren's syndrome
  D. antibodies to histones, polymyositis
  E. antibodies to DNA topoisomerase I, diffuse-type systemic sclerosis.

D is correct.
Antibodies against histones are associated with drug-induced SLE. In polymyositis, antibodies against histidyl-tRNA synthetase, called Jo-1, are commonly seen.

4.020   All of the following statements are true of SLE EXCEPT:
  A. the most prevalent clinical manifestations involve the skin, kidneys, and liver
  B. virtually every patient with SLE has antinuclear antibodies, although this finding is not specific for SLE
  C. SLE can occur at any age, but usually becomes manifest in the second and third decades of life
  D. polyclonal activation of B cells results in increased production of antibodies to both self and non-self antigens
  E. antibodies to double-stranded DNA and the so-called Smith (Sm) antigen are strongly suggestive of SLE

A is correct.
Prevalent clinical manifestations of SLE include the skin, kidneys, joints, and serosal membranes. Although virtually every organ in the body may be involved, liver involvement is relatively uncommon.

4.021   All of the following statements are true of Hashimoto's thyroiditis EXCEPT:
  A. extensive destruction of thyroid parenchyma occurs, ultimately resulting in hypothyroidism
  B. a deficiency in antigen-specific T-suppressor cells has been implicated as the basic defect resulting in the disease process
  C. the cardinal clinical feature is thyroid gland atrophy associated with hypothyroidism in elderly women
  D. patients commonly have antibodies to thyroglobulin and follicular cell membranes as well as antibodies to thyroid hormones themselves
  E. thyroid destruction occurs by a variety of mechanisms, including direct T-cell killing and immune-complex deposition

C is correct.
The cardinal clinical feature in Hashimoto's thyroiditis is goitrous enlargement of the thyroid due to an intense infiltrate of lymphocytes and plasma cells, and hypothyroidism in a middle-aged woman. There is a less common atrophic variant which exhibits fibrosis of the parenchyma with a scant lymphoid infiltrate.

4.022   Which one of the following statements is FALSE?
  A. Sjögren's syndrome is characterized by an autoimmune process resulting in destruction of the lacrimal and salivary glands
  B. mixed connective tissue disease resembles SLE and scleroderma clinically, and can exhibit high titers of antibodies to nuclear ribonucleoprotein
  C. polymyositis is characterized by symmetric muscle weakness, often accompanied by a skin rash
  D. in myasthenia gravis, antibodies to the acetylcholine receptor result in muscular weakness and fatigability
  E. scleroderma is characterized by excessive deposition of amyloid throughout the body

E is correct.
Scleroderma is characterized by excessive fibrosis throughout the body.

4.023   All of the following are possible mechanisms by which T-helper cell tolerance can be bypassed, resulting in autoimmunity, EXCEPT:
  A. presentation of cross-reacting determinants in association with self antigens
  B. emergence of sequestered antigens
  C. loss of T-suppressor cells
  D. diminished T-helper cell function
  E. generation of antibodies to bacterial determinants that react with B-cell receptors

D is correct.
A loss of T-helper cell function preserves the state of tolerance.

4.024   All of the following statements are true of each autoimmune disease EXCEPT:
  A. Sjögren's syndrome is characterized by an autoimmune process resulting in destruction of the lacrimal and salivary glands
  B. polymyositis is characterized by autoantibodies against the basement membrane of glomeruli, and is often accompanied by a skin rash
  C. scleroderma is characterized by excessive collagen deposition (fibrosis) throughout the body
  D. in myasthenia gravis, antibodies are produced against the acetylcholine receptor, resulting in decreased transmission of nerve impulses
  E. in mixed connective tissue disease, antibodies against nuclear ribonucleo-proteins are produced in high titers

B is correct.
In polymyositis, CD8$^+$ cytotoxic T cells and macrophages are found near damaged muscle fibers. There is no renal or skin involvement.

4.025 All of the following statements are true of Hashimoto's thyroiditis EXCEPT:
    A. the majority of cases present with thyroid gland enlargement and increased thyroid hormone levels
    B. extensive destruction of the thyroid parenchyma occurs
    C. the basic defect is a deficiency in antigen-specific T-suppressor cells
    D. pathogenic mechanisms include direct T-cell killing and immune-complex deposition
    E. patients commonly have antibodies against TSH receptors, thyroid hormones and thyroglobulin

A is correct.
The classic clinical presentation in Hashimoto's thyroiditis is goitrous enlargement and hypothyroidism or decreased thyroid-hormone levels. A few patients develop hyperthyroidism in mid-course which is sometimes called hashitoxicosis.

4.026 All of the following statements are true of SLE EXCEPT:
    A. clinical manifestations include involvement of the skin, joints, and kidneys
    B. antinuclear antibodies are detectable in virtually every patient
    C. tissue damage is primarily due to direct killing by cytotoxic T cells
    D. antibodies against native DNA and the so-called Sm antigen are strongly suggestive of SLE
    E. the incidence of SLE is higher among those who express certain class II major histocompatibility complex antigens

C is correct.
Tissue damage in SLE is primarily mediated by immune-complex deposition (type III hypersensitivity) in the glomeruli and small blood vessels. Autoantibodies are also directed against red cells, white cells and platelets (type II hypersensitivity). Cytotoxic T cells do not appear to play an important role in this disease.

4.027 All of the following autoantibodies are highly associated with the accompanying autoimmune disease EXCEPT:
    A. antibodies to DNA topoisomerase I, CREST variant of systemic sclerosis
    B. antibodies to histones, drug-induced SLE
    C. antibodies to ribonucleoproteins designated SS-A and SS-B, Sjögren's syndrome
    D. antibodies to histidyl-tRNA synthetase, polymyositis
    E. antibodies to double-stranded DNA, SLE

A is correct.
Antibodies against DNA topoisomerase I are associated with the diffuse type of systemic sclerosis. Antibodies against centromeric proteins, designated Scl-70, are associated with the CREST variant of systemic sclerosis.

SECTION 5: NEOPLASIA

5.001 The MOST common cancer in women in the USA begins in the:
- A. lung
- B. colon
- C. breast
- D. uterus
- E. pancreas

C is correct.

Based on 1989 incidence figures, breast cancer in women represented 28% of all cancer cases. Colorectal cancer was second at 15.4%.

5.002 The MOST frequent site of origin for a fatal cancer in the USA is:
- A. lung
- B. colon
- C. breast
- D. uterus
- E. pancreas

A is correct.

According to the 1991 figures, cancer arising in the lung was responsible for 34% of cancer deaths in men and 21% of cancer deaths in women. The second most frequent site of cancer leading to death was the prostate (12%), colon and rectum (11%) in men, and the breast (18%) in women.

5.003 Which one of the following cancers has declined markedly in incidence in the USA over the last 60 years?
- A. lung
- B. colon
- C. breast
- D. stomach
- E. pancreas

D is correct.

Stomach cancer has declined in both sexes over the past 60 years. Incidence of cancer in all of the other sites listed has either increased or remained approximately the same.

5.004 The MOST common types of primary malignant neoplasms in children age < 15 years are:
- A. brain tumors
- B. leukemias
- C. bone sarcomas
- D. urinary bladder tumors
- E. non-Hodgkin's lymphomas

B is correct.

Leukemias are the most common primary malignant neoplasms in children of both sexes under the age of 15 years. The second most common neoplasms in this age group are tumors of the central nervous system.

5.005 All of the following are among the eight MOST common primary cancer types in adult women EXCEPT:
- A. breast
- B. colorectum
- C. lung
- D. endometrium
- E. central nervous system

E is correct.

In women, cancer of the breast, colorectum, lung, and endometrium are the top four in incidence, followed by lymphomas, pancreas, cervix, and leukemia.

5.006 The highest number of cancer deaths in men in the USA is from which of the following cancer types?
  A. colorectal
  B. prostate
  C. lung
  D. pancreas
  E. leukemia/lymphoma

C is correct.
According to 1991 statistics, carcinoma of the lung accounted for 34% of cancer deaths in men. The next highest numbers were the prostate at 12% and colorectal cancers at 11%.

5.007 The major role of proteases in tumor cell invasion is to:
  A. increase cell–cell adhesion
  B. erode extracellular matrix barriers to invasion
  C. increase contractility of the cytoskeleton
  D. destroy host immune cells

B is correct.
Invasion by tumor cells involves a decrease in the cohesion of the tumor cells followed by attachment to extracellular matrix proteins such as laminin and fibronectin. Local degradation of the basement membrane and interstitial connective tissue occurs by the action of proteolytic enzymes secreted by the tumor cells.

5.008 The single MOST important environmental agent causing cancer in the USA population is/are:
  A. polychlorinated hydrocarbons
  B. nuclear power-plant radiation
  C. cigarette smoke
  D. food additives
  E. microwave emissions

C is correct.
Cigarette smoke has been implicated etiologically in lung, oropharyngeal, esophageal, pancreatic and bladder cancers.

5.009 The MOST common type of fatal cancer in patients < 15 years of age is:
  A. leukemia
  B. endocrine
  C. lung
  D. connective tissue
  E. breast

A is correct.
Leukemias, followed by cancer of the central nervous system, are associated with the highest mortality in children under the age of 15 years.

5.010 All of the following are characteristic of indirect-acting carcinogens EXCEPT:
  A. modulate secretory responses by activating protein kinase C
  B. require conversion to an electrophile
  C. are metabolized by cytochrome P-450
  D. produce permanent DNA change

A is correct.
Indirect-acting carcinogens require conversion to an electrophile before they become active carcinogens. They are believed to produce a heritable change involving DNA. Most carcinogens are metabolized by cytochrome P-450 enzymes. Promoters and not carcinogens are associated with protein kinase C activation.

5.011 Which one of the following neoplasms develops earliest after radiation exposure?
  A. lung
  B. breast
  C. acute leukemia
  D. stomach
  E. plasma cell myeloma

C is correct.
Acute leukemia, which has a mean latent period of 7 years in atomic bomb survivors, occurs before other forms of radiation-induced neoplasia.

5.012 All of the following neoplasms are associated with an oncogenic DNA virus EXCEPT:
   A. undifferentiated nasopharyngeal carcinoma
   B. Burkitt's lymphoma
   C. uterine cervical carcinoma
   D. hepatocellular carcinoma
   E. adult T-cell lymphoma/leukemia

E is correct.
Adult T-cell lymphoma/leukemia is associated with an oncogenic RNA virus.

5.013 Various serotypes of human papillomavirus are associated with all of the following neoplasms EXCEPT:
   A. deep plantar warts
   B. common cutaneous warts
   C. laryngeal squamous cell carcinoma
   D. undifferentiated nasopharyngeal carcinoma
   E. condyloma acuminatum

D is correct.
Epstein–Barr virus (EBV) is associated with undifferentiated nasopharyngeal carcinoma.

5.014 Cancer cachexia is MOST strongly related to which of the following biologic substances?
   A. tumor necrosis factor (TNF)-α
   B. interleukin-2 (IL-2)
   C. serotonin
   D. erythropoietin
   E. parathyroid hormone

A is correct.
Progressive weakness, loss of appetite, anemia, and profound weight loss (cachexia) are probably related to the production of TNF-α by macrophages.

5.015 All of the following neoplasms are frequently associated with hypercalcemia syndromes EXCEPT:
   A. multiple myeloma
   B. renal cell carcinoma
   C. pulmonary squamous cell carcinoma
   D. T-cell lymphoma
   E. pulmonary small-cell undifferentiated carcinoma

E is correct.
Of the neoplasms listed, hypercalcemia is least likely to occur in pulmonary small-cell undifferentiated carcinoma. This tumor is most likely to be associated with Cushing's or inappropriate ADH syndromes.

5.016 The carcinoid syndrome is almost always seen after metastasis of a carcinoid tumor to the:
   A. brain
   B. lung
   C. bone
   D. liver
   E. spleen

D is correct.
After metastasis to the liver, the neoplastic cells release large amounts of 5-hydroxytryptophan and 5-hydroxytryptamine directly into the systemic circulation via the hepatic veins without metabolic degradation by the hepatocytes. These substances are causative factors in the carcinoid syndrome.

5.017 Lymphokine-activated killer cells with antitumor activities develop from peripheral blood mononuclear cells stimulated by large non-physiologic doses of:
   A. IL-2
   B. IL-1
   C. IL-6
   D. TNF-α
   E. β_2-microglobulin

A is correct.
Peripheral blood lymphocytes of cancer patients may be activated with high levels of IL-2, then reinfused into the patient. These lymphokine activated cells may cause partial or complete regression of metastases in certain cancers.

5.018 An adult male patient presents with clubbing of the ends of the fingers, widespread periosteal new-bone formation on X-rays, and a painful arthritis in multiple joints. The patient should be examined for primary carcinoma of the:
    A. liver
    B. lung
    C. breast
    D. colon
    E. pancreas

B is correct.
The features listed are those of the syndrome hypertrophic osteoarthropathy, which occurs in 1–10% of patients with bronchogenic carcinoma.

5.019 The increased mortality from lung carcinoma in certain miners is strongly related to the presence of:
    A. helium
    B. radon
    C. plutonium
    D. tritium
    E. carbon-14

B is correct.
It has been found that radon gas, which emits alpha particles, is responsible for the increased frequency of lung carcinoma in miners.

5.020 The BEST criterion of malignancy is:
    A. monoclonality
    B. clinical behavior
    C. cell-cycle time of the individual tumor cells
    D. growth fraction of the tumor

B is correct.
Although most malignant neoplasms have various recognizable characteristics, the most certain criterion of malignancy is the ability of the neoplasm to invade adjacent tissue and to metastasize.

5.021 Regarding populations of tumor cells, which of the following is NOT true?
    A. most tumors are monoclonal, that is, they arise from a common ancestral cell
    B. within a given tumor, all cells are homogeneous with regard to all properties
    C. the size and growth rate of a tumor is related to the number of cells in the growth fraction weighed against cell loss
    D. tumor cells can be lost from the growth fraction by differentiation

B is correct.
Tumor cell heterogeneity is a common finding.

5.022 Regarding laminin and laminin receptors, which of the following is NOT true?
    A. laminin is a component of the basement membrane
    B. some tumor cells secrete laminin
    C. some tumor cells have laminin receptors
    D. laminin is a proteolytic enzyme that allows tumor cells to degrade and penetrate the basement membrane

D is correct.
Tumor cell enzymes capable of degrading the basement membrane or extracellular matrix include collagenases, glycosidases, proteinases, and plasmin.

5.023   Regarding the natural history of tumors, which one of the following IS true?
  A. once malignant transformation takes place, the tumor cells do not change
  B. all tumor cells have the same metastatic potential
  C. the majority of the lifespan of a tumor occurs prior to clinical detection
  D. tumor cells are genetically stable

C is correct.
Tumors have passed the majority of their life cycle by the time of clinical detection.

5.024   Regarding metastasis, which one of the following is NOT true?
  A. metastatic tumor cells tend to be less susceptible to immunologic destruction
  B. metastatic potential is decreased if tumor cells aggregate in the circulation
  C. some tumor cells have receptors that allow them to 'home in' to specific organs
  D. tumor cell motility promotes metastasis

B is correct.
Metastatic potential is increased if the tumor cells aggregate in the circulation. Aggregates of tumor cells become coated with platelets. This renders the tumor cell aggregate sticky and further protects it from immunologic attack.

5.025   Regarding oncogenes, which one of the following IS true?
  A. oncogenes are always abnormal and have no normal counterpart in normal cells
  B. oncogenes are normal cellular genes that are involved in growth control, and cancer occurs when these genes become dysregulated
  C. all cancer cells originally obtained oncogenes from viruses
  D. proteins produced by oncogenes are always structurally abnormal

B is correct.
Oncogenes are normal cellular genes that are involved in growth control. Cancer is the result when these genes become dysregulated.

5.026   Regarding the following statement, which answer is NOT true? Oncogenes mimic the action of:
  A. growth factors
  B. growth factor receptors
  C. protein kinases
  D. glycolytic enzymes

D is correct.
Oncogenes mimic the action of growth factors, growth factor receptors, guanine-binding (G) proteins, kinases, and gene regulatory phospho-proteins.

5.027   Which one of the following mechanisms has NOT been shown to cause oncogene ACTIVATION in human tumors?
  A. point mutation
  B. chromosomal translocation
  C. gene amplification
  D. gene deletion

D is correct.
Activation of oncogenes has been shown to occur from point mutations as in the *ras* gene, chromosomal translocation as in the Philadelphia chromosome, and from gene amplification through errors in DNA replication. Gene deletion has not been found to be associated with oncogene activation in human tumors.

5.028   In Burkitt's lymphoma, which one of the following mechanisms is responsible for the activation of the c-*myc* gene?
   A. point mutation
   B. gene amplification
   C. chromosomal translocation
   D. gene deletion

C is correct.
In Burkitt's lymphoma, there is one of three translocations involving chromosome 8q24, where the c-*myc* gene has been mapped.

5.029   Which one of the following mechanisms is thought to cause retinoblastoma?
   A. point mutation involving the *ras* gene
   B. amplification of the N-*myc* gene
   C. chromosomal translocation involving the c-*myc* gene and the immunoglobulin heavy chain gene locus
   D. inactivation of a tumor suppressor gene

D is correct.
There is a class of genes that normally suppress growth. In some tumors, these genes are mutated, and uncontrolled growth occurs. Retinoblastoma, an eye tumor found in children, is an example of inactivation of a tumor suppressor gene (Rb gene).

5.030   Which one of the following cancers has approximately the SAME incidence in both sexes?
   A. breast carcinoma
   B. colon adenocarcinoma
   C. lung carcinoma
   D. urinary tract carcinoma
   E. laryngeal carcinoma

B is correct.
The incidence of colon cancer is about 14% in both men and women. Breast carcinoma has a higher incidence in women, and the others listed have a higher incidence in men.

5.031   All of the following viruses are definitely associated with human neoplasms EXCEPT:
   A. Epstein–Barr virus
   B. hepatitis B virus
   C. measles virus
   D. human T-lymphocyte virus type I
   E. human papillomavirus type 16

C is correct.
Measles virus has not been proven to be etiologically involved in any human neoplasms.

5.032   Migratory venous thromboses are MOST commonly associated with:
   A. squamous cell carcinomas
   B. adenocarcinomas
   C. small-cell undifferentiated carcinomas
   D. sarcomas
   E. teratomas

B is correct.
Migratory venous thrombosis or Trousseau's syndrome may be seen with visceral cancers. Most commonly, the association is with adenocarcinomas, especially of the pancreas.

5.033   Lower income and educational status has which one of the following effects on cancer incidence and survival?
   A. incidence decreased, survival increased
   B. incidence decreased, survival decreased
   C. incidence increased, survival increased
   D. incidence increased, survival decreased
   E. no significant effects

D is correct.
The economically disadvantaged as a group have more chances of developing cancer and less chances of surviving it.

5.034 The BEST definition of malignancy is:
  A. monoclonality
  B. the ability to invade and metastasize
  C. high mitotic index
  D. chromosomal abnormalities (such as
     translocation, inversion, duplication, etc.)
  E. high nuclear-to-cytoplasmic ratio

B is correct.
Although all of the other features listed may occur in malignant neoplasms, they are not absolute criteria for malignancy. For instance, any actively growing tissue may have a high mitotic index. Cells such as normal lymphocytes have high nuclear-to-cytoplasmic ratios. By far, the best criterion for malignancy is the ability of a neoplasm to invade normal tissues and to metastasize to distant sites.

5.035 The retinoblastoma (Rb) gene is a tumor suppressor gene. Which one of the following mechanisms involving the Rb locus is NOT likely to result in tumor formation?
  A. chromosomal translocation
  B. gene deletion
  C. point mutation
  D. gene amplification

D is correct.
In retinoblastoma, a tumor suppressor gene is responsible. Tumor suppressor genes cause cancer by inactivation of the gene product, rather than activation as is seen with other oncogenes. Therefore, gene amplification is not likely to result in retinoblastoma.

5.036 Which one of the following cancers occurs with the highest incidence in men?
  A. lung
  B. prostate
  C. colorectum
  D. stomach
  E. pancreas

B is correct.
Cancer of the prostate is the most common type of cancer in men. The second most common type is lung cancer.

5.037 Which one of the following cancers occurs with the highest incidence in women?
  A. lung
  B. colorectum
  C. uterus
  D. breast
  E. liver

D is correct.
Cancer of the breast is the most common type of cancer in women. The incidence of breast cancer has been increasing for the past 80 years.

5.038 Which one of the following cancers causes the highest percentage of cancer-related deaths in men and women?
  A. breast
  B. urinary tract
  C. colorectum
  D. lung
  E. pancreas

D is correct.
Lung cancer is responsible for approximately 33% of cancer deaths in men and 23% of cancer deaths in women.

5.039   Which one of the following alterations to tumor suppressor genes, such as Rb or p53, may cause cancer to develop?
    A. both normal alleles of the tumor suppressor gene are mutated so that the protein products of these genes are inactivated
    B. one allele of the tumor suppressor gene is mutated so that its protein product is overactive
    C. one allele of the tumor suppressor gene is mutated and produces an inactive protein product
    D. both normal alleles of the tumor suppressor gene are mutated so that the protein products of these genes are overactive
    E. one normal allele of a tumor suppressor gene is deleted from the genome.

A is correct.
Both of the normal alleles of the Rb locus or the p53 locus must be inactivated to produce tumors. The Rb alteration results in retinoblastoma, and the p53 mutation has been identified in colon, breast, and lung cancers as well as other malignancies.

5.040   The *c-erb* B-2/*neu* gene encodes a tyrosine kinase of the epidermal growth factor-receptor (EGF-R) family. An abnormality of this gene is seen in >30% of all breast cancers. Which one of the following cytogenetic abnormalities is identified regarding this association?
    A. translocation of the chromosomal segment next to an active promoter, resulting in overexpression of its gene product
    B. amplification of the c-*erb* B-2/*neu* gene, resulting in overexpression of the c-*erb* B-2/*neu* gene product
    C. point mutation of the normal *c-erb* B-2/*neu* gene, causing overactivity of its protein product
    D. deletion of one allele of the c-*erb* B-2/*neu* gene, causing overexpression of the remaining allele

B is correct.
Amplification of the c-*erb* B-2 gene resulting in overexpression of its product is present in >30% of breast cancers. Such amplification is associated with a poor prognosis.

5.041   Cytogenetic analysis of chromosomes from tumor cells can identify aberrant banding patterns, indicating which one of the following genetic abnormalities?
    A. point mutations
    B. mutations caused by carcinogens
    C. gene amplification
    D. pyrimidine dimers

C is correct.
Regions of chromosomes containing amplified genes lack a normal banding pattern, a feature which can be seen on cytogenetic analysis.

5.042 Which one of the following types of cancers is characterized by early age of onset, tumors arising in two or more close relatives of the patient, and sometimes multiple or bilateral tumors, with no association with a specific marker phenotype?
    A. inherited cancer syndromes
    B. familial cancers
    C. autosomal-recessive syndromes of defective DNA repair
    D. paraneoplastic syndromes

B is correct.
Familial cancers are characterized by early age of onset, neoplasms arising in two or more close relatives that are often multiple or bilateral, and not associated with specific marker phenotypes.

5.043 Which one of the following is a small group of cancers characterized by chromosomal or DNA instability?
    A. inherited cancer syndromes
    B. familial cancers
    C. autosomal-recessive syndromes of defective DNA repair
    D. paraneoplastic syndromes

C is correct.
A group of autosomal-recessive disorders manifest chromosomal or DNA instability, such as xeroderma pigmentosum.

5.044 Which one of the following types of cancers involves specific sites and tissues, and is often associated with a specific marker phenotype?
    A. inherited cancer syndromes
    B. familial cancers
    C. autosomal-recessive syndromes of defective DNA repair
    D. paraneoplastic syndromes

A is correct.
Several cancers comprise a group known as inherited cancer syndrome. These have a single mutant gene which increases the risk of tumor development.

5.045 Acquisition of permanent changes in tumor cell characteristics such as karyotype, invasiveness, and metastatic potential is known as:
    A. excess tumor cell production relative to tumor cell loss
    B. transformation
    C. tumor progression
    D. facilitated metastasis of tumor cells
    E. host-factor effects on tumor cell growth

C is correct.
Tumor progression is defined as the acquisition of permanent changes in characteristics of selected subpopulations of the tumor, such as karyotype, invasiveness, or metastatic potential.

5.046 Which one of the following terms refers to the genetic changes in a cell that release it from normal growth control and cause it to become hyperproliferative?
    A. excess tumor cell production relative to tumor cell loss
    B. transformation
    C. tumor progression
    D. facilitated metastasis of tumor cells
    E. host-factor effects on tumor cell growth

B is correct.
When cells undergo genetic alterations which cause it to be released from normal growth control, the cells begin to proliferate. This process is called transformation.

5.047   Which one of the following determines the rate of tumor growth?
  A. excess tumor cell production relative to tumor cell loss
  B. transformation
  C. tumor progression
  D. facilitated metastasis of tumor cells
  E. host-factor effects on tumor cell growth

A is correct.
The size and growth rate of a tumor is related to the number of cells in the growth fraction of the cell cycle balanced against cell loss.

5.048   Which one of the following is associated with an immune response to tumor cells?
  A. excess tumor cell production relative to tumor cell loss
  B. transformation
  C. tumor progression
  D. facilitated metastasis of tumor cells
  E. host-factor effects on tumor cell growth

E is correct.
Many tumors contain antigens which elicit an immune response in the host. These antigens may be tumor-specific antigens, which are present only on tumor cells, or tumor-associated antigens, which may appear on tumor cells as well as on some normal cells.

5.049   Formation of platelet-coated cell aggregates in the circulation, and the presence of chemo-attractant receptors on normal cell surfaces are associated with:
  A. excess tumor cell production relative to tumor cell loss
  B. transformation
  C. tumor progression
  D. facilitated metastasis of tumor cells
  E. host-factor effects on tumor cell growth

D is correct.
Groups of tumor cells which have gained access to the circulation are vulnerable to destruction by immune processes. Tumor cells attempt to avoid this by forming platelet-coated aggregates in the circulation. Also, tumor cells may express adhesion molecules which have ligands expressed on the endothelial cells of distant organs.

5.050 Which one of the following agents is MOST closely associated with cervical carcinoma?
  A. direct-acting carcinogens
  B. ultraviolet light
  C. indirect-acting carcinogens
  D. ionizing radiation
  E. human papillomaviruses

E is correct.
DNA sequences of the human papillomavirus have been found in approximately 85% of squamous cell carcinomas of the cervix.

5.051   Which one of the following agents may cause mutations either by direct damage to DNA or DNA damage caused by free radicals formed from water or oxygen?
  A. direct-acting carcinogens
  B. ultraviolet light
  C. indirect-acting carcinogens
  D. ionizing radiation
  E. human papillomaviruses

D is correct.
The mechanism of radiation carcinogenesis involves direct interaction with DNA or indirect action mediated by free radicals generated from water and oxygen.

5.052 Which one of the following is MOST close-ly associated with squamous cell, basal cell, and melanotic carcinomas in fair-skinned subjects?
    A. direct-acting carcinogens
    B. ultraviolet light
    C. indirect-acting carcinogens
    D. ionizing radiation
    E. human papillomaviruses

B is correct.
Ultraviolet light induces squamous cell carcinoma, basal cell carcinoma, and melanotic carcinoma of the skin surface. The mechanism of carcinogenesis is related to the formation of pyrimidine dimers in DNA.

5.053 Which one of the following agents requires oxidative conversion to an electrophilic species before being able to cause damage to DNA?
    A. direct-acting carcinogens
    B. ultraviolet light
    C. indirect-acting carcinogens
    D. ionizing radiation
    E. human papillomaviruses

C is correct.
Indirect-acting carcinogens, such as polycyclic aromatic hydrocarbons, are potent carcinogens which require metabolic conversion before they can induce tumors.

5.054 Which one of the following damages DNA by causing the formation of pyrimidine dimers?
    A. direct-acting carcinogens
    B. ultraviolet light
    C. indirect-acting carcinogens
    D. ionizing radiation
    E. human papillomaviruses

B is correct.
Ultraviolet light induces squamous cell carcinoma, basal cell carcinoma, and melanotic carcinoma of the skin surface. The mechanism of carcinogenesis is related to the formation of pyrimidine dimers in DNA.

5.055 Progressive weakness, loss of appetite, anemia, and profound weight loss are an example of which one of the following?
    A. local deleterious effects of tumors on the host
    B. cancer cachexia
    C. paraneoplastic syndrome
    D. altered coagulability due to the release of tumor products

B is correct.
Many patients with cancer develop progressive weight loss, weakness, anorexia, and anemia. This syndrome is known as cachexia. It is suspected that TNF-α is a mediator of the cachexia syndrome.

5.056 Squamous cell lung cancer releasing a high level of parathyroid hormone (PTH)-like peptide is BEST described by which one of the following?
    A. local deleterious effects of tumors on the host
    B. cancer cachexia
    C. paraneoplastic syndrome
    D. altered coagulability due to the release of tumor products

C is correct.
Many tumors are associated with paraneoplastic syndromes. One such syndrome is the secretion of a PTH-like peptide by squamous cell carcinoma, especially of the lung, resulting in hypercalcemia.

5.057 Pulmonary infections due to neoplasm-blocked bronchi are due to:
    A. local deleterious effects of tumors on the host
    B. cancer cachexia
    C. paraneoplastic syndrome
    D. altered coagulability due to the release of tumor products

A is correct.
One of the local effects of a tumor is blockage of a bronchus, resulting in an inability to clear bronchial secretions. This predisposes the patient to the development of pneumonia.

5.058   Marantic endocarditis and Trousseau's sign
are examples of:
  A. local deleterious effects of tumors on the host
  B. cancer cachexia
  C. paraneoplastic syndrome
  D. altered coagulability due to the release of
     tumor products

D is correct.
Many tumors release substances that result in an
increased coagulability of the blood. Marantic endocarditis is the formation of small thrombi on heart
valves. Trousseau's sign is the migratory thrombosis
which may occur in cancer patients.

5.059   Blockage of neuromuscular transmission
caused by cross-reacting antibodies or toxins is an
example of:
  A. local deleterious effects of tumors on the host
  B. cancer cachexia
  C. paraneoplastic syndrome
  D. altered coagulability due to the release of
     tumor products

C is correct.
Tumor may induce the production of antibodies
which may then cross-react with neuronal cells,
resulting in various forms of neuropathies.

5.060   All of the following cancers most com-
monly appear in subjects > 20 years of age EXCEPT:
  A. osteosarcoma
  B. melanoma
  C. plasmacytoma
  D. clear-cell lung carcinoma
  E. colorectal

A is correct.
Approximately 75% of osteosarcomas occur in
patients < 20 years of age.

5.061   A 52-year-old woman with lung cancer has
metastases to bone, liver, brain, and adrenals. Which
one of the following BEST defines these observa-
tions?
  A. grade I
  B. grade IV
  C. stage I
  D. stage IV

D is correct.
The 'grade' of a tumor refers to the histologic
appearance of the cells. The more closely the cells
morphologically resemble normal cells, the lower
the grade (I–II). Cells that are anaplastic and have
little morphologic resemblance to normal cells are
given a high grade (IV). The clinical extent of a
tumor is reflected in the stage. The more confined
the neoplasm, the lower the stage (I–II). Tumors
with widespread metastases are given a high stage
(IV).

5.062   A biopsy of a colonic mass in a 58-year-
old man is diagnosed as adenocarcinoma. The tumor
cells are forming colonic glands resembling those
in the normal colon. Mucin secretion by the tumor
cells is evident. Which one of the following BEST
defines these observations?
  A. grade I
  B. grade IV
  C. stage I
  D. stage IV

A is correct.
The 'grade' of a tumor refers to the histologic
appearance of the cells. The more closely the cells
morphologically resemble normal cells, the lower
the grade (I–II). Cells that are anaplastic and have
little morphologic resemblance to normal cells are
given a high grade (IV). The clinical extent of a
tumor is reflected in the stage. The more confined
the neoplasm, the lower the stage (I–II). Tumors
with widespread metastases are given a high stage
(IV).

5.063   Which one of the following requires inactivation or loss of both alleles to transform cells?
   A. tumor suppressor genes
   B. proto-oncogenes
   C. genes that regulate apoptosis
   D. defective DNA-repair genes
   E. tumor progression

A is correct.
The first cancer suppressor gene discovered was the retinoblastoma (Rb) gene. It requires two mutations (one for each of the alleles of the Rb locus) to produce a retinoblastoma.

5.064   Which one of the following is implicated in the reduced cell death and consequent abnormal cell persistence observed in some slow-growing lymphomas?
   A. tumor suppressor genes
   B. proto-oncogenes
   C. genes that regulate apoptosis
   D. defective DNA-repair genes
   E. tumor progression

C is correct.
Certain lymphomas are slow-growing tumors that increase in size due to reduced tumor cell death rather than excessive proliferation. The mechanism is believed to involve alterations in a gene which regulates apoptosis.

5.065   Which one of the following statements is TRUE of tumor metastases?
   A. tumor cell motility promotes metastases
   B. tumor cells are safe from immunologic destruction
   C. metastatic potential is decreased if the tumor cells aggregate with platelets in the circulation
   D. tumor cells never exhibit preferred sites for the establishment of distant metastases

A is correct.
Normal cells have a certain degree of adhesiveness to each other. A group of transmembranous glycoproteins (cadherins) mediates adhesions in epithelial tissue. In certain epithelial tumors, there is loss of expression of these adhesion mediators, resulting in loss of the ability of cells to adhere to each other. This, in turn, allows detachment and increased motility.

5.066   The determination of the size of a primary malignant neoplasm is part of the process of:
   A. grading
   B. classification
   C. staging
   D. differentiation

C is correct.
Clinical staging of tumors is based on the size of the primary tumor, the extent of spread to nearby structures and regional lymph nodes, and the presence or absence of distant metastases.

5.067   Which one of the following terms MOST accurately describes a grade I cancer?
   A. one which has not spread beyond the site of origin
   B. one with widespread distant metastases
   C. one composed of cells that are well differentiated
   D. one composed of cells that are anaplastic
   E. one that has not penetrated the basement membrane

C is correct.
Grading of cancers is based on the degree of cellular differentiation in the tumor. Those with well differentiated cells are low-grade (I or II) tumors whereas very anaplastic tumors are high grade (IV).

SECTION 6: ENVIRONMENTAL PATHOLOGY AND NUTRITIONAL DISORDERS

6.001 Previously recognized and defined mechanisms for drug toxicity include all of the following EXCEPT:
A. increased free radical-induced covalent modification of DNA, RNA, and proteins
B. covalent modification of DNA, RNA, and proteins by electrophilic metabolites derived by phase I metabolism in the liver
C. sensitization to neoantigens produced by covalent modification of proteins by reactive metabolites of xenobiotics
D. photodynamic damage induced by compounds which spontaneously emit infrared radiation
E. altered hormonal status of the host induced by administration of synthetic compounds which resemble endogenous hormones (e.g. synthetic estrogens)

D is correct.
All of the other mechanisms listed are recognized in the pathogenesis of drug toxicity. There has never been any suggestion of infrared radiation damage related to drug toxicity.

6.002 Which one of the following phrases MOST closely defines a contusion?
A. localized loss of the stratified squamous epithelium of the skin
B. blunt-force damage with interstitial bleeding
C. a deep cut
D. accumulation of subcutaneous fibrous connective tissue
E. subcutaneous blister formation

B is correct.
A contusion is an injury caused by a blunt force that injures small blood vessels and causes interstitial bleeding, usually without disruption of the continuity of the tissue. A bruise is a contusion.

6.003 Each of the following statements concerning the effects of cold on humans is true EXCEPT:
A. cold results in a generalized decrease in the rate of temperature-dependent metabolic processes
B. the usual cause of death following overexposure to cold conditions is circulatory collapse
C. hypothermic patients display increased irritability, with overstimulation of cortical functions.
D. direct effects of cold on cells include physical dislocations and high salt concentrations due to crystallization of cell water
E. sudden sharp drops in temperature increase blood viscosity and contribute to tissue ischemia

C is correct.
When the body is exposed to excessively low temperatures, there is a slowing of metabolic processes, particularly in the brain and medullary centers.

6.004 Phase I and phase II metabolism of xenobiotics refer to metabolic processes which occur primarily in which one of the following organs?

    A. stomach
    B. liver
    C. gallbladder
    D. kidney
    E. lung

B is correct.
The term 'xenobiotic' refers to any foreign chemical substance. The majority of phase I and II metabolic processes of xenobiotics takes place in hepatocytes.

6.005 Which enzyme is primarily responsible for phase I oxidative metabolism of xenobiotics?

    A. UDP-glucuronic acid glucuronyltransferase
    B. glutathione transpeptidase
    C. aspartate aminotransferase
    D. cytochrome P-450 monooxygenase
    E. *N*-hydroxylase

D is correct.
A major phase I reaction of xenobiotics is the oxidation mediated by the microsomal cytochrome P450 isozymes. This occurs predominantly in the liver.

6.006 The extent of electrical injury to tissue following contact with a source of high-voltage alternating current is influenced by all of the following factors EXCEPT:

    A. phase of the current source
    B. magnitude of current flow
    C. path of current flow through the body
    D. surface area of tissue in electrical contact with the source
    E. voltage of the current source

A is correct.
Many variables are involved relating to the injury produced by electrical current. These include the nature of the current (direct or alternating), amperage, voltage, path of the current through the body, resistance of the intervening tissues, and duration of exposure.

6.007 Commonly encountered forms of radiation known to be capable of causing injury to cells include all of the following EXCEPT:

    A. cosmic rays
    B. gamma rays
    C. X-rays
    D. ultraviolet (UV) light
    E. UHF radio-frequency radiation

E is correct.
UHF radio-frequency radiation has not been implicated in injury to cells.

6.008 In the indirect-action theory of the interaction of ionizing radiation with cells, the primary biochemical mechanism responsible for cell injury is:

    A. free radical-induced injury of biorganic polymers
    B. UV radiation-induced formation of thymine dimers
    C. chemiluminescence
    D. immune reaction to neoantigens produced by radiation
    E. decreased synthesis of glutathione

A is correct.
The indirect-action theory proposes that radiant energy exerts its effect by producing free radicals within cells. Ultimately, these free radicals interact with critical components of the cell, such as membranes, nucleic acids, and enzymes.

6.009   The MOST clinically significant long-term complication of ionizing radiation exposure is:
  A. sterility
  B. radiodermatitis
  C. anemia
  D. neoplasia
  E. thrombocytopenia

D is correct.
Neoplasia is a well-known late complication in patients exposed to significant levels of ionizing radiation.

6.010 Lead toxicity causes anemia as a result of:
  A. inhibition of 5′-nucleotidase
  B. binding of protein sulfhydryl groups in superoxide dismutase
  C. interference with incorporation of iron into heme molecules
  D. inhibition of proximal-tubule transport function
  E. decreased sensitivity of RBC stem cells to erythropoietin

C is correct.
A microcytic hypochromic anemia is associated with lead toxicity by interfering with the enzymes aminolevulinic acid dehydratase and ferroketolase, which are involved in the incorporation of iron into the heme molecule.

6.011   The fat-soluble vitamins share all of the following characteristics EXCEPT:
  A. they are more soluble in non-polar organic solvents than in water
  B. they are derivatives of isoprenyl groups synthesized by metabolic pathways similar to those which are responsible for the synthesis of cholesterol
  C. the manifestations of a deficiency state are virtually identical for all of the fat-soluble vitamins
  D. they require bile salts and pancreatic enzymes for their absorption in the small bowel
  E. they require 'special' transport mechanisms for their distribution to tissues via the bloodstream

C is correct.
Deficiency of the fat-soluble vitamins A, D, E, and K causes widely different clinical presentations, ranging from squamous metaplasia to bleeding diathesis.

6.012 Which one of the following water-soluble vitamins can be synthesized endogenously from tryptophan?
  A. niacin (nicotinate)
  B. folate
  C. vitamin B_{12}
  D. pyridoxine
  E. thiamine

A is correct.
Niacin differs from the other B-complex vitamins in that it can be synthesized endogenously from tryptophan.

6.013   All of the following proteins require γ-carboxylation catalyzed by an enzyme which uses vitamin K as a redox cofactor EXCEPT:
   A. factor II
   B. factor V
   C. factor IX
   D. protein C

B is correct.
Proteins whose function is dependent on calcium chelation to γ–carboxyglutamate residues, requiring vitamin K, include factors II, VII, IX, and X, and proteins C and S, involved in the coagulation of blood. These calcium-dependent proteins are inactive when γ-carboxylation is inhibited. This is the mechanism for the anticoagulant effect of coumarin and related compounds.

6.014   Each of the following conditions is expected to be associated with secondary deficiency of fat-soluble vitamins EXCEPT:
   A. chronic inflammation of the jejunum and ileum
   B. pancreatic disease
   C. obstruction to bile flow from the liver
   D. surgical resection of the rectosigmoid colon
   E. chronic alcoholism with cirrhosis and end-stage liver disease

D is correct.
The rectosigmoid area is not involved in absorption or metabolism of vitamins.

6.015   Biologically active forms of vitamin A include all of the following EXCEPT:
   A. retinoic acid
   B. retinal
   C. transthyretin
   D. retinol

C is correct.
Transthyretin is a serum protein which binds and transports thyroxin and retinol.

6.016   Which combination of laboratory findings is expected to be seen in a patient who is deficient in vitamin D?
   A. decreased calcium, phosphate, and parathyroid hormone in plasma
   B. increased calcium, phosphate, and parathyroid hormone in plasma
   C. increased calcium, and decreased phosphate and parathyroid hormone in plasma
   D. decreased calcium and phosphate, and increased parathyroid hormone in plasma

D is correct.
Vitamin D in its active form $(1, 25$-dihydroxy compound) increases intestinal absorption of calcium and phosphorus, mobilizes calcium from bone, and stimulates parathyroid-dependent calcium resorption in the kidney. A deficiency leads to low calcium and phosphate levels. As a response to this, the parathyroid hormone secretes increased amounts of parathyroid hormone through the normal feedback mechanism.

6.017   The plasma vitamin B_{12} transport protein which binds to surface receptors on cells and mediates the uptake of vitamin B_{12} by receptor-mediated endocytosis is:
   A. salivary R-binder
   B. intrinsic factor
   C. apocobalamin
   D. transcobalamin II
   E. rhodopsin

D is correct.
Vitamin B_{12} (cobalamin) is released into the plasma where it binds to transcobalamin II, which is synthesized in the liver. The B_{12}-transcobalamin complex is delivered to cells where receptor-mediated endocytosis allows delivery of B_{12} to the cytosol. Intrinsic factor binds to B_{12} in the gastrointestinal tract. The B_{12}-intrinsic factor complex is absorbed in the terminal ileum.

6.018   Manifestations of vitamin A deficiency include all of the following EXCEPT:
A. glossitis
B. night-blindness
C. keratomalacia and corneal ulceration
D. hyperkeratosis of the skin
E. squamous metaplasia of the bronchial mucosa

A is correct.
Because vitamin A is necessary for cell differentiation (particularly of columnar epithelial cells), hypovitaminosis A results in replacement of normal columnar epithelium by a keratinizing squamous epithelium. Night-blindness is a typical feature of vitamin A deficiency due to its association with retinal compounds. Glossitis may be a feature of deficiencies of B_{12}, riboflavin, niacin, or pyridoxine.

6.019   The LEAST important variable in determining the degree of electrical injury in a person is:
A. nature of the current (direct or alternating)
B. age of person
C. path of the current through the body
D. resistance of intervening tissues
E. amperage

B is correct.
The age of the person is the least significant factor in determining the degree of injury from electrical injuries.

6.020   Examples of reactions which participate in the phase I metabolism of xenobiotics include each of the following EXCEPT:
A. cytochrome-P450 catalyzed hydroxylation
B. xenobiotic oxidation
C. xenobiotic reduction
D. conjugation with glucuronic acid
E. ester hydrolysis

D is correct.
Phase I metabolism of xenobiotics (foreign chemicals) typically includes hydroxylation, oxidation, reduction, and hydrolysis. Conjugation is the major phase II reaction in xenobiotic metabolism.

6.021   All of the following clinical/laboratory features are expected to occur in patients suffering from lead poisoning EXCEPT:
A. basophilic stippling of erythrocytes
B. elevated whole-blood lead concentration
C. CNS dysfunction (memory loss, cognitive dysfunction, etc.)
D. decreased erythrocyte protoporphyrin
E. hypochromic microcytic anemia

D is correct.
Lead poisons enzymes by binding to disulfide groups and by denaturing proteins. The CNS is a major target of damage by lead poisoning. Also, lead interferes with the incorporation of iron into the heme molecule, leading to a microcytic hypochromic anemia, basophilic stippling of erythrocytes and an INCREASED free erythrocyte protoporphyrin.

6.022   Catalytic function of which one of the following is involved in the conversion of methylmalonyl-CoA to succinyl-CoA, a step in the metabolism of odd chain-length fatty acids?
A. vitamin B_{12}
B. folate
C. vitamin K
D. thiamine

A is correct.
Vitamin B_{12} catalyzes two reactions. In one, it acts as a methyl group acceptor and donor in transmethylation and, in the other, it participates in the isomerization of methylmalonyl-CoA to succinyl-CoA.

6.023   Catalytic function of which one of the following is involved in the hydroxylation of proline in the synthesis of collagen?
   A. vitamin B_{12}
   B. folate
   C. vitamin C
   D. thiamine

C is correct.
Vitamin C (ascorbic acid) participates as a cofactor for hydroxylation reactions. One important reaction is the hydroxylation of proline in collagen synthesis.

SECTION 7: CARDIOVASCULAR SYSTEM

7.001 All of the following factors are thought to be associated with the antithrombotic function of the endothelial cell EXCEPT:
  A. synthesis of tissue-plasminogen activators
  B. production of prostacyclin (PGI_2)
  C. expression of tissue factor activity
  D. thrombomodulin activation of proteins C and S
  E. activity of heparin-like molecules

C is correct.
Tissue factor (thromboplastin) is present in minute amounts in normal endothelium and can promote thrombosis by activating the extrinsic clotting pathway.

7.002 Approximately how long does it take for at least 90% of patients with acute myocardial ischemia to demonstrate elevated amounts of serum activity of the MB isoenzyme form of creatine kinase (i.e. how much time must lapse after the onset of ischemia for the serum CK-MB test to have a sensitivity of $\geq 90\%$)?
  A. 30 minutes
  B. 1 hour
  C. 2 hours
  D. 12 hours
  E. 3 days

D is correct.
It takes a few hours for CK-MB to become detectable after myocardial ischemia. At 5 h, the sensitivity is only 50%. At 9 h, the sensitivity is 70%. It takes approximately 12 h before at least 90% sensitivity is reached.

7.003 The MOST common complication of acute myocardial infarction is:
  A. mural thrombosis
  B. rupture of the papillary muscle
  C. mitral insufficiency
  D. arrhythmias
  E. hemorrhagic pericarditis

D is correct.
While all of the conditions listed may be complications of acute myocardial infarction, by far the most common is the development of arrhythmias.

7.004 The MOST common cause of right heart failure is:
  A. myocarditis
  B. patent ductus arteriosus
  C. pulmonary valve stenosis
  D. tricuspid atresia
  E. left heart failure

E is correct.
While all of the other conditions listed may be a cause of right-sided heart failure, the most common cause is left-sided heart failure. The failing left side of the heart results in increasing pulmonary pressures until the right heart can no longer keep up with the increased work load.

7.005 The MOST common cause of acute cor pulmonale is:
  A. myocardial infarction
  B. intravenous drug abuse
  C. emphysema
  D. pulmonary embolism
  E. a ventricular septal defect

D is correct.
Acute cor pulmonale is almost always the result of massive pulmonary thromboembolism. Chronic cor pulmonale is the result of prolonged elevations of pulmonary vascular pressure.

7.006   Primary hemodynamic features of heart failure include decreased cardiac output and:

A. elevated systemic arterial pressure
B. decreased pulmonary venous pressure
C. elevated systemic arterial pressure and decreased pulmonary venous pressure
D. elevated systemic and pulmonary venous pressure
E. elevated systemic and pulmonary artery pressure

D is correct.
In the failing heart, venous blood pools in both the systemic and pulmonary systems, resulting in increased pulmonary and systemic venous pressures.

7.007   In chronic rheumatic heart disease, the valve(s) MOST frequently affected is / are:

A. tricuspid
B. aortic
C. mitral
D. pulmonary
E. pulmonary and aortic

C is correct.
The mitral valve alone is involved in chronic rheumatic heart disease in about 70% of cases. The next most frequent distribution is the mitral and aortic valves being affected simultaneously. This occurs in around 25% of cases of chronic rheumatic heart disease.

7.008   A 12-year-old girl presents with fever, polyarthritis, a rash, purposeless involuntary movements, and a diastolic murmur over the mitral valve area. Which one of the following cardiac histologic features is an expected finding in this child's myocardium?

A. coagulation necrosis with an infiltrate of neutrophils
B. dense deposition of collagen
C. multiple abscesses due to streptococcus group B
D. fibrinoid necrosis surrounded by lymphocytes, macrophages, and plasma cells
E. deposition of amyloid around small vessels

D is correct.
The clinical description is classic for acute rheumatic fever. During the acute stages, changes in the myocardium consist of fibrinoid necrosis, lymphocytes, macrophages, and occasional plasma cells. These focal lesions are called Aschoff bodies.

7.009   Twenty years after an episode of acute rheumatic fever, a 40-year-old man presents with fever. Several of his teeth were extracted a week prior to admission. On physical examination, he has a systolic murmur and moderate splenomegaly. Laboratory examination reveals hematuria and an elevated leukocyte count with neutrophilia. The MOST likely diagnosis is:

A. acute myocardial infarction
B. bacterial endocarditis
C. right ventricular failure
D. exacerbation of the acute rheumatic fever
E. mitral valve prolapse

B is correct.
The past history of rheumatic fever and the recent history of tooth extraction along with the clinical findings suggest a diagnosis of bacterial endocarditis. Transient episodes of bacteremia, such as from tooth extraction, may result in bacterial colonization of damaged heart valves.

7.010   Which one of the following features is NOT associated with tetralogy of Fallot?
  A. malalignment ventricular septal defect
  B. right-ventricular hypertrophy
  C. infundibular stenosis
  D. sinus venosus defect
  E. overriding aorta

D is correct.
Abnormalities of the sinus venosus are not a feature of tetralogy of Fallot.

7.011   The lipoproteins which mediate cholesterol clearance from the atheromatous plaque and are antiatherogenic are:
  A. chylomicrons
  B. very low-density lipoprotein (VLDL)
  C. intermediate-density lipoprotein (IDL)
  D. low-density lipoprotein (LDL)
  E. high-density lipoprotein (HDL)

E is correct.
High-density lipoproteins have a protective action against atheroma formation. A proposed mechanism is the facilitation of cholesterol clearance from atheromas and transport to the liver for excretion.

7.012   Which one of the following conditions is LEAST likely to have an abnormal bleeding time?
  A. thrombocytopenia
  B. hemophilia A
  C. von Willebrand's disease
  D. aspirin therapy
  E. afibrinogenemia

B is correct.
Bleeding time is a measure of platelet function. Hemophilia A (factor VIII deficiency) results in a prolonged coagulation time, but a normal bleeding time. Afibrinogenemia has a prolonged bleeding time. Platelet function is altered in the other conditions listed.

7.013   Ventricular rupture after myocardial infarction (MI) is MOST likely at which one of the following time periods after infarction?
  A. 3–4 hours
  B. 12–24 hours
  C. 4–7 days
  D. 3–4 weeks
  E. 3–4 months

C is correct.
The period of maximum necrotic softening occurs at around 4–7 days. This is the most likely time for rupture of the myocardium to occur.

7.014   A patient has had recurrent pulmonary emboli and presents with hepatomegaly, splenomegaly, and peripheral edema. The symptoms are MOST likely to be due to:
  A. right-sided heart failure
  B. left-sided heart failure
  C. systemic emboli
  D. bacterial endocarditis
  E. systemic amyloidosis

A is correct.
Recurrent pulmonary emboli may cause pulmonary vascular hypertension with resulting cor pulmonale and right ventricular failure. The clinical signs are classic for right-sided failure.

7.015 The lesions associated with acute rheumatic fever typically may include all of the following EXCEPT:
- A. myocardial inflammation
- B. acute valvulitis
- C. septic emboli
- D. inflammatory subcutaneous nodules
- E. pericardial inflammation

C is correct.
The typical case of acute rheumatic fever is not associated with concurrent bacterial infection.

7.016 The MOST common primary tumor of the heart in adults is:
- A. lipoma
- B. myxoma
- C. rhabdomyoma
- D. papillary fibroelastoma
- E. angiosarcoma

B is correct.
All primary neoplasms of the heart are rare. However, the most common is the myxoma.

7.017 Cardiomyopathy is associated with all of the following conditions EXCEPT:
- A. alcohol toxicity
- B. Adriamycin toxicity
- C. hypokalemia
- D. carcinoid heart disease
- E. Pompe's disease (acid-maltase deficiency)

D is correct.
Carcinoid heart disease primarily involves the endocardium and valves of the right heart.

7.018 Carcinoid heart disease is MOST likely to be associated with which one of the following conditions?
- A. ball-valve obstruction of mitral valve
- B. hemopericardium
- C. cardiomyopathy with failure
- D. myocarditis with mononuclear infiltrates
- E. tricuspid valvular stenosis

E is correct.
Cardiac involvement in carcinoid heart disease is predominantly of the endocardium and valves of the right heart. Plaque-like thickenings of the valvular cusps of the right heart valves may occur.

7.019 Cocaine effects on the heart include all of the following conditions EXCEPT:
- A. arrhythmias
- B. myocyte necrosis
- C. non-bacterial endocarditis
- D. infarction
- E. congestive dilated cardiomyopathy

C is correct.
Cocaine has not been implicated in non-bacterial endocarditis. It has, however, been associated with the other conditions listed.

7.020 A patient with acute myocardial infarction suddenly develops acute mitral insufficiency on the seventh day after the infarction. The BEST explanation for this is:
- A. papillary muscle rupture
- B. staphylococcal bacterial endocarditis
- C. thromboembolism
- D. extension of the infarct
- E. scarring of the mitral valve

A is correct.
Four to seven days postmyocardial infarction is a time of maximum softening of the infarcted area. Rupture of the involved myocardium may occur. Papillary muscle rupture on the left side of the heart is responsible for sudden mitral insufficiency.

7.021   Which one of the following diseases is associated with inflammation of the vasa vasorum?
   A. Kaposi's sarcoma
   B. atherosclerotic aneurysm
   C. syphilitic aneurysm
   D. cystic medial necrosis
   E. coronary artery aneurysm

C is correct.
The inflammatory reaction starts in the adventitia of the aorta with prominent involvement of the vasa vasorum and production of obliterative endarteritis. There is an infiltrate of lymphocytes and plasma cells.

7.022   Which one of the following diseases is associated with Marfan's syndrome?
   A. Kaposi's sarcoma
   B. atherosclerotic aneurysm
   C. syphilitic aneurysm
   D. cystic medial necrosis
   E. coronary artery aneurysm

D is correct.
There is a high incidence of cystic medial necrosis and dissecting aneurysm in patients with Marfan's syndrome. This is a hereditary disorder with a defect in the formation of stable collagen cross-links.

7.023   A major factor involved in the smooth muscle intimal proliferation seen in atherosclerosis is thought to be:
   A. collagen formation
   B. high-density lipoprotein stimulation
   C. platelet-derived growth factor (PDGF) stimulation
   D. viral infection
   E. colony-stimulating factor

C is correct.
PDGF is one of the principal factors implicated in smooth muscle proliferation in the intima. This factor is present in the alpha granules of platelets.

7.024   The incidence of coronary heart disease is MOST closely and directly correlated with which one of the following serum forms of cholesterol?
   A. total serum
   B. intermediate-density lipoprotein
   C. low-density lipoprotein
   D. very low-density lipoprotein
   E. postprandial

C is correct.
Around 70% of the total plasma cholesterol in normal Americans is contained in LDL. LDL is the lipoprotein most strongly correlated with athero-sclerosis.

7.025   In addition to serum cholesterol, each of the following conditions contributes an added risk for the development of atherosclerosis EXCEPT:
   A. low serum levels of high-density lipoprotein
   B. cigarette-smoking
   C. hypertension
   D. diabetes mellitus
   E. estrogen therapy

E is correct.
Estrogen does not cause an increased risk for the development of atherosclerosis.

7.026   Hypercoagulability is associated with each of the following conditions EXCEPT:
   A. protein C deficiency
   B. protein S deficiency
   C. antithrombin III deficiency
   D. factor XI deficiency
   E. presence of lupus anticoagulants

D is correct.
Factor XI is a coagulation factor in the intrinsic pathway. Apparently in contradiction to this, patients with lupus anticoagulants are prone to thrombosis. This is believed to be related to the inhibition by the lupus anticoagulants of prosta-cyclin production or release .

7.027   The incidence of congenital heart disease in the general population is:
  A. 1 case / 1000 live births
  B. 8 cases / 1000 live births
  C. most closely associated with family history
  D. variable according to race
  E. highest in the lowest socioeconomic class

B is correct.
Congenital heart disease occurs in the general population at a remarkably fixed incidence of approximately 8 cases / 1000 live births. This incidence has been found to be consistent and comparable in all socioeconomic groups and in all races, and is constant over time.

7.028   Approximately how long does it take for the enzyme activity of creatine kinase (CK) in serum / plasma to reach its highest (peak) value following uncomplicated myocardial infarction?
  A. 20–30 minutes
  B. 1–2 hours
  C. 16–24 hours
  D. 2–3 days
  E. 5–7 days

C is correct.
CK-MB isoenzyme is first to appear in the plasma, but requires 4–8 h to become detectable. Total CK serum levels peak at 18–24 h, then rapidly decline.

7.029   The MOST frequent complication of acute myocardial infarction, which often leads to a fatal outcome within the first few hours after the onset of ischemia, is:
  A. mural thrombosis
  B. acute cor pulmonale
  C. rupture of the ventricular free wall
  D. ventricular arrhythmias
  E. severe hypertension

D is correct.
Cardiac arrhythmias may appear soon after ischemia and are responsible for many sudden deaths. The arrhythmias may be in the form of sinus bradycardia or tachycardia, heart block, ventricular tachycardia or ventricular premature contractions.

7.030   In a 3-year-old child with a large isolated secundum atrial defect, a left-to-right shunt occurs because:
  A. the pulmonary vascular resistance is still elevated
  B. the left ventricle is relatively more compliant than the right ventricle
  C. there is associated anomalous pulmonary venous connection
  D. there is commonly an associated bicuspid aortic valve
  E. the right ventricle is able to accept a larger volume in diastole than the left ventricle, given the same filling pressure

E is correct.
Shunts occur from left-to-right through atrial septal defects when the compliance of the right ventricle is greater than the compliance of the left ventricle.

7.031   The MOST common cause of left heart failure is:
  A. Ebstein's anomaly
  B. patent ductus arteriosus
  C. pulmonary valve stenosis
  D. coarctation of the aorta
  E. ischemic heart disease

E is correct.
Ischemic heart disease, either chronic and / or acute, causes myocardial damage which may result in left heart failure. This is the most common cause of congestive heart failure.

7.032   In an 8-week-old infant with a large ventricular septal defect (VSD), the shunt is predicted by:
A. the location of the VSD
B. the relationship of the great vessels
C. the relationship between the systemic and pulmonary vascular resistance
D. the pulmonary arterial systolic pressure
E. the right ventricular systolic pressure

C is correct.
Whether or not there is a shunt, the direction of a shunt in VSD is related to the systemic and pulmonary vascular resistance. If the systemic vascular resistance is greater than the pulmonary vascular resistance, there will be a left-to-right shunt.

7.033   The predominant lipid constituents found in circulating lipoproteins include all of the following EXCEPT:
A. free (unesterified) fatty acids
B. free (unesterified) cholesterol
C. esterified cholesterol
D. phospholipids
E. triglycerides

A is correct.
Free fatty acids are not a significant component of circulating lipoproteins.

7.034   Which of the following is NOT associated with an increased risk of atherosclerosis?
A. smoking
B. hyperlipidemia
C. hypertension
D. factor XIII deficiency
E. diabetes mellitus

D is correct.
Factor XIII is a fibrin-stabilizing factor in the coagulation cascade. A deficiency of this factor is not associated with an increased risk of atherosclerosis.

7.035   In a typical case of coarctation of the aorta, symptoms of congestive heart failure are temporally BEST correlated with:
A. renal failure secondary to decreased distal aortic pressure
B. a fall in pulmonary vascular resistance
C. closure of the aortic end of the ductus arteriosus
D. closure of the ductus venosus
E. development of aortic stenosis due to bicuspid aortic valve

C is correct.
Coarctation usually involves the part of the aorta just distal to the origin of the left subclavian artery and proximal to the ductus arteriosus insertion. As long as the ductus is widely patent, the coarctation is usually not clinically significant. Once the ductus closes, the obstruction becomes evident.

7.036   The common sequelae of myocardial infarcts include all of the following EXCEPT:
A. mural thrombosis formation
B. ventricular rupture
C. papillary muscle rupture
D. heart failure
E. aortic valvular stenosis

E is correct.
Myocardial infarcts do not involve the heart valves directly.

7.037 Which is the MOST common congenital cardiac anomaly:
   A. tetralogy of Fallot
   B. ventricular septal defect (VSD)
   C. coarctation of the aorta
   D. atrial septal defect (ASD)
   E. tricuspid atresia

B is correct.
Ventricular septal defects are the most common congenital cardiac abnormality. Most often, these represent failures of fusion of the embryologic anlage of the ventricular septum.

7.038 A 78-year-old man presents with marked left ventricular hypertrophy, angina and syncope. Based solely on population statistics in the USA over the last 10–15 years, which one of the following findings is MOST likely?
   A. aortic regurgitation secondary to Marfan's syndrome
   B. aortic insufficiency of syphilis
   C. acute bacterial endocarditis
   D. aortic stenosis of rheumatic heart disease
   E. senile calcific stenosis of a normal or a bicuspid aortic valve

E is correct.
The symptoms of LVH, angina, and syncope are typical of aortic stenosis. The most common etiology of aortic stenosis is calcification of either a bicuspid aortic valve or a normal aortic valve in advanced age.

7.039 In patients with chronic rheumatic heart disease, which valve or valve combination is MOST commonly found to be affected?
   A. aortic
   B. mitral
   C. pulmonary
   D. tricuspid
   E. aortic and mitral valves

B is correct.
The mitral valve alone is affected in approximately 65–70% of cases of chronic rheumatic heart disease. The next most common involvement is the aortic and mitral valves together, comprising around 25% of cases.

7.040 In complete transposition of the great vessels, all of the following features are true EXCEPT:
   A. pulmonary veins drain to the right atrium
   B. aorta arises from the right ventricle
   C. pulmonary artery arises from the left ventricle
   D. the pulmonary artery is posterior to the aorta
   E. cyanosis is apparent at birth

A is correct.
The pulmonary veins are normal, draining into the left atrium. These children are intensely cyanotic and survival beyond a few days is unlikely without the presence of a large interatrial or interventricular communication or surgical intervention.

7.041 Bacterial endocarditis affecting the tricuspid valve is MOST frequently associated with:
   A. prosthetic heart valves
   B. illegal use of intravenous drugs
   C. carcinoid syndrome
   D. cardiac myxomas
   E. rheumatic heart disease

B is correct.
Drug addicts often introduce pathogenic bacteria through the use of unclean needles. These bacteria may infect the tricuspid valve. Common pathogens causing infectious endocarditis of the tricuspid valve are *Staphylococcus aureus*, *Candida*, and *Aspergillus*.

7.042   A 6-month-old infant with the tetralogy of Fallot is likely to demonstrate all of the following EXCEPT:
   A. cyanosis
   B. a systolic murmur suggesting pulmonary stenosis
   C. decreased pulmonary blood flow
   D. a right aortic arch
   E. left-to-right shunt

E is correct.
Shunting at the ventricular defect is usually from right-to-left because the right ventricular outflow obstruction presents greater resistance to flow than flow into the aorta.

7.043   A 43-year-old man presents with mild jaundice and abnormal hepatic function. He has a history of polyuria, polydipsia and polyphagia for the past 2 years. He has increased pigmentation of the skin and cardiomegaly. The MOST likely diagnosis is:
   A. amyloidosis
   B. *Trypanosoma cruzi* infection
   C. hemochromatosis
   D. cocaine cardiomyopathy
   E. hepatolenticular degeneration (Wilson's disease)

C is correct.
The findings of liver abnormalities, signs of diabetes mellitus, pigmentation of the skin, and cardiomegaly strongly suggest a diagnosis of hemochromatosis. This is an iron-overload disorder which causes organ injury.

7.044   The MOST common form of congenital left ventricular outflow obstruction is:
   A. stenotic bicuspid aortic valve
   B. hypertrophic cardiomyopathy
   C. subaortic membranous stenosis
   D. coarctation of the aorta
   E. supravalvular aortic stenosis

A is correct.
Aortic stenosis, as a congenital anomaly, is most commonly represented as a bicuspid aortic valve. Turbulence at the valve results in fibrosis and calcification and, by mid-adult life, a bicuspid valve may be severely stenotic.

7.045   All of the following are associated with acute rheumatic fever EXCEPT:
   A. button-hole stenosis of the mitral valve
   B. migratory polyarthritis of the large joints
   C. elevated antistreptolysin-O titers
   D. Aschoff bodies in the myocardium
   E. pancarditis

A is correct.
Stenosis of the mitral valve may occur in chronic rheumatic heart disease. This does not occur until years after acute rheumatic fever.

7.046   All of the following syndromes are associated with an increased incidence of congenital heart disease EXCEPT:
   A. Turner's syndrome
   B. Down syndrome
   C. Marfan's syndrome
   D. Reye's syndrome
   E. fetal alcohol syndrome

D is correct.
Reye's syndrome, an acute postviral illness (usually of children) is not associated with congenital heart disease.

7.047 The major direct role of thrombomodulin is thought to be:
  A. the generation of factor VIIIa
  B. the activation of protein C
  C. the binding of AT III
  D. the activation of protein S
  E. inactivation of factor VII

B is correct.
Thrombomodulin is a surface protein that binds thrombin, converting it into an activator of protein C. Protein C is a plasma protein that is a powerful anticoagulant when activated.

7.048 Which one of the following abnormalities is MOST likely to be associated with systemic lupus erythematosus?
  A. dissecting aneurysm of the thoracic aorta
  B. coarctation of the aorta
  C. tricuspid valve fibrosis
  D. Libman–Sacks endocarditis
  E. coronary artery aneurysm

D is correct.
In this condition, the connective tissue of the mitral or tricuspid valves become the site of fibrinoid necrosis and fibrosis. Small vegetations may form on the valve leaflets.

7.049 Which one of the following abnormalities is MOST likely to be associated with Marfan's syndrome?
  A. acute aortic dissection
  B. coarctation of the aorta
  C. tricuspid valve fibrosis
  D. Libman–Sacks endocarditis
  E. coronary artery aneurysm

A is correct.
Acute aortic dissection is pathogenetically related to a degenerative change in the aortic wall called cystic medial necrosis. There is a high incidence of cystic medial necrosis in Marfan's syndrome, in which there is a defect in collagen cross-linking.

7.050 Which one of the following abnormalities is MOST likely to be associated with Turner's syndrome?
  A. dissecting aneurysm of the thoracic aorta
  B. coarctation of the aorta
  C. tricuspid valve fibrosis
  D. Libman–Sacks endocarditis
  E. coronary artery aneurysm

B is correct.
Turner's syndrome is due to a complete or partial monosomy of the X chromosome. Such patients demonstrate hypogonadism in phenotypic females. Congenital heart disease occurs frequently in patients with Turner's syndrome, especially coarctation of the aorta and aortic stenosis.

7.051 The gross finding of 'tree-barking' of the aorta is characteristic of which one of the following diseases?
  A. luetic (syphilitic) aortitis
  B. chronic right heart failure
  C. acquired immunodeficiency syndrome
  D. pulmonary embolus
  E. myocardial infarction

A is correct.
In syphilitic aortitis, contraction of collagenous scars leads to a wrinkling effect of the aortic intima which has been called 'tree-barking'.

7.052 Kaposi's sarcoma, a vascular neoplasm, is MOST likely to be found in association with which one of the following diseases?
  A. luetic (syphilitic) aortitis
  B. chronic right heart failure
  C. acquired immunodeficiency syndrome
  D. pulmonary embolus
  E. myocardial infarction

C is correct.
Kaposi's sarcoma is frequently seen in AIDS patients. Prior to the emergence of AIDS, the neoplasm was relatively rare.

7.053 The finding of a 'nutmeg' pattern to the cut surface of the liver suggests which one of the following conditions?
  A. luetic (syphilitic) aortitis
  B. chronic right heart failure
  C. acquired immunodeficiency syndrome
  D. pulmonary embolus
  E. myocardial infarction

B is correct.
Chronic right heart failure causes increased venous pressure, which is transmitted back through the hepatic veins to the central lobular hepatic zones. This causes congestion in the centrilobular area together with hypoxic changes. This has a speckled gross appearance, resembling the inside of a nutmeg.

7.054 Which one of the following conditions is MOST likely to be associated with secondary cardiomyopathy?
  A. acute rheumatic fever
  B. tuberculosis
  C. myxoma
  D. systemic lupus erythematosus
  E. Adriamycin (doxorubicin) toxicity

E is correct.
Secondary cardiomyopathy refers to myocardial involvement due to known etiologic agents or associated with well-defined systemic diseases. Adriamycin is a recognized cause of myocardial injury. The injury is dose-dependent and believed to be due to lipid peroxidation of the myofiber membranes.

7.055 Which one of the following conditions is MOST likely to be associated with inflammation of the pericardium, myocardium, and endocardium?
  A. acute rheumatic fever
  B. tuberculosis
  C. myxoma
  D. systemic lupus erythematosus
  E. Adriamycin (doxorubicin) toxicity

A is correct.
Acute rheumatic fever affects all three layers of the heart. There is a fibrinous pericarditis, myocarditis and endocarditis.

7.056 Which one of the following conditions may be associated with 'ball-valve' obstruction?
  A. acute rheumatic fever
  B. tuberculosis
  C. myxoma
  D. systemic lupus erythematosus
  E. Aschoff body

C is correct.
Myxomas of the heart are uncommon. However, when they do occur, they tend to involve the atria. They may be pedunculated and may then fall into the valve opening, causing a ball-valve obstruction. This may result in syncope, cardiac insufficiency, or even sudden death.

7.057 Which one of the following conditions is MOST likely to cause a serosanguineous pericarditis?
  A. acute rheumatic fever
  B. tuberculosis
  C. myxoma
  D. systemic lupus erythematosus
  E. Adriamycin (doxorubicin) toxicity

B is correct.
Although acute rheumatic fever and SLE may each cause pericarditis, in these two instances, the inflammatory exudate is serous or fibrinous and not sanguineous, as it may be in tuberculous pericarditis.

7.058 Which apoprotein in the following list is found in virtually ALL atherogenic lipoproteins?
  A. lipoprotein A (LpA)
  B. apolipoprotein (apo) E
  C. apo C-II (lipoprotein lipase activator)
  D. apo B-100 (LDL-receptor ligand)
  E. apo A-I (LCAT activator)

D is correct.
All of the lipoproteins having apo B-100 (VLDL, IDL, and LDL) are atherogenic.

7.059   Tricuspid valve atresia results in cyanosis because:
   A. the pulmonary veins drain anomalously to the right atrium
   B. the ductus arteriosus remains patent
   C. a right-to-left shunt occurs at the atrial level
   D. the great vessels are transposed
   E. the ventricles are transposed

C is correct.
A patent foramen ovale provides a site for decompression of the right atrium in tricuspid atresia. This allows a right-to-left shunt at the atrial level.

7.060   Pulmonary edema may be seen in all of the following conditions EXCEPT:
   A. congestion stage of bronchopneumonia
   B. exudative phase of diffuse alveolar damage
   C. left heart failure
   D. pulmonary valve stenosis
   E. hypoalbuminemia

D is correct.
In pulmonary valve stenosis, there is a decreased pulmonary capillary pressure. The hydrostatic pressure would not be increased and, therefore, there is no etiology for pulmonary edema in such patients.

7.061   Aschoff bodies are seen histologically in which one of the following diseases?
   A. acute rheumatic fever
   B. pulmonary embolus
   C. coronary artery aneurysm
   D. systemic lupus erythematosus
   E. myocardial infarction

A is correct.
During acute rheumatic fever, distinctive inflammatory lesions called Aschoff bodies may be found in the heart. They are foci of fibrinoid necrosis surrounded by lymphocytes, macrophages, and activated histiocytes called Anitschkow's cells.

7.062   Libman–Sacks endocarditis is typically seen in which one of the following conditions?
   A. acute rheumatic fever
   B. pulmonary embolus
   C. coronary artery aneurysm
   D. systemic lupus erythematosus
   E. myocardial infarction

D is correct.
In SLE, mitral and tricuspid valvulitis may occur with the appearance of small sterile vegetations on the valves. They typically occur on the undersurface of the valves, but may appear anywhere on the valve or on the chordae tendineae. This type of endocarditis is called Libman–Sacks endocarditis.

7.063   Which one of the following conditions is associated with Kawasaki's syndrome?
   A. acute rheumatic fever
   B. pulmonary embolus
   C. coronary artery aneurysm
   D. systemic lupus erythematosus
   E. myocardial infarction

C is correct.
This syndrome is an arteritis affecting large, medium and small arteries. The coronary arteries are often affected with changes ranging from ectasia to aneurysm formation.

SECTION 8: RESPIRATORY SYSTEM

8.001 All of the following are morphologic features of asthma EXCEPT:
- A. smooth muscle hypertrophy
- B. thickened alveolar walls
- C. inflammatory infiltrate of bronchial walls
- D. bronchial mucous plugs
- E. airway eosinophils

B is correct.

Asthma is an episodic reversible bronchospasm resulting from an exaggerated bronchoconstrictor response to stimuli. Typical findings are bronchial inflammatory infiltrates, smooth muscle hypertrophy, increased size of submucosal glands, mucous plugs, and eosinophils. Alveoli are over-inflated, but thickening of alveolar walls is not a feature of asthma.

8.002 A cough productive of copious foul-smelling purulent sputum is characteristic of:
- A. asthma
- B. emphysema
- C. bronchiectasis
- D. idiopathic pulmonary fibrosis
- E. silicosis

C is correct.

Bronchiestasis is a chronic necrotizing infectious process which leads to destruction of the airway walls. Typically, patients produce large amounts of foul-smelling sputum due to the necrotizing infectious process.

8.003 The organizing stage of adult respiratory distress syndrome (ARDS) is characterized by:
- A. type II pneumocyte proliferation
- B. alveolar edema
- C. hyaline membranes
- D. sloughing of bronchiolar epithelium
- E. atelectasis

A is correct.

All of the other findings listed are characteristic of the acute stage of ARDS.

8.004 Cigarette-smoking is implicated in or is a known risk factor for the development of all of the following diseases EXCEPT:
- A. cancer of the urinary bladder
- B. chronic obstructive lung disease
- C. small-cell undifferentiated carcinoma of the lung
- D. mesothelioma
- E. coronary atherosclerosis

D is correct.

Cigarette-smoking is implicated in all of the other diseased listed. Mesothelioma, a neoplasm arising in either the visceral or parietal pleura, is related to asbestos exposure but, as yet, has not been linked to smoking.

8.005 An infant is brought to the emergency room with a 3-day history of projectile vomiting. Physical examination reveals an apparent nodule in the gastroduodenal area. A diagnosis of pyloric stenosis is made. Arterial blood gases are as follows: pH: 7.48; pCO_2: 46 (normal 35–45) mmHg; HCO_3: 28 (normal 22–26) mEq/l. These arterial blood gas results are MOST consistent with:
    A. respiratory alkalosis
    B. metabolic alkalosis
    C. compensated respiratory acidosis
    D. compensated metabolic acidosis
    E. laboratory error

B is correct.
The pH is slightly elevated, indicating the presence of alkalosis. The bicarbonate and pCO_2 are both slightly elevated, which is consistent with metabolic alkalosis. Frequently, the pCO_2 remains normal as respiratory compensation is often minimal. In respiratory alkalosis, the pCO_2 and bicarbonate are both usually decreased.

8.006 Which one of the following exposures contributes the MOST to the incidence of bronchogenic carcinoma in the USA?
    A. asbestos
    B. uranium
    C. cigarette-smoking
    D. chromium
    E. nickel

C is correct.
While all of the other substances listed may contribute to the incidence of lung cancer, cigarette-smoking is by far the most common.

8.007 Possible causes of metabolic acidosis include all of the following EXCEPT:
    A. salicylate poisoning
    B. severe diarrhea
    C. tissue hypoxia
    D. hyperventilation
    E. 'moonshine' ingestion (moonshine often contains methanol)

D is correct.
Respiratory alkalosis may result in any condition that causes respiratory-center stimulation producing hyperventilation.

8.008 In which of the following forms of pulmonary carcinoma is the classic progression of metaplasia to dysplasia to carcinoma in situ observed?
    A. small-cell carcinoma
    B. adenocarcinoma
    C. large-cell carcinoma
    D. squamous cell carcinoma
    E. metastatic carcinoma

D is correct.
All stages from squamous metaplasia to carcinoma in situ are observed in squamous cell carcinoma. Such a clear progression is not seen in the other forms of cancer listed.

8.009 The MOST common primary malignancy seen in the lung is:
    A. small-cell carcinoma
    B. adenocarcinoma
    C. large-cell carcinoma
    D. squamous cell carcinoma
    E. bronchoalveolar carcinoma

D is correct.
Squamous cell carcinoma makes up around 35–50%, small-cell carcinoma 20–25%, and adenocarcinoma 15–35%.

8.010 A 19-year-old girl who had recently been hospitalized for attempted suicide was found in a comatose state with an empty bottle of aspirin next to her. Assuming that the young girl had ingested a large amount of aspirin, the subsequent physiologic chain of events is MOST likely to be an initial:

A. respiratory acidosis, then metabolic alkalosis
B. respiratory alkalosis, then metabolic acidosis
C. metabolic acidosis, then respiratory alkalosis
D. metabolic alkalosis, then respiratory alkalosis
E. metabolic alkalosis that progressively worsens

B is correct.
Initially, there is hyperpnea which lowers the pCO_2 and causes a respiratory alkalosis. Due to a combined renal compensation for the respiratory alkalosis and the accumulation of salicylic acid, a metabolic acidosis soon appears.

8.011 Just prior to a major examination, a student develops a panic reaction with a respiratory rate of 84 chest movements/min (normal ranges: pCO_2 35–45; HCO_3 22–26). The paramedics are called and arterial blood gases are drawn. The MOST likely results are:

A. pH 7.2 pCO_2 25 HCO_3 18
B. pH 7.5 pCO_2 40 HCO_3 27
C. pH 7.2 pCO_2 40 HCO_3 18
D. pH 7.4 pCO_2 50 HCO_3 27
E. pH 7.5 pCO_2 25 HCO_3 22

E is correct.
The hyperventilation will reduce the pCO_2. Initially, the HCO_3 will be normal, but it will decrease with compensation. There is a slight increase in pH.

8.012 IgE is implicated in the pathogenesis of:
A. asthma
B. hypersensitivity pneumonitis
C. adult respiratory distress syndrome (ARDS)
D. pulmonary alveolar proteinosis
E. Goodpasture's syndrome

A is correct.
In allergic asthma, exposure of presensitized IgE-coated mast cells to the same or crossreacting antigens stimulates the release of various mediators which, in turn, trigger bronchial smooth muscle contraction, mucosal edema, and mucous hypersecretion.

8.013 Extensive pulmonary fibrosis is MOST likely to occur in:
A. pulmonary alveolar proteinosis
B. silicosis
C. emphysema
D. allergic asthma
E. Goodpasture's syndrome

B is correct.
Crystalline silica is very fibrogenic, stimulating intense collagen deposition.

8.014 The neutrophil plays a role in the morphologic reaction seen in:
A. idiopathic pulmonary fibrosis
B. bronchopneumonia
C. both
D. neither

C is correct.
The neutrophil is the predominant inflammatory cell in bronchopneumonia. In idiopathic pulmonary fibrosis, neutrophils are believed to release proteases, causing ongoing injury and repair.

8.015 The role of the alveolar macrophage is to:
   A. line the alveolar surface
   B. produce surfactant
   C. both
   D. neither

D is correct.
The primary role of the alveolar macrophage is derived from their phagocytic properties.

8.016 Bronchial epithelium contributes to:
   A. the production of granulomas
   B. the mucociliary escalator
   C. both
   D. neither

B is correct.
The bronchial epithelium contains cilia which beat rhythmically to move a mucous layer up the tracheo-bronchial tree.

8.017 Hyaline membranes indicate:
   A. substantial alveolar epithelial cell injury
   B. loss of function of the mucociliary escalator
   C. both
   D. neither

A is correct.
In severe alveolar epithelial cell injury, the necrotic cells together with edema fluid and fibrin create the hyaline membranes.

8.018 Which one of the following diseases is MOST commonly associated with asbestos exposure?
   A. hypersensitivity pneumonitis
   B. *Pneumocystis carinii* pneumonia
   C. mesothelioma
   D. squamous cell carcinoma
   E. adult respiratory distress syndrome

C is correct.
Mesothelioma is a malignant neoplasm involving either the visceral or parietal pleura. Up to 90% of mesotheliomas are believed to be asbestos-related.

8.019 Which one of the following diseases is MOST commonly seen in immunosuppressed patients?
   A. hypersensitivity pneumonitis
   B. *Pneumocystis carinii* pneumonia
   C. mesothelioma
   D. squamous cell carcinoma
   E. adult respiratory distress syndrome

B is correct.
Pneumocystis carinii is an opportunistic organism of uncertain classification. Pneumonia from this organism is only seen in severely malnourished children or in those with immunosuppressed states.

8.020 Which one of the following diseases is MOST closely related to cigarette-smoking?
   A. hypersensitivity pneumonitis
   B.*Pneumocystis carinii* pneumonia
   C. mesothelioma
   D. squamous cell carcinoma
   E. adult respiratory distress syndrome

D is correct.
There is a strong link between cigarette-smoking and squamous cell carcinoma of the lung.

8.021 Which one of the following diseases is MOST likely to occur as a complication of septic shock?
   A. hypersensitivity pneumonitis
   B. *Pneumocystis carinii* pneumonia
   C. mesothelioma
   D. squamous cell carcinoma
   E. adult respiratory distress syndrome

E is correct.
One of the clinical settings for the development of ARDS is septic shock. The basic lesion in this syndrome is diffuse damage to the alveolar epithelium and endothelium.

8.022 Which one of the following diseases may be referred to as 'farmer's lung'?
   A. hypersensitivity pneumonitis
   B. *Pneumocystis carinii* pneumonia
   C. mesothelioma
   D. squamous cell carcinoma
   E. adult respiratory distress syndrome

A is correct.
Farmer's lung results from exposure to actinomycetes which proliferate in damp, warm hay. There is an immunologically mediated interstitial lung reaction caused by exposure to the actinomycetes.

8.023 A 21-year-old woman with a history of Hodgkin's disease treated with a combination of chemotherapeutic drugs and radiation therapy presents with cough and shortness of breath. She notes that within the last month, her ability to walk even short distances has been markedly limited. Chest X-ray demonstrates diffuse reticulonodular infiltrates, with elevation of the diaphragm. Which one of the following conditions is the MOST likely?
   A. lung abscess
   B. pulmonary embolism
   C. diffuse interstitial fibrosis
   D. small-cell carcinoma
   E. adult respiratory distress syndrome

C is correct.
Certain chemotherapeutic drugs may cause diffuse interstitial fibrosis in the lungs. The clinical history and chest X-ray are compatible with this diagnosis.

8.024 A 60-year-old man is brought in by the police, who found him unconscious by the railroad tracks in Riverfront Park. When he sobers up, a history of chronic cough is elicited. Chest X-ray demonstrates a cavitary lesion in the left lower lobe. Which one of the following diagnoses is the MOST likely?
   A. lung abscess
   B. pulmonary embolism
   C. small-cell carcinoma
   D. pneumococcal pneumonia
   E. adult respiratory distress syndrome

A is correct.
Lower lobe abscesses are commonly associated with aspiration in alcoholics. None of the other conditions listed would present as a lower lobe cavitary lesion.

8.025 A 56-year-old man presents with cough and shortness of breath. For the last 5 years, he has had a cough which is productive of sputum for at least 4 months each year. Which one of the following diagnoses is the MOST likely in this patient?
   A. chronic bronchitis
   B. pulmonary embolism
   C. diffuse interstitial fibrosis
   D. small-cell carcinoma
   E. asthma

A is correct.
In chronic bronchitis, there is typically shortness of breath and a chronic cough which produces mucoid sputum due to the excessive mucous production in this condition.

8.026   A 75-year-old woman, who was previously well, presents with fever, cough, shortness of breath, and chest pain accentuated with inhalation. Her temperature is 102°F and her CBC shows a WBC of 15 000 with a mild left shift. Chest X-ray demonstrates a diffuse alveolar infiltrate involving the entire right middle lobe. The MOST likely diagnosis in this patient is:

    A. lung abscess
    B. pulmonary embolism
    C. diffuse interstitial fibrosis
    D. pneumococcal pneumonia
    E. adult respiratory distress syndrome

D is correct.
This is the classic presentation for pneumococcal pneumonia. A diagnosis of lung abscess is not supported by chest X-ray findings. The chest pain on inhalation is related to irritation of the pleura overlying the pneumonia.

8.027   All of the following situations may result in metabolic acidosis with an elevated anion gap EXCEPT:

    A. salicylate poisoning
    B. renal failure
    C. methanol intoxication
    D. thiazide diuretic therapy
    E. diabetic ketoacidosis

D is correct.
Thiazide diuretic therapy can cause metabolic alkalosis due to hypokalemia. Hypokalemia results in increased renal excretion of H^+.

8.028   Which one of the following features is MOST closely associated with the gray hepatization stage of lobar pneumonia?

    A. disintegration of alveolar neutrophils
    B. rapid bacterial multiplication
    C. 'rusty'-colored sputum
    D. prominent hyaline membranes
    E. alveolar hemorrhage

A is correct.
The stage of gray hepatization occurs later in the course of the disease. At that time, there is widespread disintegration of polymorphonuclear leukocytes in the alveolar exudate.

8.029   The principal role of the type II pneumocyte is to:

    A. act as a reserve epithelial cell
    B. phagocytose inhaled particulates
    C. produce mucin
    D. produce immunoglobulins
    E. develop cilia to aid in the mucociliary
       escalator

A is correct.
With alveolar injury, the type II pneumocyte proliferates, covering the alveolar septa, and differentiates into type I cells.

8.030   Which one of the following cell types is responsible for the production of surfactant in the lungs?

    A. endothelial cell
    B. type I pneumocyte
    C. type II pneumocyte
    D. alveolar macrophage
    E. myofibroblast

C is correct.
The type II pneumocyte produces surfactant.

8.031   A patient with α_1-antitrypsin deficiency is MOST likely to have which one of the following types of emphysema?

    A. bullous
    B. interstitial
    C. centrilobular
    D. panacinar
    E. paraseptal

D is correct.

In this type of emphysema, the acini are uniformly enlarged from the respiratory bronchiole to the terminal alveoli.

8.032   The MOST common etiologic agent in lobar pneumonia is:

    A. *Hemophilus influenzae*
    B. *Mycoplasma pneumoniae*
    C. *Streptococcus pneumoniae*
    D. *Klebsiella pneumoniae*
    E. *Staphylococcus aureus*

C is correct.

Approximately 90% of all cases of lobar pneumonia are caused by pneumococci (*Streptococcus pneumoniae*).

8.033   In the acute stage of adult respiratory distress syndrome, which one of the following is the LEAST likely?

    A. hypoxemia
    B. decreased lung compliance
    C. pulmonary edema
    D. hyaline membranes
    E. decreased pulmonary vascular resistance

E is correct.

All of the other choices are components of the acute stage of ARDS. There is increased pulmonary vascular resistance partially due to the edema and atelectasis.

8.034   All of the following laboratory values are consistent with compensated respiratory acidosis EXCEPT:

    A. decreased pH
    B. increased pCO_2
    C. decreased HCO_3
    D. decreased HCO_3/H_2CO_3 ratio

C is correct.

In respiratory acidosis, HCO_3 is retained; therefore, in the compensated state, the HCO_3 is elevated.

8.035   Cigarette-smoking is a risk factor in each of the following neoplasms EXCEPT:

    A. small-cell undifferentiated carcinoma of the lung
    B. mesothelioma of the pleura
    C. squamous cell carcinoma of the lung
    D. large-cell carcinoma of the lung
    E. transitional cell carcinoma of the urinary bladder

B is correct.

Cigarette-smoking is implicated in the etiology of all of the neoplasms listed with the exception of mesothelioma. Most patients with mesothelioma have a history of asbestos exposure.

8.036 Typical clinical presentations for bronchogenic carcinoma include all of the following EXCEPT:
   A. atelectasis
   B. hypoxemia
   C. pneumonia
   D. brain metastases
   E. focal emphysema

B is correct.
Bronchogenic carcinoma does not involve enough of the lung for patients to present with hypoxemia. Partial obstruction of bronchi by the neoplasm may predispose to atelectasis, focal emphysema, or pneumonia.

8.037 Which one of the following neoplasms originates in an intrabronchial location and is usually only locally invasive?
   A. adenocarcinoma
   B. mesothelioma
   C. small-cell undifferentiated carcinoma
   D. carcinoid tumor
   E. hamartoma

D is correct.
Bronchial carcinoids are similar to intestinal carcinoids. They originate in an intrabronchial location and, although they may occasionally metastasize, they are usually only locally invasive.

8.038 Complications of lung abscesses may include all of the following EXCEPT:
   A. brain abscess
   B. septicemia
   C. empyema
   D. hemorrhage
   E. diffuse pulmonary fibrosis

E is correct.
Abscesses by definition are localized necrotizing lesions. The only fibrosis associated with abscesses is localized to the zone of destruction.

8.039 All of the following are examples of pneumoconiosis EXCEPT:
   A. silicosis
   B. asbestosis
   C. berylliosis
   D. carcinomatosis
   E. byssinosis

D is correct.
Pneumoconiosis includes all disorders caused by the inhalation of any aerosol. This includes all of the diseases listed except for carcinomatosis.

8.040 Silicosis may predispose to the development of:
   A. asthma
   B. tuberculosis
   C. bronchogenic carcinoma
   D. lymphoma
   E. mesothelioma

B is correct.
Patients with silicosis have an increased incidence of pulmonary tuberculosis.

8.041 Each of the following conditions result in decreased pulmonary compliance EXCEPT:
   A. emphysema
   B. adult respiratory distress syndrome
   C. pulmonary sarcoidosis
   D. pulmonary damage secondary to bleomycin chemotherapy
   E. idiopathic pulmonary fibrosis (Hamman–Rich syndrome)

A is correct.
Emphysema is associated with destruction of the alveoli without significant fibrosis. There is increased lung compliance in emphysema. All of the other conditions listed are associated with either diffuse fibrosis or widespread septal edema.

8.042 Pulmonary embolism is MOST likely to result in which one of the following conditions?
- A. atelectasis
- B. bronchiectasis
- C. lung abscess
- D. cor pulmonale
- E. diffuse interstitial fibrosis

D is correct.
Massive emboli cause sudden increased pulmonary vascular resistance and acute right heart failure. Numerous small emboli over a long period of time may slowly increase the pulmonary vascular resistance, resulting in chronic right heart failure.

8.043 Which one of the following conditions is the MOST likely to be associated with decreased surfactant?
- A. atelectasis
- B. bronchiectasis
- C. chronic bronchitis
- D. bronchopneumonia
- E. thromboembolism

A is correct.
Surfactant serves as a surface tension-lowering agent and helps to keep the alveoli expanded. Decreased surfactant results in increased surface tension of the alveolar walls and an increased tendency to collapse, or atelectasis.

8.044 Patients with decreased ciliary motility are MOST likely to develop which one of the following conditions?
- A. atelectasis
- B. bronchiectasis
- C. thromboembolism
- D. bronchial carcinoid
- E. *Pneumocystis carinii* pneumonia

B is correct.
A defect in ciliary motility prevents the normal action of the mucociliary escalator. This predisposes to repeated infections, leading to destruction of the bronchial walls.

8.045 A 3-year-old girl presents to the emergency room in an obtunded state. Her mother states that she found the child with an open bottle of Bayer's orange-flavored aspirin (salicylates). Which of the following statements BEST describes the child's acid-base status?
- A. respiratory acidosis followed by metabolic alkalosis
- B. metabolic acidosis with increased anion gap followed by respiratory alkalosis
- C. isolated base-losing metabolic acidosis secondary to salicylate-induced diarrhea
- D. respiratory alkalosis followed by metabolic acidosis with increased anion gap
- E. isolated metabolic acidosis with increased anion gap

D is correct.
Early in the course of salicylate toxicity, there is hyperpnea with lowering of the pCO_2 and respiratory alkalosis. In a short period of time, a metabolic acidosis appears due to renal compensation for the respiratory alkalosis and from the accumulation of salicylic acid. There is an increased anion gap $[Na - (Cl + HCO_3)]$. Anions gaps of more than $10\,mEq/l$ above normal suggest acidic foreign substances.

8.046 All of the following disease states are associated with respiratory acidosis EXCEPT:
- A. emphysema
- B. uremia (renal failure)
- C. head trauma
- D. myasthenia gravis
- E. asthma

B is correct.
Uremia is associated with metabolic acidosis. Hydrogen ion that normally would be excreted by the kidney is retained due to loss of tubular function. All of the other conditions listed may cause decreased pulmonary function and elevated pCO_2.

8.047 Chronic bronchitis is characterized by:
   A. saccular dilatation of the airways
   B. hypersecretion of mucous
   C. thickened bronchial basement membrane
   D. defects of the cilia by electron microscopy
   E. immunologically mediated response to
      aspergillus antigen

B is correct.
Histologic changes seen in this disease include hyperemia and edema of mucous membranes, mucinous secretions collecting in airways, an increase in the size of the mucous glands, mucous plugging, inflammation, and fibrosis.

8.048 The acute stage of diffuse alveolar damage is characterized by:
   A. type I pneumocyte cell proliferation
   B. interstitial inflammation
   C. hyaline membranes
   D. prominent alveolar macrophages
   E. organization

C is correct.
The acute stage of ARDS is characterized by edema, cell sloughing, hyaline membranes and atelectasis.

8.049 All of the following findings are features of adult respiratory distress syndrome EXCEPT:
   A. pulmonary hypertension
   B. increased compliance
   C. hypoxemia
   D. pulmonary edema
   E. increased airway resistance

B is correct.
In ARDS the edema, inflammation, and hyaline membranes produce a stiff lung which is less compliant than normal.

8.050 Granulomatous tissue response may be seen in all of the following diseases EXCEPT:
   A. sarcoidosis
   B. hypersensitivity pneumonitis
   C. fungal pneumonia
   D. *Pneumocystis* pneumonia
   E. primary tuberculosis

D is correct.
Pneumocystis pneumonia presents histologically with alveolar spaces filled with a foamy amorphous material consisting of cell debris and organisms. Granulomas are not produced.

8.051 When a 5-μm carbon particle is inhaled, what is the MOST likely fate of this particle?
   A. trapped in the nasopharynx
   B. expired during the next breath
   C. trapped by the alveolar epithelium and
      translocated to the lymph nodes via the
      lymphatics
   D. phagocytosed by a macrophage, which will
      die and induce fibroblast collagen
      production
   E. impact the tracheal wall and be removed by
      the mucociliary escalator

E is correct.
Particles $> 10\,\mu m$ tend to be deposited in the nasopharyngeal areas. Particles $3–10\,\mu m$ lodge in the trachea and bronchi by impaction. Smaller particles such as bacteria are deposited in the terminal airways and alveoli.

8.052 Endogenous lipid pneumonia is frequently the result of:
  A. gastric aspiration
  B. lobar pneumonia
  C. bronchogenic carcinoma
  D. *Legionella pneumophila*
  E. empyema

8.053 Which of the following is LEAST likely to result in a cavitary lesion on chest X-ray?
  A. aspiration
  B. *Mycoplasma* pneumonia
  C. tuberculosis
  D. squamous cell carcinoma
  E. tricuspid valve endocarditis

8.054 Established risks of tobacco-smoking include all of the following EXCEPT:
  A. increased respiratory tract infections in children from homes of smokers
  B. increased risk of esophageal carcinoma
  C. increased risk of bronchogenic carcinoma in non-smoking spouses
  D. increased risk of spontaneous abortion
  E. increased risk of silicosis

8.055 Pulmonary edema may be expected to occur during the course of illness in all of the following conditions EXCEPT:
  A. nephrotic syndrome
  B. liver disease
  C. tricuspid stenosis
  D. mitral stenosis
  E. salt-water drowning

C is correct.
Endogenous or obstructive lipid pneumonia is associated with the accumulation of lipid derived from degenerating cells as well as surfactant from type II pneumocytes. The most frequent causes are obstruction due to bronchogenic carcinoma, tuberculosis, abscess formation and bronchiectasis.

B is correct.
Aspiration and tricuspid valve endocarditis may both lead to lung abscesses. Necrotic cancers may cavitate and, of course, tuberculosis frequently presents with cavitary lesions. *Myocoplasma* pneumonia presents as an interstitial inflammatory reaction. Cavitation does not occur.

E is correct.
Smoking increases the risk of all conditions listed except silicosis. The prolonged inhalation of silica particles usually encountered in the mining industry may lead to silicosis. There is no evidence that smoking increases the chances of developing silicosis.

C is correct.
In tricuspid stenosis, there is decreased blood flow to the pulmonary capillary bed and, hence, there is no pathophysiologic mechanism for the production of pulmonary edema. Nephrotic syndrome and liver disease may be associated with pulmonary edema secondary to decreased oncotic pressure. Mitral stenosis results in increased hydrostatic pulmonary pressure. Salt-water drowning produces edema by microvascular injury.

8.056   A 62-year-old male veteran comes to the emergency room with a complaint of sudden onset of severe shortness of breath. He has a long term history of chronic obstructive pulmonary disease; his usual baseline arterial blood gases are: pH: 7.36 (normal range 7.36–7.44); pO_2: 60 (normal range 83–93) mmHg; pCO_2: 55 (normal range 34–45) mmHg; HCO_3: 35 (normal range 22–26) mEq/l. His blood gas results in the emergency room without supplemental oxygen are: pH: 7.20; pO_2: 40 mmHg; pCO_2: 90 mmHg; HCO_3: 35 mEq/l. Which acid-base category BEST describes this patient?
  A. mixed acid base disorder, acute metabolic alkalosis superimposed on fully compensated chronic metabolic acidosis
  B. mixed acid base disorder, acute respiratory acidosis superimposed on fully compensated chronic respiratory acidosis
  C. isolated acute respiratory acidosis with partial compensation
  D. mixed acid base disorder, acute respiratory acidosis superimposed on partially compensated respiratory acidosis

B is correct.
This patient has a baseline normal blood pH and an elevated HCO_3. This indicates a compensated acidosis. In view of his blood gases (low pO_2 and high pCO_2), this patient has chronic respiratory disease as the most obvious cause of his compensated acidosis. The findings of acute lowering of the pO_2, elevation of the pCO_2, and the abnormally low pH at the time of his emergency room visit indicate acute respiratory acidosis.

8.057   Fetal urinary tract obstruction with oligo-hydramnios is MOST likely to be associated with which one of the following conditions?
  A. bronchopulmonary sequestration
  B. pulmonary hypoplasia
  C. bronchogenic cyst
  D. congenital emphysema

B is correct.
Oligohydramnios (insufficient amniotic fluid) is an important cause of pulmonary hypoplasia

8.058   Which one of the following statements is TRUE concerning the type I pneumocyte?
  A. produces surfactant
  B. proliferates in the repair response
  C. has a cuboidal shape
  D. covers 95% of the alveolar surface

D is correct.
The type I pneumocyte is a thin epithelial cell which covers 95% of the alveolar surface. The type II pneumocyte is more cuboidal, produces surfactant and serves as a reserve cell by proliferating when type I cells are injured.

8.059   Small-cell undifferentiated carcinoma of the lung is MOST likely to be associated with the production of which one of the following hormones?
  A. adrenocorticotropic hormone
  B. somatotropic hormone
  C. prolactin
  D. cortisol
  E. parathyroid hormone

A is correct.
Cushing's syndrome frequently occurs in patients with small-cell undifferentiated carcinoma of the lung due to production of ACTH or ACTH-like peptides by the tumor.

8.060 The decrease in FEV_1 (1 min of forced expiratory volume) seen in panacinar emphysema is primarily due to:
   A. excessive bronchial mucous secretion
   B. airway collapse due to loss of radial support
   C. bronchoconstriction
   D. alveolar interstitial fibrosis

B is correct.
In panacinar emphysema, the acini are enlarged from the respiratory bronchiole to the terminal alveoli. There is destruction of alveolar septal walls with loss of radial support to the airways. In forced expiration, the loss of support allows the airways to collapse rather than be held open during expiration.

8.061 Accumulation of epithelioid histiocytes is a histologic feature MOST likely to be seen in which one of the following diseases?
   A. bronchopneumonia
   B. viral pneumonitis
   C. fungal pneumonia
   D. pneumoconiosis

C is correct.
Many fungal organisms stimulate the formation of epithelioid histiocytes at the site of inflammation.

8.062 Alveoli filled with an inflammatory exudate are typically seen in which one of the following conditions?
   A. bacterial bronchopneumonia
   B. viral pneumonitis
   C. fungal pneumonia
   D. pneumoconiosis

A is correct.
In bacterial bronchopneumonia, there is an outpouring of fibrin and acute inflammatory cells into the alveolar spaces.

8.063 Interstitial pneumonitis is the characteristic feature of which one of the following conditions?
   A. bronchopneumonia
   B. viral pneumonitis
   C. fungal pneumonia
   D. pneumoconiosis

B is correct.
Viral pneumonitis typically presents with an interstitial inflammatory reaction. The inflammation is basically limited to the alveolar septal walls.

8.064 Macrophages with pigmented debris is a feature seen typically in which one of the following conditions?
   A. bronchopneumonia
   B. viral pneumonitis
   C. fungal pneumonia
   D. pneumoconiosis

D is correct.
Pneumoconiosis consists of pulmonary disease due to the inhalation of foreign matter. Much of this foreign material is pigmented and is phagocytized by pulmonary macrophages

8.065 A 25-year-old woman gives birth to a healthy term infant and is discharged the following day from the hospital. She felt fatigue, but her husband did not become concerned until he found her delirious and soaked in a sweat 3 days postpartum. Physical examination upon admission to the hospital demonstrated purulent drainage from her cervix which, on Gram staining, showed gram-positive cocci. Blood cultures were drawn. As her breathing was labored, a chest X-ray was performed which showed bilateral interstitial infiltrates. Which one of the following is the MOST likely cause of this patient's condition?

    A. adult respiratory distress syndrome
    B. adenocarcinoma of the lung
    C. asbestosis
    D. bronchiectasis
    E. emphysema
    F. mitral stenosis
    G. pulmonary hypoplasia
    H. silicosis
    I. small-cell carcinoma of the lung
    J. squamous cell carcinoma of the lung
    K. tricuspid stenosis

A is correct.

Adult respiratory distress syndrome (ARDS) is a term used to describe a syndrome of diffuse alveolar capillary damage with rapid onset of severe respiratory insufficiency. One of the conditions which may lead to ARDS is sepsis. This woman's clinical history strongly suggests sepsis secondary to a postpartum infection.

8.066 A 70-year-old man with no smoking history presents with a cough. Further history reveals that he has had recent significant weight loss. His occupational history fails to reveal exposure to fibrogenic dusts. Physical examination reveals a man who appears chronically ill, but is afebrile and in no acute distress. Chest X-ray demonstrates a peripheral pulmonary mass. Which one of the following is the MOST likely cause of this patient's condition?

    A. adult respiratory distress syndrome
    B. adenocarcinoma of the lung
    C. asbestosis
    D. bronchiectasis
    E. emphysema
    F. mitral stenosis
    G. pulmonary hypoplasia
    H. silicosis
    I. small-cell carcinoma of the lung
    J. squamous cell carcinoma of the lung
    K. tricuspid stenosis

B is correct.

The recent significant weight loss suggests a malignancy. Adenocarcinoma is the most common lung cancer in non-smokers. The tumors are usually peripherally located.

8.067 A 58-year-old woman with a 45-year pack-smoking history has a routine chest X-ray performed. A mass is identified in the hilar region of the left upper lobe. Routine chemistries are unremarkable except for an elevated serum calcium. What is the BEST working diagnosis for this patient?

    A. adult respiratory distress syndrome
    B. adenocarcinoma of the lung
    C. asbestosis
    D. bronchiectasis
    E. emphysema
    F. mitral stenosis
    G. pulmonary hypoplasia
    H. silicosis
    I. small-cell carcinoma of the lung
    J. squamous cell carcinoma of the lung
    K. tricuspid stenosis

J is correct.

The finding of a hilar mass in a smoker is highly suspect for lung cancer. The elevated serum calcium suggests squamous cell carcinoma. These tumors may be associated with secretion of a parathyroid hormone-related peptide.

8.068 A 53-year-old man presents with cough and shortness of breath. He notes that the dyspnea has developed gradually over many months, but has become so severe in recent days that he is unable to walk more than 50 feet without having to stop to catch his breath. His occupational history is significant as he has worked his entire life as a sandblaster. Chest X-ray demonstrates bilateral upper lobe nodules, with a reticulonodular infiltrate in the remainder of his lungs. Which one of the following is the MOST likely diagnosis for this patient?

    A. adult respiratory distress syndrome
    B. adenocarcinoma of the lung
    C. asbestosis
    D. bronchiectasis
    E. emphysema
    F. mitral stenosis
    G. pulmonary hypoplasia
    H. silicosis
    I. small-cell carcinoma of the lung
    J. squamous cell carcinoma of the lung
    K. tricuspid stenosis

H is correct.

Silicosis is caused by inhalation of crystalline silicon dioxide. Exposure to silica is high in employment such as foundry work, sandblasting, hard-rock mining and stone-cutting. Silicosis is a slowly progressive nodular fibrosing disease.

8.069   A 6-year-old boy presents with a chronic cough productive of copious amounts of foul-smelling purulent sputum. Chest X-ray demonstrates a large infiltrate involving the right lower lung field. Which one of the following is the MOST likely diagnosis in this patient?

    A. adult respiratory distress syndrome

    B. adenocarcinoma of the lung

    C. asbestosis

    D. bronchiectasis

    E. emphysema

    F. mitral stenosis

    G. pulmonary hypoplasia

    H. silicosis

    I. small-cell carcinoma of the lung

    J. squamous cell carcinoma of the lung

    K. tricuspid stenosis

D is correct.
Bronchiectasis is a chronic necrotizing infection of the bronchi and bronchioles which results in abnormal dilatation of the airways. Clinical manifestations include cough, fever, and copious amount of foul-smelling purulent sputum.

8.070   A 48-year-old woman presents with fatigue. Auscultation of the chest reveals the presence of rales. CBC and routine chemistries are within normal limits. Chest X-ray demonstrates a hazy infiltrate in the left upper lobe, and two smaller infiltrates in the right lower and right middle lobes. Which one of the following is the MOST likely diagnosis for this patient?

    A. adult respiratory distress syndrome

    B. adenocarcinoma of the lung

    C. asbestosis

    D. bronchiectasis

    E. emphysema

    F. mitral stenosis

    G. pulmonary hypoplasia

    H. silicosis

    I. small-cell carcinoma of the lung

    J. squamous cell carcinoma of the lung

    K. tricuspid stenosis

F is correct.
This woman apparently has pulmonary edema. Mitral stenosis causes pulmonary edema by obstructing the return of blood from the pulmonary veins to the left atrium. This causes elevation of pulmonary capillary pressure and transudation of fluid into the alveolar spaces.

8.071   A 4-year-old boy in a rural area develops an acute febrile illness associated with severe pain in his left ear. Due to a lack of transportation, he is not seen by a physician. Assuming he is suffering from acute otitis media, the possible complications of his illness could include all of the following EXCEPT:

    A. chronic otitis media

    B. mastoiditis

    C. conductive hearing loss

    D. otosclerosis

    E. cholesteatoma

D is correct.
Otosclerosis is a condition in which there is abnormal bone deposition in the middle ear. It usually affects both ears and is familial in most instances.

8.072 A 16-year-old boy presents to the emergency room with a nosebleed which he has been unable to stop. He reports 3–4 nosebleeds over the past 6 weeks. Physical examination revealed the source of bleeding to be a mass in the nasopharynx. The MOST likely diagnosis is:
   A. squamous cell carcinoma
   B. nasopharyngeal angiofibroma
   C. granular cell tumor
   D. adenoid cystic carcinoma
   E. Wegener's granulomatosis

B is correct.
Nasopharyngeal angiofibroma is a very vascular tumor which occurs almost exclusively in adolescent males. It may cause serious clinical problems because of its tendency to bleed profusely.

8.073 A 50-year-old male smoker presents to his physician with a complaint of hoarseness over the past 1–2 months. He has coughed up small amounts of bloody material on one or two occasions, and has also noted two firm nodules in the right side of his neck. Based on this information, which of the following is the MOST likely laryngeal lesion in this patient?
   A. squamous cell carcinoma
   B. branchial cleft cyst
   C. polyps
   D. adenocarcinoma
   E. adenoid cystic carcinoma

A is correct.
The bloody sputum along with the firm nodules in the right side of the neck raise the suspicion of malignancy. The most common malignancy of the larynx is squamous cell carcinoma.

8.074 Which of the following statements is TRUE of cholesteatoma?
   A. it is a benign neoplasm occurring in the middle ear, primarily in children
   B. it may result from metaplasia of the secretory epithelial lining of the middle ear
   C. its pathognomonic feature is cholesterol clefts
   D. typical histologic changes include amyloid deposits
   E. malignant transformation has been well described

B is correct.
Cholesteatomas are associated with chronic otitis media. It is believed that chronic inflammation and perforation of the eardrum along with ingrowth of squamous epithelium or metaplasia of secretory epithelium in the middle ear play a role in their formation.

8.075 A 50-year-old male smoker presents with a 1-year history of hoarseness, a 20-lb weight loss over the last 2 months and recent hemoptysis. Laryngoscopy reveals a large ulcerated irregular lesion on the left true vocal cord. Which of the following statements is correct concerning the disease process MOST likely to be evident upon biopsy of this lesion?
  A. Epstein–Barr virus has been implicated in its pathogenesis
  B. epidemiological evidence indicates asbestos inhalation may be a risk factor
  C. risk due to tobacco smoke is not proportional to the level of exposure
  D. death is usually due to widespread distant metastasis
  E. likely to have developed within a preexisting laryngeal polyp

B is correct.
The risk of laryngeal carcinoma is directly proportional to the level of exposure to tobacco smoke. There is also evidence of a relationship to asbestos inhalation.

8.076 The MOST common pathogen in acute otitis media is:
  A. *Enterococcus*
  B. *Meningococcus*
  C. *Staphylococcus*
  D. *Streptococcus*
  E. *Pseudomonas*

D is correct.
Otitis media is an inflammation of the ear. The most common etiologic agents are *Streptococcus pneumoniae*, *Haemophilus influenzae*, and beta-hemolytic streptococci.

8.077 Squamous cell carcinoma of the larynx is associated MOST strongly with what risk factor?
  A. cigarette-smoking
  B. excessive use (as in singers)
  C. preexisting or concomitant squamous cell carcinoma of lung
  D. previous tracheotomy
  E. thyroid radiation

A is correct.
Laryngeal carcinoma is most often related to cigarette-smoking. The risk is proportional to the amount of exposure.

8.078 All of the following statements is true of laryngeal carcinoma EXCEPT:
  A. squamous carcinoma is the most common histologic type
  B. strongly associated with cigarette-smoking
  C. prognosis is linked to location of the tumor within the larynx
  D. etiologically closely linked with the Epstein–Barr virus

D is correct.
There is no known association of laryngeal carcinoma and EBV. Human papillomavirus has been detected in some laryngeal carcinomas; however, its role has not been clearly determined.

SECTION 9: HEMATOPATHOLOGY

Lymphomas and leukemias, myelomas, and related disorders

9.001 Lacunar cells are detected in biopsy sections of the mediastinal mass of a young adult female. Of the following, the MOST likely additional finding in this patient is:
- A. generalized lymphadenopathy
- B. monoclonal B-cell phenotype
- C. t(14;18)
- D. cyclic fevers
- E. positive test for terminal deoxynucleotidyl transferase (TdT)

D is correct.
Lacunar cells are variants of Reed–Sternberg cells characteristically seen in nodular sclerosis Hodgkin's disease, the only form of Hodgkin's disease that is seen more commonly in women than in men. The majority of patients present with localized disease. Systemic complaints include fever, unexplained weight loss, pruritus, and anemia.

9.002 Endemic and non-endemic examples of small non-cleaved (Burkitt's) lymphoma differ primarily in their:
- A. age distribution
- B. propensity to involve the CNS
- C. cytogenetics
- D. immunophenotype
- E. association with Epstein–Barr virus (EBV) positivity

E is correct.
Small non-cleaved (Burkitt's) lymphoma is endemic in Africa and predominantly affects children between the ages of 5 and 10 years. Approximately 95% of children have an associated EBV infection. Non-endemic Burkitt's lymphoma occurs in the first two decades of life and is associated with EBV in only 20% of cases. Both endemic and non-endemic Burkitt's lymphoma have the same B-cell phenotype and cytogenetic translocations.

9.003 Expression of the *bcl*-2 gene product is associated MOST closely with:
- A. follicular center cell lymphoma
- B. mycosis fungoides
- C. Hodgkin's disease
- D. lymphoblastic lymphoma
- E. adult T-cell leukemia / lymphoma

A is correct.
Expression of *bcl*-2 protein is present in $>85\%$ of follicular lymphomas. Immunohistochemical staining for *bcl*-2 differentiates follicular lymphoma from reactive follicular hyperplasia in the majority of cases; *bcl*-2 is always negative in the germinal centers of reactive follicles.

9.004 CD3- and CD4-positive tumor cells may be present in each of the following lymphomas EXCEPT:
- A. adult T-cell leukemia / lymphoma
- B. mycosis fungoides
- C. small non-cleaved cell lymphoma
- D. Sézary syndrome
- E. lymphoblastic lymphoma

C is correct.
All of the disorders except small non-cleaved cell lymphoma have a T-cell origin. The cells express the pan-T cell marker CD3 and usually demonstrate a helper T-cell phenotype (CD4-positive). Approximately 20% of lymphoblastic lymphomas are of B-cell, rather than T-cell, phenotype. Small non-cleaved cell lymphoma is always of B-cell origin and expresses the B-cell antigens CD19, CD20, CD22 and CD10 (variable).

9.005 Congestive splenomegaly often accompanies all of the following EXCEPT:
  A. cardiac failure
  B. acute leukemia
  C. portal vein thrombosis
  D. cirrhosis
  E. hepatic vein thrombosis

B is correct.
Congestive splenomegaly is caused by persistent venous congestion and portal hypertension. This is present in disorders associated with systemic passive congestion, deranged intrahepatic portal venous drainage, or obstruction in the portal or splenic veins. Acute leukemia is an acute disorder without this association.

9.006 Epithelial thymomas are:
  A. seen primarily in young adult females
  B. often asymptomatic
  C. usually malignant
  D. associated with defects in cell-mediated immunity
  E. accompanied by tetany

B is correct.
Thymomas are benign or, less commonly, malignant tumors of thymic epithelial cells that are usually seen in adults >40 years of age. The widespread performance of cardiac surgery has led to the discovery of a large number of small asymptomatic tumors.

9.007 It is 6 PM Friday, and you have just admitted an acutely ill 20-year-old male patient from a hospital in a nearby small town. You receive a call from the hematology lab technologist, who has noted blasts on the peripheral smear. You review the slide and conclude that 40% of the cells are indeed blasts. You request myeloperoxidase (MP) and non-specific esterase (NSE) stains on the peripheral blood, and find that the majority of the blasts are MP-positive. You cannot detect Auer rods. What type of hematologic malignancy does the patient have?
  A. hairy-cell leukemia
  B. a severe leukemoid reaction
  C. atypical lymphocytosis associated with CMV or EBV infection
  D. acute lymphoblastic leukemia
  E. acute myelogenous leukemia

E is correct.
The French–American–British (FAB) classification of acute leukemia requires >30% blasts in the bone marrow. The subtype of leukemia depends on cytochemical stain findings. Myeloperoxidase is the most specific cytochemical stain for myeloid precursors and is therefore used to diagnose acute myelogenous leukemia (AML). Myeloperoxidase does not stain cells of lymphoid origin. Non-specific esterase stains monocytic cells.

9.008   A 6-year-old child with a peripheral blast count of 80 000 cells/μl has a bone marrow aspirate and biopsy, which reveals that nearly 100% of the nucleated cells are small blasts. The blasts are myeloperoxidase (MP)- and non-specific esterase (NSE)-negative, and Auer rods are not evident. Flow cytometric analysis confirms your suspicions about this malignancy, which you know is common in children. Your clinical colleagues want to know whether you think they should be treating an acute lymphoblastic or a myelogenous leukemia. What is the diagnosis?

    A. hairy-cell leukemia

    B. a severe leukemoid reaction

    C. atypical lymphocytosis associated with CMV or EBV infection

    D. acute lymphoblastic leukemia

    E. acute non-lymphocytic leukemia

D is correct.
The high white blood cell count with a predominance of blasts indicates an acute leukemia. More than 80% of acute leukemias in children under 15 years of age are acute lymphoblastic leukemias. The absence of myeloperoxidase and non-specific esterase staining, and the lack of Auer rods support this diagnosis. Flow cytometric studies show B-cell origin in 80–85% and T-cell origin in 15–20% of acute lymphoblastic leukemia (ALL) cases.

9.009   A marine recruit on her first furlough is admitted to your service. She is acutely ill with a tender right upper quadrant and prominent tonsillar adenopathy. You review her peripheral smear and note a lymphocytosis with 20% of the lymphoid cells having abundant blue cytoplasm, and nuclei with coarse but diffusely dispersed chromatin and indistinct nucleoli. Some of the cells have radiating basophilia of the cytoplasm and scattered azurophilic granules. You show this slide to a senior hematologist/oncologist, who informs you that they are not blasts. What is the diagnosis?

    A. hairy-cell leukemia

    B. a severe leukemoid reaction

    C. atypical lymphocytosis associated with CMV or EBV infection

    D. acute lymphoblastic leukemia

    E. acute myelogenous leukemia

C is correct.
Most benign lymphocytoses have reactive-appearing lymphocytes. These have been referred to as activated, atypical, or variant lymphocytes. This patient has symptoms of infectious mononucleosis (EBV) or infectious mononucleosis-like syndrome (CMV). These are associated with an increased number of Downy type II lymphocytes which have the morphologic characteristics described.

9.010   An acutely ill 30-year-old white man is admitted with a 120 000 cells/µl white cell count. You suspect leukemia and request a bone marrow procedure for special studies, but are unable to obtain an adequate specimen. However, therapy needs to be initiated before you can repeat the marrow evaluation. You request myeloperoxidase and non-specific esterase cytochemical stains on the peripheral blood smear. Before the stains are ready, you review the peripheral smear and find numerous blast cells, some with red needle-like structures in the cytoplasm. What is your initial diagnosis?

    A. hairy-cell leukemia

    B. a severe leukemoid reaction

    C. atypical lymphocytosis associated with CMV or EBV infection

    D. acute lymphoblastic leukemia

    E. acute myelogenous leukemia

E is correct.

Crystallization of primary (azurophilic) granules in blasts produces the distinctive red-staining needle-like structures known as Auer rods, characteristically seen in acute non-lymphocytic leukemia. These are not seen in the lymphoblasts of ALL cases and can be used to distinguish between the two entities.

9.011   A surgeon associate of yours asks you to examine one of his patients, an elderly man who has marked splenomegaly, but who is otherwise essentially asymptomatic. His peripheral white cell count is 10 000 cells/µl. You review the peripheral smear, and note small, somewhat atypical, lymphoid cells which stain positively with the tartrate-resistant acid phosphatase (TRAP) enzyme procedure. What is your initial diagnosis?

    A. hairy-cell leukemia

    B. a severe leukemoid reaction

    C. atypical lymphocytosis associated with CMV or EBV infection

    D. acute lymphoblastic leukemia

    E. acute myelogenous leukemia

A is correct.

Hairy-cell leukemia is a leukemia of B-cell phenotype characterized by cytopenias, splenomegaly, minimal lymphadenopathy, and the presence of hairy cells in the blood and bone marrow. Hairy cells have moderately abundant cytoplasm with hairy projections, and round to kidney-shaped nuclei. TRAP is the cytochemical stain most widely used to confirm the diagnosis. This is predominantly a disease of older adults and is more common seen in men than in women.

9.012   A 65-year-old woman presents with a tendency to easy bruising, a 1.2-million/mm³ platelet count, abnormal platelet function studies, and bone marrow megakaryocytosis. She has had high platelet counts for 4 months, and a physiologic cause for the thrombocytosis has been excluded. What is the MOST likely diagnosis?

    A. chronic myelogenous leukemia, myeloproliferative syndrome

    B. essential thrombocytosis, myeloproliferative syndrome

    C. polycythemia vera, myeloproliferative syndrome

    D. refractory anemia with excess blasts, myelodysplastic syndrome

    E. chronic myelomonocytic leukemia, myelodysplastic syndrome

B is correct.

The diagnosis of essential thrombocythemia requires the exclusion of other myeloproliferative syndromes (especially polycythemia vera) and reactive thrombocytoses. The peripheral blood platelet count should be >600 000 cells/µl and the blood film should show numerous giant platelets. Clusters and sheets of enlarged and hyperlobulated megakaryocytes are present in the bone marrow, in contrast to the morphologically normal megakaryocytes seen in reactive thrombocytoses. Platelet aggregation studies show hypoaggregation in the majority of cases.

9.013   A plethoric 60-year-old man presents with new-onset increased red cell mass, normal oxygen saturation, iron deficiency, and splenomegaly. The patient shows no apparent reason for iron loss, has never smoked, and denies a recent attempt to climb Mount Everest. What is the MOST likely diagnosis?
    A. chronic myelogenous leukemia, myeloproliferative syndrome
    B. essential thrombocytosis, myeloproliferative syndrome
    C. polycythemia vera, myeloproliferative syndrome
    D. refractory anemia with excess blasts, myelodysplastic syndrome
    E. chronic myelomonocytic leukemia, myelodysplastic syndrome

C is correct.
Definitive criteria for the diagnosis of polycythemia vera were established by the Polycythemia Vera Study Group in 1971. The three major criteria required to make the diagnosis are: 1) increased red blood cell volume (>36 ml/kg in men); 2) normal arterial oxygen saturation (>92%); and 3) splenomegaly. Iron stores are often decreased or absent due to the increased requirement for erythropoiesis.

9.014   A leukemoid reaction is MOST likely to be seen in:
    A. viral infection
    B. fungal infection
    C. bacterial infection
    D. protozoal infection

C is correct.
Inflammatory reactions with very high white cell counts suggesting leukemia are called leukemoid reactions. Infections causing leukemoid reactions are usually bacterial in origin with the peripheral blood smear showing a predominance of segmented neutrophils and some band neutrophils.

9.015   Which of the following is LEAST likely to be accompanied by a lymphocytosis in the peripheral blood?
    A. viral infection
    B. fungal infection
    C. bacterial infection
    D. protozoal infection

C is correct.
Bacterial products (endotoxins) stimulate macrophages to produce the cytokine interleukin-1 and tumor necrosis factor. These factors have numerous effects, including induction of acute-phase reactions and increasing circulating neutrophils. Thus, bacterial infections are most commonly associated with a reactive neutrophilia.

9.016   A patient presents with plasmacytosis in the bone marrow, osteolytic bone lesions and a monoclonal immunoglobulin in the serum. The MOST likely diagnosis is:
    A. follicular center cell lymphoma
    B. multiple myeloma
    C. acute lymphocytic leukemia
    D. chronic lymphocytic leukemia

B is correct.
In a patient with lytic bone lesions and a monoclonal gammopathy, the presence of >10% plasma cells in the bone marrow is diagnostic of multiple myeloma.

9.017   A 70-year-old man presents for routine physical examination. Laboratory tests reveal a monoclonal IgG immunoglobulin in the serum. Physical examination reveals no adenopathy. Serum IgA and IgM are within normal levels. Skeletal X-ray survey reveals no osteolytic lesions and examination of the bone marrow reveals no increase in plasma cells. The MOST likely diagnosis is:

    A. atypical IgG-secreting multiple myeloma

    B. monoclonal gammopathy of undetermined significance

    C. atypical IgG-secreting B-cell lymphoma

    D. Hodgkin's disease

B is correct.

For a diagnosis of monoclonal gammopathy of undetermined significance, a monoclonal immunoglobulin is required, but it is less than that associated with multiple myeloma. Bone marrow plasma cells are < 10% of the bone marrow cellularity and no lytic bone lesions or myeloma-related symptoms are present.

9.018   A patient with a 40 000 cells/µl white cell count, predominantly composed of band and segmented neutrophils, MOST likely has which of the following conditions?

    A. leukemoid reaction

    B. chronic myelogenous leukemia (CML)

    C. acute myelogenous leukemia (AML)

    D. acute lymphoblastic leukemia (ALL)

    E. chronic lymphocytic leukemia (CLL)

A is correct.

Leukemoid reactions are associated with mature neutrophils consisting predominantly of polymorphonuclear leukocytes with some band neutrophils, usually < 10%. Basophilia or eosinophilia, suggesting a myeloproliferative disorder, is absent and platelets are small.

9.019   A patient with headaches and intermittent episodes of blindness has a 200 000 cells/µl white cell count, comprising 5% blasts, 20% promyelocytes, 10% metamyelocytes, 15% myelocytes, 20% band neutrophils, 20% polymorphonuclear leukocytes, 5% basophils and 5% eosinophils, is MOST likely to have which of the following conditions?

    A. leukemoid reaction

    B. chronic myelogenous leukemia (CML)

    C. acute myelogenous leukemia (AML)

    D. acute lymphoblastic leukemia (ALL)

    E. chronic lymphocytic leukemia (CLL)

B is correct.

The leukocyte count in CML commonly exceeds 100 000 cells/µl. The circulating cells are mainly neutrophils and immature granulocytes. Basophilia and eosinophilia are common in CML and unusual in a reactive condition. Circulating blasts (< 10%) are typical of the 'chronic phase' of CML. Higher blast counts reflect transformation to an 'accelerated phase' or acute leukemia (blast crisis).

9.020   A 5-year-old child has a 35 000 cells/µl white cell count consisting predominantly of blasts. Anemia, generalized malaise, ecchymosis, and lymphadenopathy are present. This patient MOST likely has which of the following conditions?

    A. leukemoid reaction

    B. chronic myelogenous leukemia (CML)

    C. acute myelogenous leukemia (AML)

    D. acute lymphoblastic leukemia (ALL)

    E. chronic lymphocytic leukemia (CLL)

D is correct.

The high blast count is consistent with acute leukemia. More than 80% of cases of acute leukemia in patients < 15 years of age are ALL, making this the most likely diagnosis. The blasts accumulate in the bone marrow and replace normal hematopoietic elements. This child's presenting signs and symptoms are related to the resulting blood cytopenias.

9.021   A patient has a 35 000 cells/μl white cell count comprising 90% blasts with prominent Auer rods. He MOST likely has which of the following conditions?

   A. leukemoid reaction
   B. chronic myelogenous leukemia (CML)
   C. acute myelogenous leukemia (AML)
   D. acute lymphoblastic leukemia (ALL)
   E. chronic lymphocytic leukemia (CLL)

C is correct.
With 90% circulating blasts, the patient most likely has >30% blasts in the bone marrow (required for a diagnosis of acute leukemia by FAB classification criteria). ALL is excluded by the presence of Auer rods in the blasts and, therefore, one of the subtypes of AML must be considered.

9.022   The characteristics of myeloproliferative syndromes (excluding CML) include all of the following EXCEPT:

   A. <10% progress to acute leukemia
   B. indolent course
   C. origination at the stem cell level
   D. evolution to blast crisis in >90% of cases

D is correct.
Transformation to blast crisis (>30% blasts in bone marrow) occurs in >90% of cases of CML, and is uncommon in the other myeloproliferative disorders. When present, it is often associated with the use of radioactive phosphorus or alkylating agent chemotherapy.

9.023   Myelofibrosis with myeloid metaplasia is characterized by all of the following EXCEPT:

   A. progressive pancytopenia in the peripheral blood
   B. progressive bone marrow fibrosis
   C. a leukoerythroblastic response in the peripheral blood
   D. progressive increase in bone marrow cellularity

D is correct.
The bone marrow may show trilineage hyperplasia with minimal fibrosis early in the course of myelofibrosis with myeloid metaplasia (cellular phase). With disease progression, marrow fibrosis occurs secondary to the secretion of fibroblast growth factors by abnormal megakaryocytes. Diffuse fibrosis results in marrow hypocellularity.

9.024   Patients with immunoglobulin-producing B-cell neoplasms often experience all of the following EXCEPT:

   A. renal failure
   B. infections
   C. hypercalcemia
   D. elevation of normal serum immunoglobulins

D is correct.
Uninvolved immunoglobulins may be decreased in patients with monoclonal gammopathies. In particular, it is a feature of multiple myeloma, where severe depression of normal immunoglobulins pose major clinical problems with infections.

The following case history relates to questions 9.025–9.029. A 58-year-old man presents to the emergency room in profound shock. The patient was obtunded; his blood pressure was 90/40 mmHg, his temperature 40°C, and his extremities were cold and cyanotic. Splenomegaly was present. The patient's wife states that he has undergone a recent transurethral prostatectomy for benign prostatic hypertrophy and has had recurrent urinary tract infections with *Escherichia coli* since the surgery. You suspect that the patient has *E. coli* sepsis. You order blood cultures and a complete blood count.

9.025 Which of the following white cell counts and differentials are MOST consistent with your impressions?
  A. WBC 29 000: 75% polymorphs (PMNs), 10% band neutrophils, 10% metamyelocytes, 5% myelocytes
  B. WBC 110 000: 98% lymphocytes, 2% PMNs
  C. WBC 2900: 80% lymphocytes, 20% monocytes
  D. WBC 79 000: 90% blasts with Auer rods, 10% PMNs

A is correct.
In a reactive neutrophilia, the WBC count rarely exceeds 30 000 cells/µl. In addition to an increase in mature neutrophils, immature granulocytes are present with the exception of circulating blasts. A neoplastic disorder should be considered when the WBC is > 50 000 cells/µl.

9.026 As the patient has splenomegaly, you are concerned that he has a neoplasm involving the spleen (such as chronic myelogenous leukemia) *vs* septic splenitis. Which one of the following tests allows you to distinguish between a leukemoid reaction due to primary infection and a CML complicated by secondary infection?
  A. tartrate-resistant acid phosphatase stain (TRAP)
  B. leukocyte alkaline phosphatase stain (LAP)
  C. flow cytometry
  D. myeloperoxidase stain

B is correct.
LAP is an enzyme present in the secondary granules of granulocytes which is often increased in activated cells. The LAP score in a leukemoid reaction secondary to a primary infection is high. In contrast, the enzyme score is low in the abnormally maturing clonal granulocytes of CML. A concurrent infection may slightly raise the low LAP score in CML.

9.027 If the patient has primary sepsis and not CML, the granulocytic series in the peripheral blood is MOST likely to exhibit which of the following?
  A. hypersegmented nuclei
  B. hypogranularity
  C. toxic granulation
  D. Pelger–Huët anomaly

C is correct.
Toxic granulation represents a toxic change in the cytoplasm of reactive neutrophils. The etiology of the granulation is controversial, but most likely represents either retained primary granules or altered uptake of stain by secondary granules.

9.028 The following laboratory values are returned. WBC 98 000: 30% PMNs; 30% band neutrophils; 10% metamyelocytes; 5% myelocytes; 10% promyelocytes; 10% basophils; and 5% blasts. The LAP score is 0. Blood cultures are positive for *E. coli*. What is the MOST likely diagnosis now?

   A. acute non-lymphocytic leukemia, M2 type

   B. chronic myelogenous leukemia with *E. coli* sepsis

   C. primary *E. coli* sepsis with a leukemoid reaction

   D. myelodysplastic syndrome

B is correct.

The high WBC with a left-shifted granulocytosis, basophilia, and low LAP score is characteristic of CML. The positive blood culture confirms a concurrent *E. coli* infection.

9.029 The patient is treated with massive doses of antibiotics and is stabilized. However, the peripheral blood findings remain the same (high WBC count, increased granulocytes with a left-shifted differential, increased basophils and decreased LAP). You now are almost certain that the patient has CML. Which of the following tests is the BEST for confirming your diagnosis?

   A. cytogenetics

   B. flow cytometry

   C. myeloperoxidase stain

   D. DNA studies for immunoglobulin gene rearrangements

A is correct.

The Ph (Philadelphia) chromosome is observed in approximately 90–95% of patients with the typical clinical and hematologic findings of CML. The Ph chromosome results from a reciprocal translocation between chromosomes 9 and 22 [t(9;22)]. A hybrid 210 kD protein is formed with enhanced tyrosine kinase activity.

The following case history relates to questions 9.030–9.032. A 23-year-old white woman presents to the emergency room with uncontrollable epistaxis. Laboratory tests reveal a WBC of 45 000 cells/μl with abnormal cells containing irregular nuclei and numerous Auer rods. Her hemoglobin is 9.2 g/dl, hematocrit is 27 ml/dl, and platelets 5000/mm³. The patient is admitted to the hospital. Five days later, a cytogenetics report shows a t(15;17) chromosomal translocation.

9.030 What is the MOST likely diagnosis?

   A. acute myelogenous leukemia (AML), M2 type

   B. AML, M4 type

   C. AML, M3 type

   D. myelodysplastic syndrome

C is correct.

Acute promyelocytic leukemia (AML-M3) is a clinically distinct form of leukemia found in young adults. Patients may present with either leukopenia or leukocytosis and usually have laboratory evidence of disseminated intravascular coagulation. The majority of leukemic cells are abnormal promyelocytes that often exhibit marked nuclear irregularities. The cells are usually hypergranular with numerous Auer rods, but may have small difficult-to-visualize granules (microgranular variant). The identification of a t(15;17) cytogenetic translocation is diagnostic.

9.031   The patient is treated with chemotherapy, resulting in a dramatic decrease in the number of abnormal cells in the blood and bone marrow. During treatment, which of the following is the MOST serious life-threatening complication in this patient?

   A. fungal infection
   B. disseminated intravascular coagulation
   C. bacterial infection
   D. bone marrow aplasia

B is correct.

Disseminated intravascular coagulation (DIC) is a significant complication of AML-M3. Laboratory evidence of DIC is present in approximately 80% of patients. It is caused by degranulation of the leukemic cells with release of tissue factors and mediators. Chemotherapy-induced cell damage increases granule release and the risk of DIC.

9.032   Recent advances in the understanding of the molecular biology of this disease have led to new treatment strategies. Which of the following would be MOST useful (based on the molecular biology of this tumor) in the treatment of this patient's disease?

   A. interleukin-2
   B. retinoic acid
   C. granulocyte–macrophage colony-stimulating factor (GM-CSF)
   D. erythropoietin

B is correct.

Treatment with all-transretinoic acid (vitamin A) overcomes the block in differentiation and maturation of the abnormal promyelocytes. When differentiation of the promyelocytes into mature myeloid forms has occurred after retinoic acid administration, chemotherapy can be initiated with a significantly decreased risk of DIC (due to decreased promyelocyte granule release).

9.033   A 58-year-old man presents to the Family Practice Clinic with extreme fatigue. The patient is found to be pancytopenic. Examination of the peripheral blood reveals hypogranular neutrophils with the pseudo-Pelger–Hüet anomaly. Examination of the bone marrow reveals a hypercellular marrow with hyperplasia of the erythroid, myeloid and megakaryocytic elements. Cytologic abnormalities in all three cell lineages in the bone marrow and ringed sideroblasts are noted. Myeloblasts are 18%. Cytogenetics reveals a deletion of the long arm of chromosome 5 (5q-). The MOST likely diagnosis is:

   A. acute myelogenous leukemia, FAB-M2
   B. aplastic anemia
   C. myelodysplastic syndrome
   D. chronic myelogenous leukemia in blast crisis

C is correct.

Myelodysplastic syndromes are bone marrow stem cell disorders that lead to ineffective and disorderly hematopoiesis. Both quantitative and qualitative defects of hematopoiesis are present. Granulocyte hypogranulation and hyposegmentation (pseudo-Pelger–Hüet anomaly) is a common finding. The FAB classification system defines five subtypes of myelodysplasia based on the percentage of blasts in blood and bone marrow, Auer rods, ringed sideroblasts, and monocytosis. Approximately 80% of patients have chromosomal abnormalities; 5q-, monosomy 7 and trisomy 8 are common.

9.034   A 78-year-old woman presents to the hematology clinic with marked fatigue and a herpetic rash over the right side of her face. Physical examination reveals splenomegaly and adenopathy. The WBC count is 540 000 cells/µl with 89% mature lymphocytes and 11% prolymphocytes. Anemia and thrombocytopenia are noted. Flow cytometric analysis reveals that the peripheral blood lymphocytes are positive for surface immunoglobulin and CD5+. The MOST likely diagnosis is:
  A. hairy-cell leukemia
  B. prolymphocytic leukemia
  C. chronic lymphocytic leukemia
  D. reactive lymphocytosis to the herpes
     infection

The following case history relates to questions 9.035 and 9.036. A 19-year-old college student presents to the student health clinic with fatigue. Physical examination reveals slight splenomegaly, cervical adenopathy, hyperemia of the oropharynx and a fever of 39°C. The WBC count is 8000 cells/µl with 90% reactive lymphocytes. Flow cytometry reveals predominantly T-cell markers on the peripheral blood lymphocytes. The platelet count, hemoglobin and hematocrit are normal as is the examination of the bone marrow.

9.035   The MOST likely diagnosis is:
  A. acute lymphocytic leukemia
  B. chronic lymphocytic leukemia (T-cell type)
  C. infectious mononucleosis
  D. hairy-cell leukemia

9.036   The etiologic agent of this disease is:
  A. Epstein–Barr virus
  B. HIV
  C. papillomavirus
  D. Ebola virus (Zaire subtype)

C is correct.
Approximately 95% of chronic lymphocytic leukemia is of B-cell phenotype with expression of B-cell antigens, weak monotypic surface immunoglobulin light chain, and T-cell-associated antigen CD5. The FAB proposal for diagnosis includes a persistent lymphocytosis $>10 \times 10^9/1$ with $<10\%$ prolymphocytes. Clinical symptoms are secondary to bone marrow, splenic and lymph node involvement.

C is correct.
Infectious mononucleosis classically occurs in adolescents and young adults living in good socio-economic conditions in developed countries. Fatigue, sore throat, fever, and lymphadenitis are the most common clinical symptoms. The peripheral blood shows a lymphocytosis with distinctive large atypical lymphocytes bearing T-cell markers.

A is correct.
Epstein–Barr virus, a gamma-group herpesvirus, infects B lymphocytes, causing polyclonal activation and proliferation. A symptomatic infection presents as infectious mononucleosis. In many developing countries, primary EBV infection occurs during childhood and is asymptomatic.

The following case history relates to questions 9.037–9.039.   A 3-year-old girl presents to the hematology clinic because of fever and spontaneous bruising without trauma. Physical examination reveals a temperature of 39°C, mild splenomegaly, and a pale, acutely ill, child. The WBC count is 330 000 cells/μl with 98% small blasts and 2% lymphocytes. Flow cytometry reveals pre-B-cell markers and the cells are positive for CD10 (CALLA). The patient is significantly anemic and thrombocytopenic.

9.037 The MOST likely diagnosis is:
    A. reactive lymphocytosis due to viral infection
    B. acute lymphocytic leukemia
    C. chronic lymphocytic leukemia
    D. non-Hodgkin's lymphoma, Burkitt's type

B is correct.
A child with a large number of small blasts is most likely to have an acute lymphocytic leukemia of B-cell origin. Approximately 20% of B-cell ALL have a pre-B-cell phenotype characterized by the presence of cytoplasmic immunoglobulin and lack of surface immunoglobulin.

9.038 The MOST common cytogenetic abnormality likely to be seen in this child is:
    A. t(11;14)
    B. t(14;18)
    C. t(8;14)
    D. t(1;19)

D is correct.
The t(1;19) chromosomal translocation is present in 30% of cases of ALL of pre-B-cell phenotype and portends a worse prognosis within this subgroup.

9.039 Because of the high blast count, the physicians considered this child's condition to be a medical emergency. Why?
    A. the incidence of DIC is significantly increased
    B. leukostasis could result in widespread organ infarction
    C. congestive heart failure could result from increased blood viscosity
    D. the blasts produce cytokines that induce profound immunosuppression resulting in life-threatening infection

B is correct.
This child has a hyperleukocytosis syndrome and needs to be treated promptly to significantly lower the leukocyte count to < 100 000 cells/μl to avoid thrombotic complications.

9.040 A 60-year-old man is referred to a hematologist due to an elevated hemoglobin. Physical examination reveals marked rubor of the skin and splenomegaly. Adenopathy is not noted. The hemoglobin is 19 g/dl, hematocrit is 58 ml/dl, RBC count 7.5×10^6/ml and WBC count is 12 000 cells/μl with a normal differential. Platelets are elevated at 600 000/mm^3 with occasional large bizarre forms noted. The patient denies smoking and the pO_2 is normal. LAP is elevated as is the serum B_{12} level. The bone marrow is hypercellular with trilineage hyperplasia. The MOST likely diagnosis is:
   A. myelofibrosis myeloid metaplasia
   B. polycythemia vera
   C. reactive polycythemia
   D. essential thrombocythemia

The following case history relates to questions 9.041–9.043. An 8-year-old boy is referred to an oncologist because of a large abdominal mass. Physical examination reveals a 10-cm mass in the center of the abdomen. Hepatosplenomegaly is not prominent. Adenopathy is not noted. The child is febrile, and petechiae are noted over the trunk and extremities. The WBC count is 45 000 cells/μl, with 95% blasts having prominent basophilic vacuolated cytoplasm. Flow cytometry of the peripheral blood reveals mature B-cell markers on the peripheral blasts. A biopsy of the abdominal mass reveals a group of matted lymph nodes with complete, diffuse effacement of the architecture with intermediate-sized blast-like cells with prominent vacuoles. A 'starry-sky' pattern is noted and numerous mitotic figures are seen. Flow cytometry on the cells from the abdominal mass reveals markers identical to those found in the peripheral blood. Cytogenetics reveals the presence of a t(8;14) chromosomal translocation.

9.041 The MOST likely diagnosis is:
   A. follicular lymphoma (low-grade)
   B. lymphoblastic lymphoma (high-grade)
   C. Burkitt's lymphoma (high-grade)
   D. mantle-cell lymphoma
      (intermediate-grade)

B is correct.
Diagnostic criteria for polycythemia vera have been established by the Polycythemia Vera Study Group and are: 1) increased red cell mass; 2) normal arterial O_2 saturation (>92%); and 3) splenomegaly. Two of the following minor criteria can be substituted if splenomegaly is absent: 1) thrombocytosis; 2) leukocytosis; 3) increased LAP, serum B_{12}; or 4) elevated or unbound B_{12}-binding capacity.

C is correct.
Sporadic Burkitt's lymphoma (small non-cleaved cell lymphoma) is a B-cell lymphoma that occurs primarily in the first two decades of life, more commonly in boys than in girls. Over 90% of patients have abdominal disease. Large reactive histiocytes intermixed with the smaller malignant cells impart the 'starry-sky' pattern, which is associated with high-grade lymphomas in general, but is particularly prominent in Burkitt's lymphoma.

9.042 The t(8;14) translocation is associated with activation of which of the following genes?
  A. c-*abl*
  B. c-*myc*
  C. *bcl*-2
  D. *bcl*-1

9.043 Although the significance is unknown, this disease is often associated with which of the following viruses?
  A. Epstein–Barr virus
  B. papillomavirus
  C. varicella–zoster virus
  D. Rous sarcoma virus

9.044 A 67-year-old black man presents with pneumonia. Laboratory evaluation reveals an elevated serum and urinary protein. Serum protein electrophoresis reveals a monoclonal immunoglobulin 'spike' (IgA type) and skeletal X-ray reveals numerous osteolytic lesions. Bone marrow examination reveals 80% plasma cells with an immature nuclear chromatin pattern and prominent nucleoli. The MOST likely diagnosis is:
  A. follicular lymphoma involving the bone marrow
  B. Waldenstrom's macroglobulinemia
  C. multiple myeloma
  D. monoclonal gammopathy of unknown significance

9.045 A 44-year-old man presents with fatigue. Laboratory examination reveals a monoclonal IgM 'spike' on serum protein electrophoresis. Physical examination reveals generalized adenopathy and mild splenomegaly. Examination of the lymph nodes and bone marrow reveals replacement by cells with a lymphoplasmacytic morphology. Normal serum immunoglobulins are decreased, but osteolytic bone lesions are not noted. The MOST likely diagnosis is:
  A. multiple myeloma (IgM type)
  B. follicular lymphoma
  C. chronic lymphocytic leukemia
  D. Waldenstrom's macroglobulinemia

B is correct.
The c-*myc* gene at 8q24 is juxtaposed to the immunoglobulin heavy chain gene at 14q32, creating t(8;14). The translocation is thought to cause deregulation of c-*myc* gene function in normal cell proliferation and differentiation.

A is correct.
Evidence of EBV infection in association with Burkitt's lymphoma is present in approximately 20% of sporadic cases and 95% of endemic cases.

C is correct.
Diagnostic criteria for multiple myeloma are divided into major and minor criteria, depending on the degree of bone marrow plasmacytosis, level of monoclonal immunoglobulin, presence of lytic bone lesions, and presence of reduced normal immunoglobulins. The findings of >30% bone marrow plasma cells (major criteria) in conjunction with either the monoclonal immunoglobulin or lytic bone lesions fulfill the criteria for diagnosis in this case.

D is correct.
Waldenstrom's macroglobulinemia is an immunoproliferative disorder with morphologic and clinical features of mixed lymphoma and multiple myeloma. Lymphadenopathy, hepatosplenomegaly and bone marrow involvement without osteolysis simulate a lymphoma. The monoclonal gammopathy and decreased serum immunoglobulin are more characteristic of multiple myeloma.

9.046   Patients with IgM-producing tumors often experience retinal hemorrhages. The MOST likely cause of this is:
   A. hypertension
   B. hyperviscosity syndrome
   C. blood vessel wall degeneration due to deposition of IgM
   D. platelet dysfunction due to interaction with IgM

The following case history relates to questions 9.047 and 9.048. A 23-year-old man presents with chronic diarrhea and weight loss. Biopsy of the small intestine reveals significant villous atrophy with an infiltrate of IgA-producing plasma cells in the lamina propria of the villi. The patient is treated with a course of antibiotics and improves. However, the symptoms return and he becomes unresponsive to any therapeutic intervention. Testing for food allergies is negative.

9.047   The MOST likely diagnosis in this case is:
   A. occult lymphoma involving the small intestine
   B. multiple myeloma (IgA type)
   C. alpha heavy-chain disease
   D. monoclonal gammopathy of unknown significance (IgA type)

9.048   The natural history of this disease includes:
   A. evolution to multiple myeloma (IgA type)
   B. evolution to chronic lymphocytic leukemia (IgA type)
   C. evolution to high-grade immunoblastic lymphoma
   D. evolution to low-grade follicular center cell lymphoma

The following case history relates to questions 9.049 and 9.050. A 1-year-old boy presents with a 2-cm mass protruding from the skull. X-ray analysis reveals a solitary osteolytic lesion, and biopsy reveals Langerhans histiocytes, eosinophils, lymphocytes and plasma cells. Extensive physical examination fails to reveal disease in any other location.

B is correct.
Because of the large molecular size of IgM, an increased concentration in the blood tends to form large aggregates. This increases the viscosity of the blood, giving rise to a hyperviscosity syndrome. Clinical manifestations of such a syndrome include visual impairment, retinal hemorrhage, neurologic problems and bleeding due to immunoglobulin interference with clotting factors and platelet function.

C is correct.
Alpha heavy-chain disease, otherwise known as Mediterranean lymphoma, typically involves patients in the second or third decades of life. The marked lymphoplasmacytic infiltration of the small intestine leads to villous atrophy and severe malabsorption.

C is correct.
Antibiotic therapy may stop the lymphoplasmacytic proliferation in the early phases of alpha heavy-chain disease but, more frequently, the disease progresses to a high-grade lymphoma.

9.049 The MOST likely diagnosis is:
  A. solitary eosinophilic granuloma of bone
  B. Hand–Schüller–Christian disease
  C. Letterer–Siwe disease
  D. Hodgkin's disease

A is correct.
Three clinical variants of Langerhans cell histiocytosis (LCH) have been identified: eosinophilic granuloma; multifocal eosinophilic granulomas with diabetes insipidus and exophthalmos (Hand–Schüller–Christian disease); and progressive disseminated LCH (Letterer–Siwe disease). The three variants differ in their clinical severity, but share the same histologic features. The most common of the three is eosinophilic granuloma, which usually presents as expanding accumulations of Langerhans cells in medullary cavities of bones, often in association with a lytic bone lesion, pain and swelling.

9.050 The natural history of this lesion is:
  A. progression to systemic disease and death
  B. progression to high-grade histiocytic
     lymphoma
  C. spontaneous remission
  D. progression to osteogenic sarcoma

C is correct.
Unifocal eosinophilic granuloma is an indolent disorder that may heal spontaneously or be cured by local excision or irradiation.

9.051 Acute myelogenous leukemia is LEAST often associated with which of the following?
  A. leukocytosis
  B. >30% blasts or leukemic cells in the bone
     marrow
  C. thrombocytosis
  D. Auer rods

C is correct.
Anemia, thrombocytopenia, and neutropenia occur in the majority of patients with AML due to bone marrow replacement by leukemic cells. In contrast to leukocytosis and Auer rods, only rare cases of thrombocytosis have been described. Thrombosis is associated with the inv(3) chromosomal abnormality.

9.052 All of the following are characteristic of multiple myeloma EXCEPT:*
  A. increased levels of normal immunoglobulins
  B. bone marrow plasmacytosis
  C. renal failure
  D. osteolytic bone lesions

A is correct.
Normal non-neoplastic immunoglobulin is usually depressed in multiple myeloma, resulting in an increased susceptibility to bacterial infections.

9.053 A leukemoid reaction is MOST likely to be seen with:
  A. *E. coli* sepsis
  B. Epstein–Barr virus infection
  C. hepatitis B infection
  D. *Candida* infection

A is correct.
A neutrophilic leukocytosis is a feature of inflammatory reactions, especially those induced by bacterial infections. Bacterial products (endotoxins) stimulate macrophages to produce cytokines that induce acute-phase reactions and increase circulating neutrophils. Extreme increases in the leukocyte count are referred to as leukemoid reactions.

9.054 Which of the following is common to all of the myeloproliferative disorders?
   A. lymphocytosis
   B. splenomegaly
   C. increased erythrocyte mass
   D. decreased leukocyte alkaline phosphatase activity

B is correct.
Splenomegaly is most common in myelofibrosis with myeloid metaplasia (>80%) and least common in essential thrombocythemia (40–50%). Splenomegaly is caused by extramedullary hematopoiesis or, less frequently, tumor infiltration (CML).

9.055 All of the following cells are seen in Hodgkin's disease. Which one of the following is considered to be the malignant cell?
   A. T lymphocyte
   B. plasma cell
   C. eosinophil
   D. Reed–Sternberg cell

D is correct.
The Reed–Sternberg cell is now widely accepted as the neoplastic, or transformed, cell in Hodgkin's disease. These large cells are binucleate or multinucleate, or have lobulated nuclei. Distinctive large acidophilic nucleoli, at least one-fourth the size of the nucleus, are classically present. Cells with variant morphology are characteristic of specific morphologic subtypes, such as lacunar cells in nodular sclerosing Hodgkin's disease or L and H cells in Hodgkin's disease with lymphocyte predominance. T lymphocytes, plasma cells, and eosinophils may also be seen in tissue involved by the disease; however, they are reactive in nature.

9.056 An 18-year-old male college freshman presents to the student health clinic with a 1-week history of flu-like symptoms. Physical examination reveals that the patient is febrile with pronounced cervical adenopathy and a hyperemic oropharynx. Hepatosplenomegaly is not noted. Laboratory examination reveals: hemoglobin 15.2 (normal range: 13.5–18) g/dl; hematocrit 45 (normal range: 40–50) ml/dl; WBC count 4500 (normal range: 4000–11 000) cells/μl; platelets 254 000 (normal range: 150 000–350 000)/mm^3. The WBC differential shows 89% 'atypical reactive-looking lymphocytes' and 11% PMNs. An overanxious medical resident orders a bone marrow test, which is interpreted as normal. What is the MOST likely diagnosis?
   A. acute lymphoblastic leukemia
   B. viral infection
   C. bacterial sepsis
   D. allergic reaction

B is correct.
Lymphocytosis is present when the absolute lymphocyte count is >4000 in adults. Medium and large lymphocytes are referred to as 'activated' forms. Activated lymphocytes have been given various descriptive names such as variant lymphocytes, atypical lymphocytes, and plasmacytoid lymphocytes. The most common cause of a lymphocytosis is a viral infection. If the lymphocytosis is marked, infectious mononucleosis must be considered. The peripheral blood in acute lymphoblastic leukemia contains neoplastic blasts of lymphocytic origin. The peripheral blood in bacterial sepsis and in allergic reaction reveals granulocytosis and eosinophilia, respectively.

9.057 You are called to the emergency room to see a 50-year-old man in acute discomfort due to apparent fever and infection. You find that the peripheral smear reveals a WBC of 95 000 (normal range: 4000–11000) cells/µl, consisting mostly of mature neutrophils, band neutrophils, metamyelocytes, myelocytes, promyelocytes, and rare blasts. Eosinophils and basophils are not increased. The resident thinks that this patient has chronic myelogenous leukemia. However, you think that the patient may have a leukemoid reaction due to infection. You quickly order the test that will prove the resident wrong. Which test do you order?

   A. tartrate-resistant acid phosphatase (TRAP) stain of peripheral blood smear

   B. leukocyte alkaline phosphatase (LAP) stain of the peripheral blood smear

   C. flow cytometry on the peripheral blood which reveals increased myeloid cell markers

   D. examination of the peripheral blood smear for Auer rods

The following case history relates to questions 9.058 and 9.059. A 32-year-old white woman presents to the emergency room with uncontrollable menstrual bleeding. Laboratory tests reveal: WBC: 45 000 (normal range: 4000–11 000) cells/µl with 90% hypergranular promyelocytes containing numerous Auer rods; hemoglobin 7.2 (normal range: 12–16) g/dl, hematocrit 21 (normal range: 38–47) ml/dl; and platelets 7000 (normal range: 150 000–350 000)/mm^3. The patient is admitted to the hospital. Five days later, a cytogenetics report shows a t(15;17) chromosomal translocation.

9.058 What is the MOST likely diagnosis?

   A. acute monocytic leukemia

   B. acute myelomonocytic leukemia

   C. acute promyelocytic leukemia

   D. acute megakaryocytic leukemia

B is correct.

LAP activity is normal or elevated in the leukemoid reaction whereas it is decreased in chronic myelogenous leukemia (CML). Therefore, the LAP stain is helpful in distinguishing these two entities.

C is correct.

Acute promyelocytic leukemia (AML-M3) is characterized by a proliferation of abnormal promyelocytes, with increased numbers of these cells in the peripheral blood and bone marrow. The neoplastic promyelocytes may have multiple Auer rods in their cytoplasm. A t(15;17) translocation is found in the majority of cases of AML-M3. This disease is associated with disseminated intravascular coagulation, and most patients present with anemia and thrombocytopenia.

9.059 The t(15:17) translocation is associated with which of the following?
   A. BCR–Abl fusion protein activation
   B. E2A–PBX fusion protein activation
   C. c-*myc* activation
   D. PML–RAR-alpha fusion protein activation

D is correct.

The t(15;17) translocation results in the fusion of a shortened version of the retinoic acid receptor-alpha (RAR-alpha) gene on chromosome 17 to a transcription unit called PML (for promyelocytic leukemia) on chromosome 15. The PML–RAR-alpha rearrangement produces a hybrid mRNA that can be detected in virtually all cases of M3 leukemia. The fused gene encodes for an abnormal RAR that in some manner blocks cell differentiation.

9.060 A 67-year-old man is evaluated in the hematology clinic for pancytopenia. Physical examination reveals a pale-looking patient with oral candidiasis and marked splenomegaly. Laboratory examination reveals a WBC count of 2100 (normal range: 4000–11 000) cells/μl; hemoglobin 7.8 (normal range: 13.5–18),g/dl; hematocrit 24 (normal range: 40–50) ml/dl; and platelets 34 000 (normal range: 150 000–350 000)/mm^3. Abnormal cells with cytoplasmic projections are noted on the peripheral smear. Evaluation of the abnormal cells reveals that the cells are CD5-negative, CD25-positive and tartrate-resistant acid phosphatase (TRAP)-positive. What is the MOST likely diagnosis:
   A. chronic lymphocytic leukemia
   B. prolymphocytic leukemia
   C. non-Hodgkin's lymphoma
   D. hairy-cell leukemia

D is correct.

Hairy-cell leukemia occurs mainly in older men. Splenomegaly is the most common, and sometimes the only, abnormal physical finding. The leukemic cells are one to two times the size of a normal lymphocyte with fine hair-like cytoplasmic projections. These cells contain tartrate-resistant acid phosphatase (TRAP) and express CD25. (In contrast to the leukemic cells in CLL, the cells in hairy-cell leukemia lack CD5.)

The following case history relates to questions 9.061–9.064. A 17-year-old high school senior presents to his local physician for a routine physical prior to the start of the football season. During the physical examination, a non-tender single cervical lymph node, measuring approximately 2 cm in diameter, is noted. Upon questioning, the patient complains of a 10-lb weight loss over the past summer and occasional night sweats. He also complains of generalized pruritus with no evidence of any rash or skin irritation. The remainder of the physical examination is unremarkable with the exception of a palpable spleen 5 cm below the left costal margin. A biopsy of a lymph node revealed effacement of the node, with nodules composed of mature lymphocytes, plasma cells, eosinophils, and Reed–Sternberg cells (lacunar type). The nodules are separated by large bands of collagen.

9.061 What is the MOST likely diagnosis?
  A. non-Hodgkin's lymphoma, small lymphocytic type
  B. Hodgkin's disease, lymphocyte-predominance type
  C. non-Hodgkin's lymphoma, follicular, predominantly large-cell, type
  D. Hodgkin's disease, nodular sclerosing type

D is correct.

The nodular sclerosing type of Hodgkin's disease (NSHD) is characterized histologically by the presence of neoplastic Reed–Sternberg variant cells, namely, lacunar cells, in a background of inflammatory cells, and broad bands of collagen dividing the tissue into circumscribed nodules. NSHD is the most common form of Hodgkin's disease and often occurs in adolescents or young adults. It has a marked propensity to involve the lower cervical, supraclavicular, and mediastinal lymph nodes.

9.062 Subsequent evaluation revealed that the patient's spleen and bone marrow were involved by this process. What is the stage of this patient's disease?
  A. I
  B. IIB
  C. IV
  D. IVB

D is correct.

According to the Ann Arbor Staging Classification for Hodgkin's Disease, involvement of one or more extralymphatic organs and the presence of systemic symptoms indicates stage IVB. This patient has bone marrow involvement (stage IV) with weight loss and night sweats (B).

9.063 The malignant cell in Hodgkin's disease is the:
  A. plasma cell
  B. lymphocyte
  C. Reed–Sternberg cell
  D. eosinophil

C is correct.

The Reed–Sternberg cell is now widely accepted as the neoplastic, or transformed, cell in Hodgkin's disease. The origin of this cell remains controversial. T lymphocytes, plasma cells, and eosinophils may also be seen in tissue involved by the disease; however, they are reactive in nature.

9.064 All of the following are 'B' symptoms EXCEPT:
  A. weight loss
  B. fever
  C. night sweats
  D. pruritus

D is correct.

According to the Ann Arbor Staging Classification for Hodgkin's Disease, systemic (or B) symptoms include fever, night sweats, and weight loss of >10% of normal body weight. The absence (A) or presence (B) of systemic symptoms is added to the numeric (I–IV) staging.

9.065 All of the following are consistent with *E. coli* sepsis EXCEPT:
  A. leukemoid reaction in the peripheral blood
  B. elevated leukocyte alkaline phosphatase level (LAP)
  C. toxic granulation in peripheral blood neutrophils
  D. elevated lymphocytes in the peripheral blood

D is correct.

Bacterial infection is one of the most common causes of neutrophilia. The magnitude of the neutrophil response varies and, if marked, is considered a leukemoid reaction. Activated neutrophils have increased 'toxic' granulation and elevated LAP enzyme levels. Lymphocytosis is common in chronic inflammatory states and in viral infections.

9.066   All of the following are consistent with a diagnosis of acute myelogenous leukemia EXCEPT:
- A. elevated WBC count
- B. <30% blasts in the bone marrow
- C. Auer rods in the blasts
- D. neutropenia, anemia, and thrombocytopenia

B is correct.
Acute myelogenous leukemia is characterized by the presence of $\geq 30\%$ blasts in the bone marrow or blood. The latter results in an elevated WBC count. The blasts in acute myelogenous leukemia may contain Auer rods in their cytoplasm. These neoplastic cells often crowd out the normal hematopoietic elements in the bone marrow, resulting in neutropenia, anemia, and thrombocytopenia.

9.067   All of the following are characteristic of hairy-cell leukemia EXCEPT:
- A. positive tartrate-resistant acid phosphatase (TRAP) test
- B. positive for the CD5 marker by flow cytometry
- C. splenomegaly
- D. pancytopenia

B is correct.
Hairy-cell leukemia occurs mainly in older men. Splenomegaly is the most common, and sometimes the only, abnormal physical finding. The leukemic cells have fine hair-like cytoplasmic projections. These cells contain TRAP and express CD25. (In contrast to the leukemic cells in CLL, the cells in hairy-cell leukemia lack CD5.) Pancytopenia resulting from bone marrow failure and splenic sequestration is seen in over half of all cases.

9.068   All of the following are characteristic of multiple myeloma EXCEPT:
- A. bone marrow plasmacytosis
- B. osteolytic bone lesions
- C. adenopathy
- D. monoclonal serum immunoglobulin (IgG or IgA)

C is correct.
Multiple myeloma is a monoclonal proliferation of plasma cells characterized by bone marrow plasmacytosis, associated osteolytic bone lesions, and monoclonal serum immunoglobulin. Although it may spread to many extraosseous sites, infiltration of the lymphoid tissues is uncommon.

9.069   In the myeloproliferative disorders, splenomegaly is caused by:
- A. infiltration by leukemic cells
- B. extramedullary hematopoiesis
- C. fibrosis in the spleen
- D. infarction of the spleen

B is correct.
The myeloproliferative disorders are a group of disorders with similar clinical and hematologic manifestations at some stage in the disease process. All have splenomegaly, ranging from mild in essential thrombocythemia to marked in myeloproliferative myeloid metaplasia. Extramedullary hematopoiesis in the spleen is part of the myeloproliferative process.

9.070 Myelodysplastic syndromes are characterized by all of the following EXCEPT:
  A. cellular dysplasia
  B. bone marrow hypercellularity
  C. bone marrow fibrosis
  D. peripheral blood cytopenias
  E. ringed sideroblasts

C is correct.
The myelodysplastic syndromes are bone marrow disorders characterized by dysplastic changes in cells of the myeloid, erythroid, and megakaryocytic lineages, with or without a concurrent increase in myeloblasts. Generally, in these disorders, bone marrow is hypercellular and there is peripheral blood cytopenia. Ringed sideroblasts are seen in a specific subtype of myelodysplastic syndrome (refractory anemia with ringed sideroblasts). Bone marrow fibrosis is seen in myeloproliferative disorders, but is unusual in the myelodysplastic syndromes. Fibrosis is secondary to fibroblast growth factors released from abnormal megakaryocytes.

9.071 Manifestations of the hyperviscosity syndrome seen in association with Waldenstrom's macroglobulinemia include all of the following EXCEPT:
  A. hypercalcemia
  B. visual impairment
  C. coagulation disorders
  D. altered mental status
  E. rouleaux formation

A is correct.
Hyperviscosity syndrome in Waldenstrom's macroglobulinemia is due to the large molecular size and increased concentration of macroglobulins in the blood, causing the IgM macroglobulin to form large aggregates that greatly increase the viscosity of the blood. This may lead to visual impairment, coagulation disorders, altered mental status, and rouleaux formation (the erythrocytes stick together like stacks of coins). Hypercalcemia is the result of bony destruction and erosion of bone. This is commonly seen in multiple myeloma, but not in Waldenstrom's macroglobulinemia.

9.072 The lymphoid neoplasms encountered most frequently in children and young adults include all of the following EXCEPT:
  A. acute lymphoblastic leukemia, B-cell type
  B. small non-cleaved cell lymphoma
  C. acute lymphoblastic leukemia, early pre-B-cell type
  D. small lymphocytic lymphoma
  E. acute lymphoblastic leukemia, T-cell type

D is correct.
Acute lymphoblastic leukemia (ALL) is primarily a disease of children and young adults. ALL originates from either B or T lymphocytes, and is subtyped accordingly. Similarly, small non-cleaved cell lymphomas (including Burkitt's lymphoma) are found predominantly in children and young adults. Small lymphocytic lymphoma (and the related chronic lymphocytic leukemia) are seen mostly in elderly patients.

9.073 Parafollicular hyperplasia in a lymph node is MOST likely caused by which of the following?
  A. adjacent cancer
  B. bacterial infection
  C. collagen–vascular disease
  D. Hodgkin's disease
  E. viral infection

E is correct.
The parafollicular or paracortical area of a lymph node is populated predominantly by small lymphocytes. Viral infections cause expansion of this area secondary to proliferation of small and large lymphocytes and immunoblasts.

9.074 Which of the following two cells are derived from the same progenitor cell in myelopoiesis?
    A. megakaryocyte, monocyte
    B. eosinophil, neutrophil
    C. megakaryocyte, erythrocyte
    D. monocyte, neutrophil
    E. basophil, erythrocyte

D is correct.
Granulocytic and monocytic differentiation proceed from the same progenitor cell, CFU-GM.

9.075 A patient presents to the emergency room with asthma. What cell is MOST likely to be increased in the peripheral blood smear?
    A. basophil
    B. eosinophil
    C. lymphocyte
    D. monocyte
    E. neutrophil

B is correct.
Eosinophilic leukocytosis is characteristic of allergic disorders, such as bronchial asthma, hay fever, and parasitic infections. In hospitalized patients, the most likely cause of eosinophilia is an allergic drug reaction.

9.076 Which of the following disorders is NOT associated with a peripheral blood neutrophilic leukocytosis?
    A. chronic myelogenous leukemia
    B. leukemoid reaction
    C. essential thrombocythemia
    D. polycythemia vera
    E. refractory anemia

E is correct.
Refractory anemia, one of the myelodysplastic syndromes, is usually associated with peripheral blood cytopenias, including neutropenia. In contrast, neutrophilic leukocytosis (neutrophilia) is commonly seen in the myeloproliferative disorders, including chronic myelogenous leukemia, essential thrombocythemia, and polycythemia vera, and is characteristic of the leukemoid reaction.

9.077 Which of the following findings is MOST definitive for rendering a diagnosis of acute myelogenous leukemia?
    A. Auer rods in blasts
    B. >3% myeloblasts in the peripheral blood
    C. >30% myeloblasts in bone marrow
    D. neutropenia, thrombocytopenia, and anemia
    E. abnormal cytogenetic karyotype

C is correct.
The FAB Cooperative Group published a universally accepted classification of AML in 1976. The classification was made in an attempt to improve standardization and accuracy of AML diagnoses. The classification requires >30% bone marrow blasts for a diagnosis of AML.

9.078 A bone marrow aspirate smear shows an increase in immature cells. The patient is reported to have subcutaneous skin nodules and a high urine lysozyme level. The MOST likely diagnosis is:
    A. acute myeloblastic leukemia without maturation (FAB-M1)
    B. acute myeloblastic leukemia with maturation (FAB-M2)
    C. acute promyelocytic leukemia (FAB-M3)
    D. acute monocytic leukemia (FAB-M5)
    E. acute megakaryocytic leukemia (FAB-M7)

D is correct.
The leukocyte count in acute monocytic leukemia is typically elevated and, therefore, patients have a high incidence of tissue infiltration by leukemic blasts. Extramedullary tumor is relatively common in acute monocytic leukemia (FAB-M5). Sites of involvement include the orbit, skin, paraspinal tissue, and testes. The serum lysozyme level is increased in approximately half the patients with this disease.

9.079 Which of the following laboratory findings is MOST often seen in polycythemia vera?
  A. increased platelets
  B. decreased red blood cells
  C. increased reticulocytes
  D. decreased leukocyte alkaline phosphatase
  E. decreased serum vitamin B_{12}

A is correct.
Polycythemia vera, one of the myeloproliferative disorders, often produces increased platelets (thrombocytosis) together with erythrocytosis and neutrophilia. One of the minor criteria for making a diagnosis of polycythemia vera is thrombocytosis with a platelet count $>400\,000\,mm^3$.

9.080 Which of the following statements about myelofibrosis with myeloid metaplasia is TRUE?
  A. it is a neoplastic disorder of the CFU-GEMM stem cell
  B. the fibrotic stage is characterized by bone marrow hypercellularity
  C. extensive extramedullary hematopoiesis is present
  D. cytogenetic abnormalities include trisomy 8, trisomy 9, and trisomy 10
  E. the leukocyte alkaline phosphatase (LAP) is decreased

C is correct.
Myelofibrosis with myeloid metaplasia (agnogenic myeloid metaplasia) is a clonal disorder arising from an abnormal multipotent hematopoietic stem cell. No specific cytogenetic abnormalities have been described. Abnormal bone marrow megakaryocytes release growth factors which stimulate fibroblasts, causing bone marrow fibrosis and secondarily decreased cellularity in the spleen, liver, and lymph nodes. Extramedullary hematopoiesis occurs.

9.081 Features characteristic of adult T-cell leukemia/lymphoma include:
  A. hypercalcemia, CD3 positivity, skin lesions
  B. human T-cell lymphotrophic virus (HTLV)-1 positivity, cerebriform nuclei, mediastinal mass
  C. CD4 and CD8 positivity, TdT positivity, hypercalcemia
  D. TdT positivity, HTLV-1 positivity, circulating abnormal cells
  E. hypercalcemia, Pautrier's microabscesses, CD3 positivity

A is correct.
Adult T-cell leukemia/lymphoma is an aggressive disease caused by infection with HTLV-1. It is clinically characterized by skin lesions, generalized lymphadenopathy, hepatosplenomegaly, and hypercalcemia. The leukemic cells have marked lobulation of the nucleus, leading to the description of 'flower-like' cells. The cells are CD3+ and usually CD4+. TdT is negative. Pautrier's microabscesses are seen in the skin of patients with mycosis fungoides, but not in adult T-cell leukemia/lymphoma.

9.082 You determine the differential diagnosis in an elderly woman with splenomegaly and circulating abnormal lymphoid cells to be chronic lymphocytic leukemia *vs* hairy-cell leukemia. To resolve this differential, you order:
  A. genotypic analysis to detect a clonal IgH gene rearrangement
  B. cytogenetic studies
  C. cytochemistry for TRAP
  D. phenotypic analysis for CD10 and HLA-DR
  E. phenotypic analysis for CD19 and CD20

C is correct.
Hairy-cell leukemia is a chronic lymphoproliferative disorder in which the neoplastic cells characteristically stain positively for tartrate-resistant acid phosphatase (TRAP). Acid phosphatase reactivity is present in neutrophils, monocytes, platelets, and lymphocytes, and in chronic lymphocytic leukemia in addition to hairy cells. However, only hairy cells show reactivity after tartrate treatment (TRAP positive). The phenotypic marker CD5 best differentiates between CLL (positive) and hairy-cell leukemia (negative).

9.083   What peripheral blood finding is MOST commonly associated with drug-induced bone marrow suppression?
  A. hypochromic microcytic anemia
  B. lymphopenia
  C. monocytopenia
  D. neutropenia

D is correct.
Numerous drug treatments have been associated with the development of neutropenia. Although the precise mechanism of neutropenia varies, it is most commonly due to a granulocyte production defect in the bone marrow.

9.084   The FAB classification for acute myelogenous leukemia is based on cellular morphology in conjunction with:
  A. cytochemical evidence of cellular differentiation
  B. flow cytometric evidence of cellular differentiation
  C. cytogenetic evidence of abnormal chromosomes
  D. molecular evidence of abnormal chromosomes

A is correct.
An important determinant in the FAB classification of AML is the cytochemical reactivity pattern of the blasts. The most useful cytochemical stains are myeloperoxidase and Sudan black B for evidence of myeloid differentiation, and non-specific esterase for evidence of monocytic differentiation.

9.085   Monoclonal gammopathy of undetermined significance:
  A. is usually of the IgM type
  B. rarely predates multiple myeloma
  C. usually exhibits only mild hypercalcemia
  D. is seen in 10% of elderly adults

D is correct.
Monoclonal gammopathy of undetermined significance (MGUS) is the term used to describe the presence of a monoclonal immunoglobulin in the serum or urine of a patient who shows no evidence of a hematopoietic malignancy. The immunoglobulin is usually IgG, but may be IgA or IgM. The marrow plasmacytosis is $<10\%$ and no lytic bone lesions are present.

9.086   A 26-year-old woman presents for evaluation of malaise, recurring drenching night sweats, and an unplanned 15-lb weight loss, and is found to have a right supraclavicular lymphadenopathy; lymph node biopsy reveals Hodgkin's disease. There is no additional palpable peripheral lymphadenopathy. Following an unrevealing bone marrow biopsy, a staging laparotomy is performed; biopsies of the liver, bilateral iliac and lower aortic lymph nodes, and spleen are negative. Sections of one upper abdominal periaortic lymph node reveal involvement by Hodgkin's disease. This patient's disease is therefore:
  A. stage IB
  B. stage IIB
  C. stage IIIB
  D. stage IVB

C is correct.
The Ann Arbor staging classification of Hodgkin's disease includes four stages. Stage III is involvement of lymph node regions on both sides of the diaphragm or localized involvement of an extra-lymphatic organ or site and/or spleen. The numeric stage is combined with either A, indicating absence of clinical symptoms, or B, indicating presence of fever, sweats and/or weight loss. This patient had lymph node involvement on both sides of the diaphragm and was symptomatic.

9.087 Tumor cells were obtained from a patient by bone marrow aspiration and were submitted for special laboratory evaluation. Cytogenetic studies revealed karyotype 46, XY, t(14;18). Immunophenotypic analysis by flow cytometry revealed a predominating cell which was positive for CD10, CD19, CD20, and kappa light chain. Molecular studies revealed clonal rearrangement of the IgM heavy chain and kappa light chain genes. What is the diagnosis?

A. acute lymphoblastic leukemia, pre-B-cell type

B. malignant lymphoma, small lymphocytic type

C. lymphoblastic lymphoma

D. malignant lymphoma, follicular center cell type

E. hairy-cell leukemia

D is correct.

Follicular lymphomas are monoclonal B-cell lymphomas. The presence of CD10 positivity excludes hairy-cell leukemia and small lymphocytic lymphoma. Kappa light chain expression (surface immunoglobulin) excludes a pre-B-cell acute lymphoblastic leukemia or lymphoblastic lymphoma of B-cell phenotype. Only follicular lymphoma is associated with the chromosomal translocation t(14;18). The tumor cells in almost all patients with follicular center cell lymphoma reveal a characteristic t(14;18) translocation. The breakpoint on chromosome 18 involves 18q21, where the antiapoptosis gene *bcl*-2 has been mapped. This translocation causes overexpression of *bcl*-2. The neoplastic cells express pan-B-cell markers, such as CD19 and CD20. In addition, the more restricted B-cell marker CD10 is expressed in many cases of follicular center cell lymphoma.

9.088 Peripheral blood was submitted for immunophenotypic studies in the work-up of a patient with an abnormal WBC count and differential. Due to technical difficulties, only the following results were obtained: CD5 positivity, TdT negativity. What is the diagnosis?

A. acute lymphoblastic leukemia, pre-B-cell type

B. malignant lymphoma, small lymphocytic type

C. lymphoblastic lymphoma

D. malignant lymphoma, follicular center cell type

E. hairy-cell leukemia

B is correct.

Virtually all lymphoblastic lymphomas and pre-B-cell acute lymphoblastic leukemias express the enzyme terminal deoxynucleotidyl transferase (TdT). Follicular center cell lymphoma and hairy-cell leukemia are monoclonal B-cell neoplasms that, unlike small lymphocytic lymphoma, do not aberrantly coexpress the T-cell-associated antigen CD5.

9.089 A 32-year-old woman presented to the emergency room following the development of swelling of her face and neck accompanied by respiratory difficulty. Mediastinal widening was appreciable on chest X-ray, accompanied by evidence of a right pleural and pericardial effusion. What is the diagnosis?

A. acute lymphoblastic leukemia, pre-B-cell type

B. malignant lymphoma, small lymphocytic type

C. lymphoblastic lymphoma

D. malignant lymphoma, follicular center cell type

E. hairy-cell leukemia

C is correct.

Approximately 65% of patients with lymphoblastic lymphoma present with an anterior mediastinal mass and associated symptoms, including superior vena cava syndrome, large airway obstruction, and pericardial or pleural effusions.

9.090 A 12-year-old boy in remission following chemotherapy for his neoplasm returns to the clinic with a 2-day history of headache, which has worsened and is accompanied by nausea and vomiting. Papilledema is detected on ophthalmic examination. CSF is obtained by spinal tap and is found to contain numerous atypical cells. Immunophenotypic studies of these cells reveal positivity for CD3, CD4 and CD8. What is the diagnosis?
    A. acute lymphocytic leukemia, pre-B-cell type
    B. malignant lymphoma, small lymphocytic type
    C. lymphoblastic lymphoma
    D. malignant lymphoma, follicular center cell type
    E. hairy-cell leukemia

C is correct.
Lymphoblastic lymphoma is closely related to T-cell acute lymphoblastic leukemia. It has a male predominance (2 : 1), and most patients are < 20 years of age. Lymphoblastic lymphoma accounts for approximately 40% of cases of childhood lymphoma. The disease is rapidly progressive, and early dissemination to the bone marrow, blood, and meninges leads to a picture resembling T-ALL. The phenotype of the neoplastic cells resembles intrathymic T cells; in some patients, the cells are CD1-, CD2-, CD5-, and CD7-positive whereas, in others, they coexpress CD4 and CD8.

9.091 A 63-year-old man presents for evaluation of decreased stamina, a sense of abdominal fullness, and early satiety. Physical examination reveals a left upper quadrant mass. Pallor is present. A CBC reveals pancytopenia. What is the diagnosis?
    A. acute lymphoblastic leukemia, pre-B-cell type
    B. malignant lymphoma, small lymphocytic type
    C. lymphoblastic lymphoma
    D. malignant lymphoma, follicular center cell type
    E. hairy-cell leukemia

E is correct.
Pancytopenia and splenomegaly are the predominant clinical findings of hairy-cell leukemia. The left upper quadrant mass is most likely an enlarged spleen. Abdominal symptoms are frequently reported due to the splenomegaly.

9.092 A relative paucity of Reed–Sternberg cells is seen in which of the following types of Hodgkin's disease?
    A. nodular sclerosis type
    B. lymphocyte-predominance type
    C. mixed cellularity type
    D. lymphocyte-depletion type

B is correct.
The lymphocyte-predominance type of Hodgkin's disease is characterized by complete or partial effacement of the lymph node by small lymphocytes and varying numbers of histiocytes. The pattern is usually vaguely nodular. Classical Reed–Sternberg cells are extremely difficult to find; however, Reed–Sternberg variants called 'L and H cells' ('popcorn cells') are often plentiful. (Note: It may also be difficult to find classical Reed–Sternberg cells in the nodular sclerosis type.)

9.093 Lacunar variants are an important cytologic feature in which of the following types of Hodgkin's disease?
    A. nodular sclerosis type
    B. lymphocyte-predominance type
    C. mixed cellularity type
    D. lymphocyte-depletion type

A is correct.
Nodular sclerosis Hodgkin's disease is characterized histologically by bands of collagen fibrosis and the presence of a particular variant of the Reed–Sternberg cell, the lacunar cell. In formalin-fixed tissue, the cytoplasm of these cells often retracts, giving rise to the appearance of cells lying in clear spaces or 'lacunae'.

9.094 Patients are more likely to present with stage IV disease in which of the following types of Hodgkin's disease?
A. nodular sclerosis type
B. lymphocyte-predominance type
C. mixed cellularity type
D. lymphocyte-depletion type

D is correct.
The lymphocyte-depletion type of Hodgkin's disease is rare in the United States. A majority of patients with the lymphocyte-depletion pattern of Hodgkin's disease are older men, have disseminated involvement, and present with systemic manifestations. Approximately 50–75% of patients have bone marrow involvement at diagnosis in contrast to <25% in other types of Hodgkin's disease.

9.095 The lowest incidence of systemic 'B' symptoms is seen in which of the following types of Hodgkin's disease?
A. nodular sclerosis type
B. lymphocyte-predominance type
C. mixed cellularity type
D. lymphocyte-depletion type

B is correct.
Lymphocyte-predominance Hodgkin's disease is an uncommon variant, accounting for approximately 5% of Hodgkin's disease. The majority of these patients are male, usually <35 years of age, and present with limited disease, such as low-stage without 'B' symptoms. The prognosis is excellent.

9.096 There is a strong association with mediastinal involvement in which of the following types of Hodgkin's disease?
A. nodular sclerosis type
B. lymphocyte-predominance type
C. mixed cellularity type
D. lymphocyte-depletion type

A is correct.
Nodular sclerosis Hodgkin's disease is the most common form of Hodgkin's disease. It has several distinctive features, including a predominance in women and a propensity to involve the lower cervical, supraclavicular, and mediastinal lymph nodes. It is also the type most commonly affecting the lungs. Most patients with this disease are adolescents or young adults; the prognosis is excellent.

9.097 A patient with which of the following neoplastic disorders is MOST likely to develop acute leukemia?
A. myelofibrosis with myeloid metaplasia
B. chronic myelogenous leukemia
C. essential thrombocythemia
D. polycythemia vera
E. refractory anemia

B is correct.
More than 90% of patients with CML progress to blast crisis (acute leukemia). The development of a blast crisis usually occurs between 2 and 6 years from the time of diagnosis. Blast crisis is usually myeloid (60%), but lymphoid or mixed lineage blasts may also occur. That different types of acute leukemias arise from CML is not surprising as it is a clonal disorder originating from the multipotential hematopoietic stem cell.

9.098 What is the mechanism of action for retinoic acid in the treatment of acute promyelocytic leukemia (FAB-M3)?
A. inhibits DNA synthesis
B. enhances gene-targeting sites
C. induces differentiation
D. reverses the t(15;17) chromosomal
    translocation

C is correct.
The t(15;17) translocation characteristic of acute promyelocytic leukemia results in the fusion of a portion of the retinoic acid receptor gene on chromosome 17 to a transcription unit called PML on chromosome 15. This hybrid gene encodes an abnormal retinoic acid receptor that blocks cell differentiation. High doses of all-transretinoic acid are able to overcome this block in differentiation both *in vivo* and *in vitro*, and this agent has been used to induce remission in patients with AML-M3.

9.099   A benign axillary lymph node is removed from a woman with breast cancer. Which of the following is MOST likely to be seen in the lymph node?

    A. parafollicular hyperplasia
    B. necrosis in germinal centers
    C. neutrophils in sinuses
    D. sinus histiocytosis

9.100   While performing differential counts on a set of peripheral blood smears, an astute medical technologist notices that one smear contains atypical lymphoid cells with cerebriform nuclear folding. He suspects that the patient has:

    A. Hodgkin's disease, nodular sclerosis type
    B. follicular center cell lymphoma
    C. small non-cleaved cell lymphoma
    D. acute lymphoblastic leukemia, pre-B-cell type
    E. cutaneous T-cell lymphoma

9.101   Evaluation of a 10-year-old girl for abdominal pain of recent onset reveals a right lower quadrant mass. Exploratory laparotomy is scheduled; preoperative blood tests reveal mild anemia with thrombocytopenia and a markedly elevated LDH. Review of the peripheral blood smear reveals occasional abnormal lymphoid cells with prominent nucleoli and moderately abundant vacuolated basophilic cytoplasm. The surgeon suspects:

    A. Hodgkin's disease, nodular sclerosis type
    B. follicular center cell lymphoma
    C. small non-cleaved cell lymphoma
    D. acute lymphoblastic leukemia, pre-B-cell type
    E. cutaneous T-cell lymphoma

9.102   A 27-year-old medical student becomes aware she is experiencing persistent low-grade fever and occasional drenching night sweats. She has felt unusually fatigued and has lost her appetite. Pruritus becomes troublesome. Self-examination reveals firm 1-cm lymph nodes in her lower neck bilaterally and in her right axilla. She becomes concerned that she may have:

    A. Hodgkin's disease, nodular sclerosis type
    B. follicular center cell lymphoma
    C. small non-cleaved cell lymphoma
    D. acute lymphoblastic leukemia, pre-B-cell type
    E. cutaneous T-cell lymphoma

D is correct.

Sinus histiocytosis refers to distention of the lymphatic sinusoids, and is seen in lymph nodes draining cancers, particularly carcinoma of the breast. This pattern of reaction is thought to represent an immune response on the part of the host against the tumor or its products.

E is correct.

In cutaneous T-cell lymphomas, including mycosis fungoides, focal skin lesions are characterized histologically by infiltration of the epidermis and upper dermis by neoplastic T-cells with cerebriform-shaped nuclei. In a related condition, Sézary syndrome, there is generalized involvement of the skin by this neoplastic process, and an associated leukemia with lymphocytes with cerebriform-shaped nuclei ('Sézary' cells).

C is correct.

Small non-cleaved (Burkitt's) lymphoma is a high-grade lymphoma composed of a relatively monomorphic population of cells with blastic-like nuclei and a moderate rim of deeply basophilic cytoplasm. In smear preparations, cytoplasmic vacuolation is characteristic. Sporadic Burkitt's lymphoma occurs in the first two decades of life and often presents with abdominal disease. Involvement of the mandible and maxilla is often seen in Burkitt's lymphoma.

A is correct.

Nodular sclerosis Hodgkin's disease differs from the other subtypes in that it is the only type that is more common in women. Furthermore, most patients are adolescents or young adults. Hodgkin's disease is frequently associated with constitutional symptoms such as fever, night sweats, pruritus, and weight loss. These symptoms in a young woman with enlarged lymph nodes (particularly in the lower cervical, supraclavicular area) are suggestive of nodular sclerosis Hodgkin's disease.

9.103 A clinical pathologist, interpreting a batch of immunophenotypic analyses in the flow cytometry laboratory, reviews a case with these results: CD10+, CD19+, sIg-, HLA-DR+. He suspects that the patient has:
  A. Hodgkin's disease, nodular sclerosis type
  B. follicular center cell lymphoma
  C. small non-cleaved cell lymphoma
  D. acute lymphoblastic leukemia, pre-B-cell type
  E. cutaneous T-cell lymphoma

D is correct.
Immunophenotypic analysis shows a B-cell process (CD19+) with coexpression of CD10 and the activation antigen HLA-DR. This phenotype can be seen in both follicular center cell lymphoma and acute lymphoblastic leukemia, pre-B-cell type. Follicular lymphomas usually have surface immunoglobulin; the exception is rare cases that are undergoing transformation into aggressive disease. In contrast, acute lymphocytic leukemia of pre-B-cell type always lacks surface immunoglobulin.

9.104 Bone marrow transplantation may correct the underlying defect in:
  A. severe combined immunodeficiency disease (SCID)
  B. DiGeorge syndrome
  C. both of the above
  D. neither of the above

A is correct.
SCID is characterized by combined T-cell and B-cell defects, and bone marrow transplantation is the current mainstay of treatment. In contrast, DiGeorge syndrome is a selective T-cell deficiency due to failure of development of the third and fourth pharyngeal pouches, with subsequent thymic hypoplasia. T-cell function improves with age in children affected by this disorder. In patients with complete absence of thymus, transplant of fetal thymus may be beneficial.

Anemias

9.105 Which of the following laboratory tests would you order to distinguish between an anemia due to decreased production of erythrocytes *vs* increased destruction of erythrocytes?
  A. serum bilirubin level
  B. serum iron level
  C. reticulocyte count
  D. red blood cell count

C is correct.
A reticulocyte is a red blood cell that has recently left the bone marrow and has an increased amount of RNA. They are manually counted on peripheral blood smears after supravital staining with, for example, new methylene blue. Because of the low numbers of cells counted, the manual reticulocyte count lacks precision; a manual reticulocyte percentage of 3% after counting 1000 RBCs may have a true reticulocyte percentage of 2–5%. Flow cytometric reticulocyte counts are more precise because of the increased numbers (30 000) of RBCs counted.

9.106   You suspect that a patient has sickle cell anemia. Which of the following laboratory tests confirms your diagnosis?
  A. serum B_{12} level
  B. hemoglobin electrophoresis
  C. bone marrow aspirate examination
  D. measurement of mean corpuscular volume (MCV) and mean corpuscular hemoglobin concentration (MCHC)

B is correct.
Hemoglobin electrophoresis is a qualitative and semiquantitative technique performed on serum. It separates the commonly seen hemoglobins based on their net charge at a given pH. The method is commonly used to confirm sickle cell disease and sickle cell trait. Electrophoretic gels include cellulose acetate and citrate agar. It is being replaced in some institutions by quantitative hemoglobin studies using high-performance liquid chromatography.

9.107 If a patient has sickle cell disease, which of the following would NOT exacerbate symptoms?
   A. mountain climbing
   B. nasal oxygen administration
   C. diarrhea
   D. vomiting

B is correct.
Any phenomenon which causes the patient with sickle cell disease to be more hypoxemic (mountain climbing) or acidotic (diarrhea/vomiting) may exacerbate symptoms. Under these conditions, increased sickling occurs with its varied consequences.

9.108   If you do not supplement a pregnant patient's diet with vitamins, which of the following is MOST likely to develop during the course of the pregnancy?
   A. folate deficiency
   B. vitamin B_{12} deficiency
   C. glucose-6-phosphate dehydrogenase (G6PDH) deficiency
   D. polycythemia

A is correct.
The pregnant woman has an increased requirement for several vitamins, including iron and folic acid. Folate is a water-soluble vitamin for which humans have no storage reservoir. Thus, the pregnant woman is at risk of folate deficiency without folate supplementation. Vitamin B_{12} is stored in the liver in quantities sufficient for 1–4 years on a B_{12}-deficient diet. Supplementation with B_{12} during normal pregnancy, although given, is probably not necessary. G6PDH deficiency is a hereditary enzyme deficiency and not dependent on vitamin intake. The pregnant woman becomes hemodiluted due to an increased plasma volume rather than hemoconcentrated with associated polycythemia.

9.109 The BEST frequently used laboratory test to measure erythrocyte production is:
   A. reticulocyte count
   B. red blood cell count
   C. mean corpuscular volume (MCV)
   D. hematocrit

A is correct.
The reticulocyte count is a crude measure of the ability of bone marrow to manufacture erythrocytes. The resultant reticulocyte percentage may be imprecise and, after correction for both the degree of anemia and the patient's hematocrit, an apparent reticulocytosis may 'correct' itself into the normal range.

9.110 Which of the following is NOT important for proper erythrocyte development?
   A. stem cells
   B. appropriate microenvironment (i.e. bone marrow)
   C. interleukin-2
   D. erythropoietin

C is correct.
In addition to the general growth factors (granulocyte–monocyte colony-stimulating factor, interleukin-3 and interleukin-11), the primary growth factor necessary for RBC production is erythropoietin. This glycoprotein is produced by renal cells in response to hypoxia. It acts as both a mitogen and survival factor on erythroid precursors. All erythroid, granulocytic, and megakaryocytic cells arise from stem cells. Differentiation of the stem cell into any of these three lineages and maturation of the precursors within these lineages is dependent on an appropriate microenvironment with an appropriate stromal breakdown and cytokine availability.

9.111 Erythrocytes are biconcave disks. Which of the following is MOST important in maintaining the erythrocyte shape?
    A. glycolytic enzymes
    B. glutathione
    C. cytoskeletal proteins
    D. hemoglobin

C is correct.

The membrane skeleton is formed by a number of proteins, including spectrin, actin, ankyrin, and protein 4.1. When one or more of these proteins is qualitatively or quantitatively abnormal, the normal biconcave shape may be lost. The prototypical example of this phenomenon involves a quantitative decrease in RBC spectrin, yielding a spherical, rather than biconcave, shape. The disease is appropriately termed 'hereditary spherocytosis'.

9.112 Which of the following provides the majority of adenosine triphosphate (ATP) for mature erythrocytes?
    A. glycolytic pathway (Embden–Meyerhof pathway)
    B. mitochondrial citric acid cycle (Krebs' cycle)
    C. hexose monophosphate shunt
    D. glutathione pathway

A is correct.

As RBCs lack mitochondria, they are completely dependent on anaerobic glycolysis as a source of their ATP. The hexose monophosphate shunt provides NADPH which, in turn, provides reducing equivalents necessary for enzymatic and cytoskeletal integrity. NADPH maintains glutathione in its reduced form (GSH). Reduced glutathione is an important molecule in the maintenance of an appropriate intraerythrocytic redox potential.

9.113 Which of the following is NOT an example of anemia caused by a decreased production of erythrocytes?
    A. aplastic anemia
    B. myelophthisic anemia (e.g. metastatic carcinoma)
    C. hemolytic anemia due to glucose-6-phosphate dehydrogenase (G6PDH) deficiency
    D. iron-deficiency anemia

C is correct.

In aplastic anemia, the bone marrow is markedly hypocellular or acellular and lacks the erythroid progenitor mass necessary for erythrocyte production. Metastatic carcinoma replacing large amounts of marrow also destroys the stem cell and precursor population necessary for erythropoiesis. Iron deficiency results in quantitatively smaller numbers of erythrocytes, which are also relatively deficient in the iron-containing protein hemoglobin. G6PDH deficiency leads to increased destruction of peripheral RBCs and normally results in a compensatory increased production of erythrocytes.

9.114 Which of the following is NOT a likely cause of megaloblastic anemia?
    A. vitamin B_{12} deficiency
    B. folate deficiency
    C. intrinsic-factor deficiency
    D. iron deficiency

D is correct.

Megaloblastic anemia represents a 'nuclear' defect characterized by the inability of bone marrow cells to synthesize adequate amounts of DNA. This DNA synthesis defect is secondary to the lack of either vitamin B_{12} or folate. Intrinsic factor, produced by gastric parietal cells, is requisite to absorption of dietary vitamin B_{12} in the ileum. Thus, any deficiency or impairment of absorption of vitamin B_{12} and folate, and their absence in the bone marrow, will yield megaloblastic anemia. In contrast, iron deficiency represents a 'cytoplasmic' defect that yields hemoglobin-poor erythrocytes.

9.115   Hereditary spherocytosis (HS) is due to a defect in which of the following?
    A. cytoskeletal proteins
    B. glutathione pathway
    C. hexose monophosphate shunt
    D. globin chain protein structure

9.116   Polymerization of hemoglobin within erythrocytes in sickle cell anemia is caused by:
    A. a single amino acid substitution in the alpha chain
    B. a single amino acid substitution in a cytoskeletal protein
    C. a single amino acid substitution in the beta chain
    D. a single amino acid substitution in an ion pump protein

The following case history relates to questions 9.117–9.120.   A 25-year-old black woman is referred by her family physician to a neurologist for a disturbance in her balance and gait. The patient had been healthy until 20 years of age, when she developed Crohn's disease (a chronic inflammatory disease of the small bowel and terminal ileum). Due to extensive disease, she underwent resection of her terminal ileum and a portion of the small bowel at age 21 years. Postoperatively, she experienced no further symptoms and was lost to follow-up until the present. Laboratory examination at this time reveals a WBC count of 3800 cells/μl with 61% PMNs (polymorphonuclear leukocytes) and 39% lymphocytes. Hypersegmented PMNs and macro-ovalocytes were noted on the peripheral smear. Hemoglobin was 9.2 g/dl and hematocrit 27 ml/dl. The MCV was 141 μM^3 and MCHC 32%. The reticulocyte count was <1% (low).

A is correct.

Most cases of HS are due to quantitative decreases in the amount of a cytoskeletal protein called spectrin. The RBCs lose their biconcave shape and become spherocytic, with a decreased surface-to-volume ratio. The spherocytes become more fragile and damaged. The spleen sequesters these damaged spherocytes and, thus, these patients often present with splenomegaly. Splenectomy will correct the anemia in HS, and this correction is considered diagnostic of HS.

C is correct.

Several hemoglobinopathies are due to single point mutations in the β chain of hemoglobin, for example, HbS, HbC, HbE. Hemoglobin A, or 'normal' hemoglobin, contains glutamate at position 6 of the β chain. When valine is substituted for glutamate at this position, sickle cell hemoglobin results. This HbS is unstable under hypoxic, acidotic conditions and polymerizes. With polymerization , the erythrocyte loses its biconcavity and becomes sickle-shaped.

9.117 The MOST likely diagnosis is:
   A. iron-deficiency anemia
   B. aplastic anemia
   C. megaloblastic anemia
   D. sickle cell anemia

C is correct.

Megaloblastic anemia is a macrocytic anemia (usually MCV $> 115\,\mu M^3$) and, in this case, due to impaired vitamin B_{12} absorption secondary to loss of the terminal ileum. Without the terminal ileum, the intrinsic factor–B_{12} complex is not absorbed and cobalamin (B_{12}) is not available for DNA synthesis in the bone marrow. Hypersegmented neutrophils (characterized by six or more segmented nuclear lobes) are one of the earliest features of either vitamin B_{12} or folate deficiency. Macro-ovalocytes are also classical features of vitamin B_{12}/folate deficiency, but may be seen in other non-related anemias such as myelodysplasia.

9.118 Which of the following laboratory tests is LEAST likely to be abnormal?
   A. serum iron
   B. Schilling test
   C. serum B_{12} levels
   D. bone-marrow morphologic examination

A is correct.

Iron is not a direct causal factor in pure megaloblastic anemia secondary to vitamin B_{12} deficiency. Decreased serum B_{12} levels are expected in megaloblastic anemia. Bone marrow examination classically reveals megaloblastic cellular features in erythroid and granulocytic precursors, and giant myelocytes and metamyelocytes are also seen. Megaloblastosis is characterized by nuclear cytoplasmic dyssynchrony. Although the cytoplasm continues to mature normally with normal hemoglobinization, the nuclear features remain immature due to deficient DNA synthesis. The three-part Schilling test is a cumbersome and somewhat outdated test, which uses radioactive B_{12} as a marker for impaired gastrointestinal absorption of the vitamin.

9.119 This patient's anemia is due to:
   A. inhibition of mRNA synthesis and/or processing
   B. inhibition of iron absorption
   C. inhibition of DNA synthesis
   D. oxidation of hemoglobin

C is correct.

DNA synthesis requires the synthesis of thymidylic acid (TMP) which, in turn, is converted from deoxyuridylic acid (dUMP) by thymidylate synthetase, an enzyme requiring the coenzyme 5,10-methylene-tetrahydrofolate reductase. Vitamin B_{12} is involved in the synthesis of this tetrahydrofolate coenzyme. Thus, a lack of vitamin B_{12} ultimately leads to impaired TMP synthesis and subsequent DNA synthesis.

9.120 Which of the following will NOT resolve if the patient is treated with folate alone?
  A. anemia
  B. bone marrow morphological abnormalities
  C. macrocytosis and hypersegmentation of PMNs
  D. neurological signs

D is correct.

The folate derivative 5-methyltetrahydrofolate is an important cofactor in the vitamin B_{12}-mediated reaction of homocysteine to methionine. This reaction is crucial to normal central nervous system methylation reactions and biochemical neurologic integrity. Thus, although folate may correct the megaloblastic anemia, it would not correct the deficient CNS methylation and accompanying neurologic signs.

The following case history relates to questions 9.121–9.127. A 6-year-old black boy presents to the hematology clinic with acute abdominal pain. The patient's mother states that he has had the flu for 4 days with vomiting 4–5 times a day. Physical examination reveals tender, warm, and swollen ankles, knees and interphalangeal joints. A 3-cm ulcer is present over the right calf. Scleral icterus is noted, and the spleen is not palpable. Chest X-ray is normal. Laboratory tests reveal a metabolic alkalosis, decreased potassium, hemoglobin 6.3 g/dl, hematocrit 20 ml/dl, MCV 110 μM^3, MCHC 35% and a reticulocyte count of 35% (increased). Abnormal erythrocytes were noted on the peripheral smear. Erythrocytes and renal epithelial cells were noted upon microscopic examination of the urine; however, WBC and bacteria were not noted. Serum bilirubin was elevated.

9.121 What is the MOST likely diagnosis?
  A. sickle cell disease in crisis
  B. megaloblastic anemia due to vitamin B_{12} deficiency
  C. megaloblastic anemia due to acute gastritis
  D. glucose-6-phosphate dehydrogenase (G6PDH) deficiency

A is correct.

Acute musculoskeletal pain is the most prevalent symptomatic manifestation of sickle cell anemia and accounts for most hospital admissions in these patients. The majority of attacks are both unexplained and unpredictable. Any event in which acidosis, hypoxia or dehydration prevails may be a triggering mechanism for a sickle cell crisis. In young children, painful crises often occur in association with infection.

9.122 The acute arthritis and leg ulcers are MOST likely due to:
  A. autoimmune disease
  B. plugging of microcapillaries with subsequent acute ischemia
  C. trauma with chronic bleeding due to an inherited disorder of coagulation
  D. chronic infection due to immune deficiency

B is correct.

The crisis is termed 'vaso-occlusive' secondary to sickle cell plugging of microcapillaries with associated hypoxic injury and infarction.

9.123 The erythrocytes and renal epithelial cells in the urine are MOST likely due to:
   A. chronic glomerulonephritis
   B. acute pyelonephritis
   C. plugging of capillaries with subsequent renal papillary necrosis
   D. urinary tract infection

C is correct.
Infarction secondary to vascular occlusion occurs in a number of organs, including bone, brain, kidney, spleen, liver, and retina. Erythrocytes in the urine define hematuria and this sign is abnormal. In the setting of sickle cell disease or trait, hematuria represents a marker of renal infarction. Renal epithelial cells in the urine are also abnormal and are a marker of renal tubular necrosis.

9.124 The MOST likely immediate cause of this patient's acute illness is:
   A. dehydration due to vomiting
   B. hypoxia due to pneumonia
   C. splenic sequestration of abnormal erythrocytes
   D. bone marrow aplasia due to acute viral infection

A is correct.
Vomiting leads to both dehydration and metabolic acidosis. Dehydration, in turn, leads to intravascular hemoconcentration with increased 'crowding' of normal and sickled erythrocytes. The acidosis promotes further sickling of erythrocytes. Both result in hypoxic tissue injury.

9.125 Assume that the osmotic fragility test is abnormal and that the hemoglobin electrophoresis, Coombs' test and vitamin B_{12} levels are normal. What is the MOST likely diagnosis?
   A. autoimmune hemolytic anemia (AIHA)
   B. hereditary spherocytosis
   C. sickle cell anemia
   D. α-thalassemia

B is correct.
The osmotic fragility test is a confirmatory test for hereditary spherocytosis (HS). The test is based on the fact that the spherocyte lyses at more hypertonic saline solutions compared with normal erythrocytes. Spherocytes found in both HS and AIHA show increased osmotic fragility due to decreased surface-to-volume ratio. In hypotonic solution, as water enters the spherocyte, its ability to expand and accommodate the increased water is compromised, causing lysis. In AIHA, a positive direct Coombs' test is expected. Neither the Coombs' test nor vitamin B_{12} levels are expected to be abnormal in either sickle cell anemia or α-thalassemia. The normal hemoglobin electrophoresis rules out sickle cell anemia.

9.126 Assume that the Coombs' test is abnormal, but that the osmotic fragility, hemoglobin electrophoresis and vitamin B_{12} levels are normal. What is the MOST likely diagnosis now?
   A. autoimmune hemolytic anemia (AIHA)
   B. hereditary spherocytosis
   C. sickle cell anemia
   D. α-thalassemia

A is correct.
AIHA is caused by destruction of erythrocytes secondary to coating of the erythrocytes by antibody against the patient's own surface antigens. AIHA is divided into either warm or cold types, according to whether the antibody attaches to the surface at body temperature or colder temperatures, respectively. Cold-type antibodies are IgM and the destruction is complement-mediated. Warm-type antibodies are IgG and destruction occurs in the spleen. An abnormal Coombs' test is not part of the pathogenesis in either hereditary spherocytosis, sickle cell anemia or α-thalassemia.

9.127 If the osmotic fragility test is abnormal and all other tests are normal, what then is the MOST likely molecular abnormality of this child's anemia?
   A. an abnormality in DNA synthesis
   B. deletion of one or more α-globin genes
   C. a defect in erythrocyte cytoskeletal proteins
   D. autoantibodies directed against erythrocyte cell surface determinants

9.128 Myelophthisic anemia can be caused by all of the following EXCEPT:
   A. metastatic carcinoma
   B. myelofibrosis
   C. disseminated tuberculosis
   D. antierythrocyte autoantibodies

9.129 A positive direct Coombs' test is MOST likely to be associated with:
   A. hereditary spherocytosis
   B. glucose-6-phosphate dehydrogenase deficiency
   C. autoimmune hemolytic anemia
   D. sickle cell anemia

The following case history relates to questions 9.130 and 9.131). A 43-year-old white man is referred to the outpatients clinic for evaluation of chronic fatigue. The patient has never been anemic and states that he has followed a normal diet and not lost any weight. However, he reveals that he has routinely passed black, tarry stools for the past 6 months. Physical examination reveals pallor of the mucous membranes and the sclera. No hepatosplenomegaly or adenopathy is noted. Laboratory tests reveal: hemoglobin 6.7 (normal: 13.5–18) g/dl; hematocrit 20 (normal: 40–50) ml/dl; MCV 70 (normal: 80–96) μM^3; MCHC 23% (normal: 32–36%); WBC 5000 (normal: 4000–11 000) cells/ μl; platelet count 500 000 (normal: 150 000– 300 000)/mm^3. The differential is normal, although hypochromic microcytic erythrocytes are noted on the peripheral blood smear. The stool guaiac test is positive.

C is correct.
Hereditary spherocytosis is characterized by an abnormal osmotic fragility test. The primary defect in most cases of HS is deficient quantities of the RBC protein spectrin. Defects in other cytoskeletal proteins are the causative factors in hereditary elliptocytosis, hereditary stomatocytosis and hereditary acanthocytosis.

D is correct.
Myelophthisis is the replacement of bone marrow by cells that normally do not reside there. Common examples of this include metastatic carcinoma, malignant lymphoma and miliary tuberculosis. (The latter is the most common non-cancerous cause of myelophthisis.) Because normal marrow cells are replaced, anemia, leukocytopenia and/or thrombocytopenia ensue. A positive Coombs' test reflecting antierythrocytic antibodies is not part of the pathogenesis of myelophthisis.

C is correct.
The direct Coombs' test is also called the direct antiglobulin test (DAT). It detects self-produced antibodies (antiglobulins) directly adsorbed to the patient's erythrocyte membrane self-antigens, hence the term 'autoimmune'. If antibodies are detected, they are often eluted (stripped) from the membrane and specifically identified with other techniques. In this way, the patient may receive RBC transfusions lacking the identified antigen and avoid intravascular hemolysis of the transfused RBCs.

9.130 What is the MOST likely diagnosis?
   A. megaloblastic anemia due to malabsorption
      of vitamin B_{12}
   B. thalassemia
   C. infiltration of bone marrow by acute
      myelogenous leukemia
   D. iron deficiency anemia due to chronic blood
      loss

D is correct.

Iron deficiency is the most common cause of anemia and is seen in infants, children, and adults. Iron deficiency anemia in the adult is almost always due to blood loss, and a careful and thorough search for obvious or occult blood loss is mandatory before ruling out iron deficiency as the cause of anemia in adults. Patients with iron deficiency are often mildly thrombocytotic.

9.131 Of the following, which is the MOST likely cause of this patient's anemia?
   A. gastrointestinal bleeding
   B. vitamin B_{12} deficiency
   C. folate deficiency
   D. antiparietal cell autoantibodies

A is correct.

The gastrointestinal and urogenital tracts are the most common sources of blood loss in an adult with iron deficiency. Vitamin B_{12} deficiency (in which antiparietal cell autoantibodies may play a role) and folate deficiency lead to megaloblastic anemia, not iron deficiency anemia. The primary mechanism in these latter anemias is not bleeding.

The following case history relates to questions 9.132–9.134. You are a general medical officer in the army. A 22-year-old black male private is referred to you because of the recent onset of cola-colored urine. Upon questioning the soldier, you discover that he has consumed a normal diet and not lost any weight. His physical performance status has been reported as excellent. He states that he has never been anemic, has never experienced hemoglobinuria in the past, and has otherwise been healthy. You also discover that he has been given quinine recently as a prophylaxis for malaria. Physical examination reveals icterus of the sclera and mucous membranes. The remainder of the examination is normal. Laboratory tests reveal: hemoglobin 11.0 (normal: 13.5–18) g/dl; hematocrit 33 (normal: 40–50) ml/dl; MCV 98 (normal: 80–96) μ^3; MCHC 32% (normal: 32–36%); platelet count 267 000 (normal: 150 000–300 000)/mm^3. Bleeding time, prothrombin time (PT) and activated partial thromboplastin time (APTT) are normal. Examination of the urine reveals a positive test for hemoglobin, although no cells are noted on microscopic examination of the urine.

9.132 Which of the following is the MOST likely diagnosis?

    A. sickle cell anemia

    B. hereditary spherocytosis

    C. glucose-6-phosphate dehydrogenase (G6PDH) deficiency

    D. microangiopathic hemolytic anemia

C is correct.

G6PDH deficiency is the most prevalent inborn metabolic error of RBCs, affecting 100 million people worldwide. This X-linked recessive disease is seen in approximately 11% of black men who carry the variant isoenzyme G6PDA-. Women who are heterozygotes are also sometimes affected, depending on which of their two X chromosomes is inactivated, as per the Lyon hypothesis. Overall, the enzyme deficiency renders the patient's RBCs more susceptible to oxidative stress (usually oxidative drugs). The prototype of this process is the patient who is undergoing hemolytic anemia while taking antimalarial drugs.

9.133 Regarding this case, all of the following are likely EXCEPT:

    A. increased reticulocytes

    B. Heinz bodies on the peripheral blood smear

    C. increased serum bilirubin

    D. numerous sickle cells on the peripheral blood smear

D is correct.

As the anemia progresses, the bone marrow attempts to compensate by extruding more immature RBCs (reticulocytes) into the peripheral blood. Damage to the RBCs causes precipitation of hemoglobin and RBC membrane fragments in the form of Heinz bodies, which are seen with supravital stains such as new methylene blue. Hemolysis leads to increased hepatic catabolism of hemoglobin to biliverdin and bilirubin.

9.134 The pathogenesis of this patient's anemia is due to:

    A. decreased DNA synthesis

    B. oxidative damage of hemoglobin and RBC membrane proteins

    C. decreased α-globin chain synthesis

    D. polymerization of hemoglobin due to low arterial pO_2

B is correct.

Through the hexose monophosphate shunt, G6PDH produces NADPH-reducing equivalents. NADPH, in turn, keeps glutathione in its reduced state (GSH) and GSH keeps low levels of spontaneously generated oxygen radicals from destroying the RBC proteins. G6PDH-deficient RBCs are unable to maintain glutathione in its reduced state, thereby impairing RBC ability to cope with oxidative stress.

The following case history relates to questions 9.135–9.137. A 60-year-old black man, hospitalized with pneumonia, develops septic shock from an infected central line. Laboratory tests reveal: hemoglobin 9.8 (normal: 13.5–18) g/dl; hematocrit 30 (normal: 40–50) ml/dl; MCV 99 (normal: 80–96) μM^3; and MCHC 32% (normal: 32–36%). Examination of the peripheral blood smear reveals the presence of schistocytes. There are increased fibrin degradation products and hypofibrinogenemia.

9.135 What is the MOST likely diagnosis?
A. microangiopathic hemolytic anemia
B. megaloblastic anemia
C. iron deficiency anemia
D. glucose-6-phosphate dehydrogenase (G6PDH) deficiency

A is correct.

Microangiopathic hemolytic anemia is characteristic of diseases such as disseminated intravascular coagulation, thrombotic thrombocytopenic purpura, hemolytic uremic syndrome, and severe burns. The pathogenesis is of microthrombi formation within small blood vessels. As erythrocytes attempt to pass through the web of microthrombi and fibrin strands, they are deformed and destroyed. The *sine qua non* of microangiopathic hemolytic anemia is the schistocyte. It is important to realize that most hemolytic anemias are not associated with schistocytes, but only those with the pathologic microvascular abnormalities mentioned above.

9.136 In this patient, which of the following laboratory abnormalities is MOST likely to be found?
A. elevated bilirubin levels
B. decreased vitamin B_{12} levels
C. decreased folate levels
D. presence of Heinz bodies on the peripheral smear

A is correct.

Any hemolytic anemia may cause hyperbilirubinemia. If the hemolytic rate is relatively slow, thereby allowing the liver to conjugate the bilirubin, levels of direct bilirubin will be greater than indirect bilirubin levels. As with most hemolytic anemias, however, the liver cannot keep up the pace of glucuronide conjugation of bilirubin presented to it and, thus, indirect hyperbilirubinemia prevails. Vitamin status and unstable hemoglobin (with the formation of Heinz bodies) are not part of the pathogenesis of microangiopathic hemolytic anemias.

9.137 Examination of the bone marrow in this patient is MOST likely to show:
A. granulocytic hyperplasia
B. erythroid hyperplasia
C. lymphocytosis
D. hyperplasia of the eosinophil series

B is correct.

The bone marrow compensates for anemia and the attendant hypoxemia by manufacturing more RBCs. This response is secondary to increased erythropoietin levels. Erythropoietin is secreted from the kidney in response to hypoxemia. A normal bone marrow shows a $3:1$–$5:1$ ratio of granulocytic-to-erythroid cells. However, in compensated hemolytic anemia, the ratio may be $1:1$ or even reversed, such that erythroid cells are present in greater numbers than are granulocytic cells, hence the term 'erythroid hyperplasia'.

9.138 Which of the following is the MOST likely cause of megaloblastic anemia?
A. vitamin B_6 deficiency
B. deficiency of erythropoietin
C. vitamin B_{12} deficiency
D. interleukin-3 deficiency

C is correct.

Megaloblastic anemia is classically caused by either vitamin B_{12} and/or folic acid deficiency. Vitamin B_6 (pyridoxine) deficiency is essentially non-existent in the United States. Pyridoxine is used in the treatment of the sideroblastic anemia arising from antituberculous drug treatment. These drugs interfere with pyridoxine metabolism. In the absence of renal disease, serum erythropoietin levels are elevated in megaloblastic anemia.

9.139 A patient is receiving methotrexate chemotherapy for treatment of her malignancy. The agent is known to selectively block DNA synthesis. From your knowledge of the changes seen in vitamin B_{12}/folate deficiency, you expect to see all of the following peripheral blood and bone marrow findings EXCEPT:

   A. peripheral blood macrocytosis
   B. peripheral blood granulocyte hypersegmentation
   C. delayed nuclear maturation in the marrow erythroid precursors
   D. giant myelocytes and metamyelocytes
   E. delayed hemoglobinization

E is correct.

Megaloblastic anemia secondary to vitamin B_{12}/folate deficiency is characterized by nuclear/cytoplasmic dyssynchrony. Nuclear maturation is delayed due to defective DNA synthesis; however, cytoplasmic maturation continues with normal hemoglobinization. Hemoglobin synthesis is not directly dependent on either vitamin B_{12} or folate. The peripheral blood macrocytes are not round but oval, an important distinction. Hypersegmented PMNs are one of the earliest blood findings in megaloblastic anemia. Giant myelocytes and metamyelocytes are seen in the bone marrow in this disorder.

9.140 A frail elderly woman presents with peripheral blood hypersegmentation of neutrophils with an MCV of $120\,\mu M^3$. She is pale, and her diet is sparse in dairy foods and meats. Proprioception is deficient on neurologic examination. The MOST likely cause of her anemia is:

   A. iron deficiency
   B. vitamin B_{12} deficiency
   C. vitamin K deficiency
   D. folate deficiency
   E. bone marrow aplasia

B is correct.

Those most susceptible to vitamin B_{12} deficiency are the elderly, the alcoholic and the strict vegetarian whose diets are deficient in vitamin B_{12}-rich dairy foods and meats. This patient, who most likely has pernicious anemia, reveals the classical peripheral blood smear findings of megaloblastic anemia, namely, oval macrocytosis (MCV $120\,\mu M^3$) and granulocytic hypersegmentation. Her deficient proprioception is a sign of her subacute combined degeneration, due to degeneration of the white matter in the posterior and lateral columns of the spinal cord caused by the vitamin B_{12} deficiency.

9.141 A paper-plant worker, who has cleaned out a chemical tank containing benzene, presents with malaise and petechiae 2 months later. His peripheral WBC count is 300 (normal: 3000–12 000) cells/μl, with a hematocrit of 10 (normal: 40–52) ml/dl and a platelet count of 10 000 (normal: 150 000–300 000)/mm³. His MCV is 90 (normal: 80–100)μM^3. A reticulocyte count is reported to be undetectable. The bone marrow is markedly hypocellular. The BEST diagnosis for this patient is:

   A. aplastic anemia
   B. iron deficiency anemia
   C. vitamin B_{12} deficiency
   D. folate deficiency
   E. hereditary spherocytosis

A is correct.

Aplastic anemia is characterized by complete or nearly complete, loss of erythroid, granulocytic, and megakaryocytic precursors in the marrow. The result is pancytopenia, as described in the case history. Seventy per cent of cases are of undetermined etiology. Drug- and chemical-related causes account for 10–20% of cases, and infectious hepatitis for approximately 6% of cases. Benzene exposure is a well-known cause of marrow toxicity with its attendant aplastic anemia.

9.142 A 19-year-old marine recruit has some difficulty completing her basic training in Florida. She recently had infectious mononucleosis. You review her CBC count, and note that her hematocrit is 27 (normal: 34–47) ml/dl and her MCV is 104 (normal: 80–100) μM^3. Her granulocyte and platelet counts are essentially unremarkable. A reticulocyte count is reported to be 5% (normal: 0.5–1.5%). Manual review of the peripheral smear reveals that the RBCs are normal in size, but are agglutinated. What is the MOST likely diagnosis?

A. aplastic anemia

B. vitamin B_{12} deficiency anemia

C. paroxysmal cold hemoglobinuria

D. autoimmune hemolytic anemia, cold type

E. iron deficiency anemia

D is correct.

Cold agglutinin-associated disease is characterized by acute onset in young people who often have self-limited infections due to *Mycoplasma pneumoniae*, cytomegalovirus or Epstein–Barr virus (etiologic agent of infectious mononucleosis). The antibodies are attached to the RBC membranes and cause the RBCs to clump together at temperatures below body temperature, hence the agglutination noted on the peripheral smear. Acute postinfectious cold auto-antibody formation leads to intravascular hemolysis in 40% of cases. The bone marrow compensates with reticulocytosis. This, in turn, causes the mildly increased MCV. (Reticulocytes are larger than normal RBCs.)

9.143 A patient presents with a history of episodic hematuria after a viral syndrome. The patient reports the puzzling finding that his house had lost heat for several hours, and that the hematuria occurred after the heat had been restored. A blood-bank evaluation reveals that the patient has an IgG-type antibody, with anti-P specificity. A reticulocyte count is elevated. What is the MOST likely diagnosis?

A. paroxysmal nocturnal hemoglobinuria

B. (soldier) march-induced hemoglobinuria

C. paroxysmal cold hemoglobinuria

D. warm autoimmune hemolytic anemia

E. aplastic anemia

C is correct.

Paroxysmal cold hemoglobinuria is a self-limited disease usually treated by keeping the patient warm. The Donath–Landsteiner antibody is an IgG complement-dependent biphasic antibody which binds to RBCs at cold temperatures and lyses RBCs at warm temperatures. The specificity of the antibody is usually against RBC antigens in either the P or I systems. The bone marrow compensates for the anemia with a reticulocytosis.

9.144 A patient receives the oxidizing agent dapsone for a presumed brown recluse spider bite. Unfortunately, the patient responds with a serious hemolytic event because of G6PDH deficiency. If the patient is otherwise healthy, how long does it take for the reticulocyte count to begin to rise?

A. 30 minutes

B. 6 hours

C. 6 days

D. 6 weeks

E. 6 months

B is correct.

A normal bone marrow can increase erythroid production 4- to 6-fold in response to a hemolytic anemia. This response is rapid and efficient, and reticulocytosis is noted within hours of the hemolytic event. The reticulocytosis may reach levels of 60–70%.

9.145 All of the following are characteristic of iron deficiency EXCEPT:
   A. red cell microcytosis
   B. low serum ferritin levels
   C. normal nuclear, but delayed cytoplasmic, maturation
   D. elevated reticulocyte count

D is correct.
Because iron-deficient RBCs are hemoglobin-poor, they are small in size (microcytic). This is an expression of delayed cytoplasmic maturation and inadequate hemoglobin synthesis. Iron is not directly involved in DNA synthesis and nuclear maturation (as are B_{12} and folate). Ferritin is an excellent marker of body iron stores. As iron stores are depleted, ferritin levels decrease. However, because ferritin is an acute-phase reactant, patients with conditions such as neoplasia or inflammation may not manifest with decreased serum ferritin levels in the face of true iron deficiency anemia. Without iron for hemoglobin synthesis, erythroid precursors stay in the bone marrow longer than normal before being extruded into the peripheral blood. Thus, reticulocyte counts are decreased.

9.146 A very pale pregnant young woman comes to your office for evaluation. You do a CBC, and the hemoglobin is 7 (normal: 11.5–16) g/dl, hematocrit is 20 (normal: 34–47) ml/dl, MCV is 72 (normal: 80–100) μM^3. The serum iron and serum ferritin are low: What single diagnosis is the MOST likely?
   A. aplastic anemia
   B. iron deficiency anemia
   C. paroxysmal nocturnal hemoglobinuria (PNH)
   D. paroxysmal cold hemoglobinuria (PCH)

B is correct.
Iron deficiency anemia is common in the pregnant woman who previously was losing blood through monthly menstrual periods and lacked iron supplementation. Iron deficiency is characterized by low serum iron and serum ferritin, the latter acting as a serum marker of body iron stores. Because of erythrocyte destruction and the body's efficiency in preserving heme iron, iron stores are usually increased in PNH and PCH. Iron stores are often normal or increased in aplastic anemia because erythropoiesis is arrested and iron is not needed for hemoglobinization.

9.147 A patient with achlorhydria undergoes a Schilling test. Which of the following results are seen in typical pernicious anemia associated with gastric atrophy?
   A. most of the radioactive vitamin B_{12} is detected in the urine within a week without any other treatment
   B. radioactive vitamin B_{12} is not detected in the urine, not even after addition of oral porcine intrinsic factor
   C. radioactive vitamin B_{12} is not detected in the urine, but is after addition of oral porcine intrinsic factor
   D. radioactive vitamin B_{12} is detected in the urine only when repeated after antibiotic administration

C is correct.
Patients with pernicious anemia possess antiparietal cell antibodies. Their gastric parietal cells cannot produce either hydrochloric acid or intrinsic factor. Intrinsic factor is necessary for binding vitamin B_{12} and transporting it to the terminal ileum where the vitamin is normally absorbed. Without endogenous intrinsic factor the vitamin cannot be absorbed. A Schilling test in a patient with pernicious anemia reveals previously ingested radiolabeled vitamin B_{12} in the patient's urine only if exogenous intrinsic factor is given simultaneously. Ingested radiolabeled vitamin B_{12} without exogenous intrinsic factor results in lack of vitamin B_{12} absorption. Thus, no radiolabeled vitamin B_{12} is excreted in the urine.

9.148 You review the records of a patient who you suspect has β-thalassemia trait. The peripheral smear shows microcytosis, a mildly elevated RBC count, and target cells. Iron studies are normal. Which of the following hemoglobin electrophoresis results is MOST characteristic of β-thalassemia trait?

   A. HbC is present
   B. HbA₂ is elevated
   C. HbS is present
   D. HbH is present

B is correct.

The classical findings of a patient with β-thalassemia trait are a microcytic hypochromic anemia with a mildly elevated RBC count and target cells on the peripheral blood smear. Basophilic stippling may also be seen. Hemoglobin electrophoresis reveals increased HbA_2 levels (up to around 9%). β-thalassemia is an anemia secondary to inadequate production of normal hemoglobin β-chains. HbH is an α-thalassemia in which three of the four α–chain genes are either missing or non-functional. HbS and HbC represent qualitative mutational changes in the β chain of hemoglobin rather than quantitative changes.

9.149 A patient has anemia with the following laboratory results: hemoglobin 10 (normal: 13.5–17.5) g/dl; hematocrit 30 (normal: 40–52) ml/dl; RBCs 3.5 (normal: 4.5–6) million/mm³; MCV 77 (normal: 80-100) µM³. You evaluate the peripheral blood smear and find that the RBCs are hypochromic and microcytic. The RBC distribution width (RDW) is 21 (normal: 12–14.5). Which of the following diagnoses is the MOST appropriate?

   A. megaloblastic anemia
   B. anemia of chronic disease
   C. iron deficiency anemia
   D. aplastic anemia
   E. leukoerythroblastic anemia

C is correct.

In iron deficiency anemia, the MCV is decreased in proportion to the hemoglobin level. Elliptocytes may be seen on the peripheral smear in addition to the microcytic hypochromic cells. Anisocytosis (as measured by the RDW) may be moderate to marked. A few target cells may be seen. In the other common microcytic hypochromic anemia, β-thalassemia minor, the MCV is far more decreased than the hemoglobin level, for example, Hb 10 g/dl *vs* MCV 68 µM³. In addition, numerous target cells are usually seen as well as basophilic stippling. Anisocytosis is not seen or only mildly present (normal or mildly increased RDW).

9.150 A patient of Oriental extraction has heterozygous α-thalassemia-1 trait. He marries another Oriental with the identical trait. Assuming they both have one allele with deletion of both α-globin genes, what are the odds that their progeny will have the fatal disorder hydrops fetalis?

   A. < 10%
   B. 15%
   C. 25%
   D. 50%
   E. 75%

C is correct.

The normal α-chain hemoglobin genotype is aa/aa. In this case, both parents are genetically labeled aa/--. Based on normal Mendelian genetics, 25% of the progeny will be aa/aa (with no α-thalassemia), 50% would be aa/-- (α-thalassemia trait and associated mild hypochromic anemia) and 25% would be --/--. With the latter phenotype, the fetus is not able to produce any normal HbA, HbA₂ or HbF (fetal hemoglobin). All HbF becomes Bart's hemoglobin, characterized by a tetramer of γ chains. Bart's hemoglobin avidly binds oxygen and is unable to transport oxygen to fetal tissues. Fetal death due to hydrops follows.

9.151   Which of the following does NOT cause sickling in a sickle cell patient?

A. low oxygen levels
B. acid pH
C. vomiting and diarrhea with dehydration
D. elevated HbF

D is correct.

Sickling occurs in the presence of hypoxemia and acidosis. Without adequate intraerythrocytic oxygen pressure and an intraerythrocytic pH to maintain normal tertiary and quarternary hemoglobin protein structure, the point mutation of HbS renders this hemoglobin susceptible to polymerization, denaturation and precipitation. Vomiting and diarrhea can cause dehydration with associated metabolic acidosis. Elevated HbF levels protect against sickling presumably by interfering with HbS polymerization.

Coagulation

9.152   Which of the following is NOT associated with hypercoagulability?

A. heparin-associated thrombocytopenia
B. lupus anticoagulants
C. protein C deficiency
D. antithrombin III (AT III) deficiency
E. factor VIII deficiency

E is correct.

Factor VIII deficiency is hemophilia A which is associated with bleeding. A hypercoaguable tendency may be due to heparin-associated thrombocytopenia, lupus anticoagulants, protein C deficiency, and AT III deficiency.

9.153   von Willebrand's factor (vWF) is thought to have each of the following properties and functions EXCEPT:

A. binds to collagen
B. binds to glycoprotein (GP) Ib on platelets
C. binds to GP IIb / IIIa on platelets
D. binds to factor XIII
E. binds to factor VIII

D is correct.

vWF functions in hemostasis by mediating adhesion of platelets to exposed subendothelial collagen through binding at the platelet GP Ib and IIb / IIIa sites, forming the basis for the hemostatic plug. In addition, vWF forms a non-covalent complex with factor VIII, thus stabilizing and protecting it against rapid removal from the circulation. The vWF does not bind to factor XIII.

9.154   Factors which favor the thrombotic state include all of the following EXCEPT:

A. decreased protein C
B. decreased AT III
C. decreased protein S
D. increased tissue-plasminogen activator (t-PA)
E. increased activated protein C (APC) resistance [decreased APC – activated partial thromboplastin time (APTT)]

D is correct.

t-PA release from adjacent endothelial cells is stimulated by the deposition of fibrin following vascular injury. t-PA binds to fibrin and converts adsorbed plasminogen to plasmin, accompanied by lysis of fibrin and formation of soluble fibrin-degradation products. t-PA is inhibited by plasminogen-activator inhibitor (PAI). Accumulation of excessive amounts of t-PA in the blood leads to systemic fibrinolysis, a bleeding disorder.

9.155 A patient 10 days after his second coronary artery bypass-graft operation has been doing well until this morning, when the nurse tells you that his right leg is pulseless. The patient has an intravenous line still in place and you notice that his platelet count has dropped from 250 000 to 50 000/mm^3. Over the past 3 days, his PT has been normal and APTT slightly elevated. His D-dimer and fibrin split products (FSP) are within normal limits. WBC is normal, hematocrit is 37 ml/dl, and CK and LDH are within normal limits. The MOST likely diagnosis is:

    A. bone marrow failure secondary to metastatic cancer

    B. disseminated intravascular clotting

    C. protein C deficiency

    D. heparin-associated thrombocytopenia (HAT)

    E. thrombotic thrombocytopenic purpura (TTP)

D is correct.

The HAT syndrome is to be suspected in patients receiving heparin when there is an unexpected fall in platelets to $< 100 000/mm^3$ or by 50% over 24–48 h. Heparin leads to the formation of IgG antibodies that react with heparin to form immune complexes that bind to platelet Fc receptors and trigger platelet aggregation, the release reaction, and the subsequent decrease in circulating platelets. Platelet aggregates cause occlusion of the microvasculature. The HAT antibody binds to heparin on the endothelial cell surface, and stimulates the synthesis and expression of tissue factor by endothelial cells.

9.156 Hypercoagulability is associated with which of the following?

    A. von Willebrand's disease

    B. hemophilia A

    C. Bernard–Soulier syndrome

    D. activated protein C (APC) resistance

    E. uremia

D is correct.

APC resistance is the most common laboratory-based cause of deep vein thrombosis (DVT). A single amino-acid substitution is found in the coagulation factor V gene. An example of familial thrombosis and APC resistance via this mutation has been identified. The other diseases listed are associated with bleeding.

9.157 A 30-year-old woman has a history of extensive epistaxis (nose bleeds), and very heavy periods (menorrhagia) except when she was pregnant and when she was taking oral contraceptives. Her father also has nose bleeds and had bled profusely (requiring blood transfusions) during a herniorrhaphy. The patient's 12-year-old daughter has symptoms similar to her mother's, but the son is asymptomatic. The patient is currently asymptomatic. Which of the following tests is MOST likely to be normal?

    A. prothrombin time (PT)

    B. activated partial thromboplastin time (APTT)

    C. bleeding time (BT)

    D. von Willebrand's antigen level (vWF)

    E. ristocetin cofactor assay

A is correct.

vWD is characterized by predominantly mucous membrane hemorrhage such as epistaxis, gastrointestinal hemorrhage, menorrhagia, or postoperative bleeding of variable severity in both men and women. Type I vWD has a pattern of a prolonged BT, normal platelet count, decreased level of factor VIII (hence a prolonged APTT and normal PT), decreased level of vWF, and decreased ristocetin cofactor activity.

9.158 After being hit by a railroad train, a 44-year-old man receives 8 units of packed RBCs as well as the usual and customary fluid replacement. There is oozing from the surgical incision site only and the laboratory results include hemoglobin 13.2 g/dl, platelets 53 000 (normal: 150 000–350 000)/mm^3, hematocrit 40.2 ml/dl, fibrinogen 85 (normal: 150–350) mg/dl, prothrombin time 15 (normal: 10–13) s, and partial thromboplastin time 55 (normal: 27–37) s; the D-dimer is markedly elevated. The MOST likely etiology of this patient's problem is:

    A. disseminated intravascular coagulation

    B. dilutional decrease in factor concentration

    C. factor VII deficiency

    D. von Willebrand's disease

    E. heparin administration

A is correct.

The pattern of laboratory results in acute disseminated intravascular coagulation includes prolongation of PT and PTT, decreases in platelets and fibrinogen, and marked increases in the D-dimer.

9.159 A 75-year-old patient chronically receiving warfarin is brought to the emergency room with acute profuse, bright red, rectal bleeding. The initial impression is that the cause of the bleeding is a large overdose of warfarin. Which of the following tests is LEAST expected to be abnormal?

    A. prothrombin time (PT)

    B. hemoglobin

    C. partial thromboplastin time (PTT)

    D. factor VII level

    E. thrombin time (TT)

E is correct.

The hemoglobin level falls because of bleeding. Warfarin inhibits the synthesis of vitamin K-dependent proteins by the liver, including factors II, VII, IX, and X. Shortly after initiation of warfarin therapy, the PT becomes prolonged because of the rapid fall in factor VII activity. Several days later, there is then an increase in APTT as factors II, IX, and X are decreased. Thrombin (clotting) time remains unaffected by treatment with warfarin, but is prolonged with heparin treatment.

9.160 Which of the following inactivates factors Va and VIIIa?

    A. protein C

    B. protein S

    C. factor XIII

    D. factor VII

    E. factor VIII

    F. factor III

    G. factor XI

    H. factor IV

    I. plasmin

A is correct.

Factors Va and VIIIa are inactivated by protein C. Protein C is activated by thrombin bound to endothelial cell-associated thrombomodulin. Protein S is a cofactor for the anticoagulant function of activated protein C.

9.161 Which of the following cross-links fibrin molecules?

    A. protein C

    B. protein S

    C. factor XIII

    D. factor VII

    E. factor VIII

    F. factor III

    G. factor XI

    H. factor IV

    I. plasmin

C is correct.

Factor XIII, the fibrin-stabilizing factor, when activated by thrombin in the presence of calcium ions, may cause several cross-linked complexes such as the fibrin–fibrin and fibrin–fibrinogen complexes. The 5 M urea screening test is able to determine severe deficiency of factor XIII. If the plasma clot dissolves in 5 M urea, then the fibrin has not been cross-linked by factor XIII.

9.162   Which of the following is a cofactor for protein C?

   A. protein C
   B. protein S
   C. factor XIII
   D. factor VII
   E. factor VIII
   F. factor III
   G. factor XI
   H. factor IV
   I. plasmin

B is correct.
Protein S is a vitamin K-dependent plasma glycoprotein synthesized in hepatocytes and endothelial cells. It is a cofactor for the anticoagulation function of activated protein C in the inactivation of factors Va and VIIIa. A hereditary deficiency of protein S is associated with a thrombotic tendency.

9.163   Which of the following releases D-dimers by acting on cross-linked fibrin?

   A. protein C
   B. protein S
   C. factor XIII
   D. factor VII
   E. factor VIII
   F. factor III
   G. factor XI
   H. factor IV
   I. plasmin

I is correct.
Plasmin acts on cross-linked fibrin to produce D-dimers. The D-dimer test detects the action of plasmin on cross-linked fibrin, but not on fibrinogen or the monomer complexes.

9.164   Which of the following binds to von Willebrand's factor?

   A. protein C
   B. protein S
   C. factor XIII
   D. factor VII
   E. factor VIII
   F. factor III
   G. factor XI
   H. factor IV
   I. plasmin

E is correct.
vWF binds to factor VIII in a non-covalent complex to stabilize and protect factor VIII against rapid removal from the circulation.

9.165   A 22-year-old man is brought to the emergency room because of chest pain, mild hemoptysis, and shortness of breath. Examination reveals a positive Homans' sign. This is the third episode of deep vein thrombosis for this patient. His family history reveals that his father had a mesenteric vein thrombosis at age 45 years and the patient's brother had DVT at age 20 years. All of the following diagnoses need to be eliminated from the differential diagnosis EXCEPT:

   A. decreased protein C
   B. decreased protein S
   C. resistance of activated protein C
   D. increased factor VII
   E. decreased antithrombin III

D is correct.
Factor VII is part of the procoagulant system whereas proteins C and S, and antithrombin III, belong to the inhibitor system. Therefore, resistance to activated protein C, or decreases in protein C, protein S or antithrombin III are all associated with a thrombotic tendency. Reduced levels of factor VII are associated with bleeding.

9.166 A 30 year-old man with deep vein thrombosis is also heterozygous for protein C deficiency. He is at increased risk for purpura fulminans when initially treated with:
  A. aspirin
  B. thromboxane
  C. coumarin
  D. desmopressin (DDAVP)
  E. protamine

C is correct.

Coumarin-induced skin necrosis is associated with heterozygous protein C deficiency. The syndrome involves progressive purpuric necrotic skin lesions that appear during the first few days after large loading doses of coumarin (warfarin) due to the rapid depletion of protein C before depression of the other vitamin K-dependent proteins (except factor VII). Acute DVT in known protein C-deficient heterozygotes is treated by, first, giving heparin followed by gradual doses of warfarin until the desired response is achieved before stopping the heparin and, second, transfusion of fresh-frozen plasma as a source of protein C when administering the loading doses of warfarin.

9.167 A 17-year-old woman arrives at the emergency room at 1:00 AM with massive vaginal bleeding as the result of a 'botched' abortion performed the day before. She has petechiae, red urine (hematuria) and fever. You order all of the following laboratory tests on admission EXCEPT:
  A. CBC (with manual smear)
  B. PT and PTT
  C. type and cross-match
  D. blood culture
  E. proteins C and S

E is correct.

The work-up for bleeding and sepsis includes a CBC (with manual smear), PT, PTT, type and cross-match, and blood culture. A deficiency of both protein C and protein S is associated with a thrombotic tendency. As the patient has vaginal bleeding, evaluation of protein C and protein S is not necessary.

9.168 Which of the following is LEAST likely to lead to arterial thrombosis?
  A. lupus anticoagulants
  B. antithrombin III deficiency
  C. homocystinemia
  D. heparin-associated antibody
  E. atherosclerosis

B is correct.

Both hereditary and acquired antithrombin III deficiencies cause thrombosis with subsequent embolization and extension of the venous system, usually the deep veins of the lower extremities, and the iliofemoral, venacaval, renal, axillary, and retinal veins. Arterial thromboses rarely occur with antithrombin III deficiency. Arterial thrombosis may be associated with lupus anticoagulant, homocystinemia, heparin-associated antibody, and atherosclerosis.

9.169 A patient has the following results: platelets 300 000 (normal: 150 000–350 000)/mm^3; bleeding time 12 (normal: 4–8) min. Based on these findings, the MOST likely etiology is:
  A. von Willebrand's disease (vWD)
  B. idiopathic thrombocytopenic purpura (ITP)
  C. factor XII deficiency
  D. factor V deficiency
  E. factor VII deficiency

A is correct.

vWD may present as a normal platelet count, but with a prolonged bleeding time. ITP is associated with a low platelet count. A prolonged bleeding time may be the result of defects in specific components of platelet–vessel interaction and/or platelet–fibrin plug formation.

9.170   Which of the following is NOT a cause of
a. prolonged thrombin time?
    A. heparin
    B. hypofibrinogenemia
    C. disseminated intravascular coagulation
    D. factor XII deficiency
    E. dysfibrinogenemia

D is correct.
The thrombin (clotting) time is assessed by adding
thrombin to citrated plasma (with or without calcium), then measuring the amount and quality of
fibrinogen and the rate of conversion of fibrinogen
to fibrin. Prolongation of thrombin time is seen
in both hypofibrinogenemia and dysfibrinogenemia.
Heparin causes a prolonged thrombin time by
interfering with the thrombin-induced conversion of
fibrinogen to fibrin. DIC produces fibrin degradation products which accumulate in the circulation
and inhibit fibrin formation, thereby causing prolongation of thrombin time. Factor XII deficiency is
not associated with a prolonged thrombin (clotting)
time.

9.171   A 28-year-old man was referred to the special
coagulation laboratory because of the following
clinical history. At ages 21, 24, and 26 years, he was
treated for myocardial infarction secondary to coronary vessel occlusions. At age 27 years, his left leg
was amputated below the knee because of an arterial occlusion. In a work-up for his condition, which
of the following tests are you LEAST likely to
order?
    A. serum homocysteine
    B. APTT
    C. factor V levels
    D. protein S levels
    E. serum cholesterol levels

C is correct.
Hereditary factor V deficiency is a mild-to-moder-
ately severe bleeding disorder and not part of the
thrombosis work-up. An elevated serum cholesterol
level is associated with atherosclerosis, and elevated serum homocysteine results in premature atherosclerosis and arterial or venous thromboembolism.
Protein S deficiency is associated with recurrent
deep vein and arterial thromboses. An APTT test
is prolonged in the presence of fibrin–fibrinogen
degradation products due to DIC and should be
included in the work-up. APTT is also prolonged in
the presence of a lupus anticoagulant, which is associated with thrombosis.

9.172   Which of the following mediates anticoagulant activity by activating protein C?
    A. antithrombin III
    B. thrombomodulin
    C. heparin
    D. tissue factor
    E. nitric oxide

B is correct.
Protein C is activated by thrombin bound to endothelial cell-associated thrombomodulin. As a result
of the binding of thrombin to thrombomodulin,
thrombin can no longer act on its usual substrates –
factors VIII, V, I (fibrinogen) and XIII – but its
activation of protein C is increased by more than a
thousand-fold. Activated protein C has a anticoagulant effect.

9.173   Protein C together with protein S inactivates
which of the following coagulation factors?
    A. Ia and VIIa
    B. IIa and IXa
    C. Va and VIIIa
    D. VIIIa and Xa
    E. XIa and Iva

C is correct.
Activated protein C inactivates factors Va and VIIIa.
Protein C is activated by thrombin bound to endothelial cell-associated thrombomodulin. Protein S is
a cofactor for the anticoagulant function of activated
protein C.

9.174   Activated protein C resistance is associated with a mutation in which of the following factors?

   A. factor X
   B. factor IX
   C. factor V
   D. factor IV
   E. factor XI

C is correct.

Activated protein C resistance is the most common laboratory-based cause of deep vein thrombosis and is associated with a mutation involving a single amino-acid substitution in the coagulation factor V gene. Familial thrombosis has been associated with such APC resistance.

9.175   In the work-up of patients with thrombophilia (thrombotic tendencies), which of the following is the MOST likely finding?

   A. increased antithrombin III
   B. increased protein C
   C. resistance to activated protein C
   D. prolonged PT
   E. loss of platelet glycoprotein (GP) Ib/IX

C is correct.

Resistance to APC is the most common laboratory-based cause of deep vein thrombosis. Decreases in antithrombin III and protein C are associated with a thrombotic tendency. A prolonged PT and the loss of platelet GP Ib are associated with a bleeding tendency.

9.176   The following are frequently associated with bacterial endocarditis EXCEPT:

   A. *Staphylococcus aureus* septicemia
   B. polycythemia
   C. rheumatic heart disease
   D. prosthetic heart valves
   E. intravenous drug abuse

B is correct.

Bacterial endocarditis is associated with *S. aureus* septicemia, rheumatic heart disease, prosthetic heart valves, and intravenous drug abuse. Polycythemia is not associated with bacterial endocarditis.

9.177   All of the following statements regarding von Willebrand's factor (vWF) are true EXCEPT:

   A. vWF is composed of subunits (molecular weight ranging from 250 000 to 20×10^6 daltons)
   B. vWF binds to GP Ib
   C. vWF binds to collagen
   D. vWF binds to factor VIII
   E. vWF is a serine esterase

E is correct.

vWF is a large glycoprotein composed of subunits and is not a serine esterase. vWF causes adhesion of platelets to exposed subendothelial collagen by binding at the platelet GP Ib and IIb/IIIa sites. vWF binds to factor VIII in a non-covalent complex which stabilizes and protects factor VIII against rapid removal from the circulation.

9.178   Antithrombin III has all of the following properties EXCEPT:

   A. binds to heparin
   B. produced in the liver
   C. vitamin K-dependent and requires carboxylation
   D. inactivates factor Xa
   E. inactivates factor IIa

C is correct.

Antithrombin III is made in the liver and is a serine protease inhibitor. It inactivates thrombin (factor IIa), and serine protease factors IXa, Xa, XIa, and XIIa, by irreversibly binding to the active serine protease site via an arginine residue. Heparin and vessel wall heparan sulfate bind to the lysine residue on the AT III molecule, causing a conformational change in the AT III molecule, resulting in an instantaneous inactivation of thrombin (factor IIa). AT III is not a vitamin K-dependent protein whereas factors II, VII, IX, and X, and proteins C and S, are. Vitamin K is an essential cofactor for the synthesis of these coagulation proteins.

9.179 The most common type of von Willebrand's disease (vWD) is:

A. pseudo-vWD
B. type IIa
C. type IIb
D. type I
E. type Normandy

D is correct.
The most common type of vWD is type I, in which all vWF multimers are present, but with a quantitative multimer deficiency. Type I vWD responds to desmopressin (DDAVP), which causes a rise in the level of vWF and factor VIII. DDAVP is contraindicated in type IIb vWD.

9.180 Major contributions to the anticoagulant properties of endothelial cells are thought to be related to the function of all of the following molecules EXCEPT:

A. antithrombin III
B. thrombomodulin
C. heparin
D. tissue factor
E. nitric oxide

D is correct.
Tissue factor is part of the extrinsic pathway of the procoagulant system and is not involved in the anticoaguant properties of endothelial cells. Tissue factor is expressed on damaged endothelial cells and, in the presence of factor VII and calcium ions, initiates fibrin formation. An anticoagulant mechanism limits and localizes the hemostatic plug to the site of blood vessel injury. Heparin increases AT III inactivation of factors IIa, IXa, Xa, XIa, and XIIa, which inhibits clot formation. Nitric oxide is generated by the smooth muscle in many blood vessels, and allows the vessels to relax and dilate and, thus, does not favor clot formation. Thrombomodulin, associated with endothelial cells, binds thrombin and prevents thrombin from forming clots.

In general, there is a relationship between bleeding time (BT) and platelet count. This relationship is shown in the diagram below.

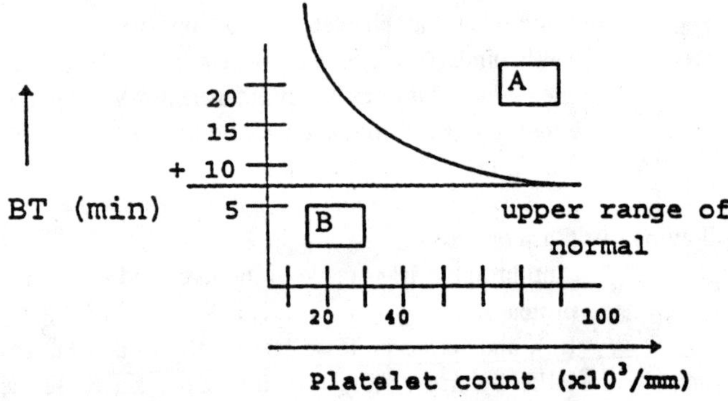

9.181 A patient falls into area A on this graph. His diagnosis is LEAST likely to be consistent with:

A. a healthy subject
B. postcardiac bypass surgery
C. uremia with renal failure
D. aspirin therapy
E. von Willebrand's disease (type I)

A is correct.
Area A includes a platelet count of approximately 100 000 with a markedly prolonged bleeding time of approximately 20 min (range 4–8 min). Such an abnormal bleeding time is not seen in a healthy subject. A prolonged bleeding time may be due to aspirin therapy, postcardiac bypass surgery, uremia with renal failure, and vWD. Aspirin therapy is the most common cause of a prolonged bleeding time when the platelet count is normal.

9.182 Another patient falls into area B on the graph. Her diagnosis is MOST likely to be:
    A. healthy subject
    B. chronic idiopathic thrombocytopenic purpura
    C. uremia with renal failure
    D. acute leukemia with thrombocytopenia (post-chemotherapy)
    E. Bernard–Soulier syndrome

B is correct.
Area B of the graph shows a markedly decreased platelet count with a normal BT (range 4–8 min). This is characteristic of chronic idiopathic thrombocytopenic purpura, wherein the number of blood platelets is decreased, but the platelets are functional. Bernard–Soulier syndrome, uremia with renal failure, and good health are conditions which may show a normal platelet count. Acute leukemia with thrombocytopenia after chemotherapy is associated with a low platelet count with or without non-functional platelets.

9.183 A 78-year-old man presents to the emergency room with atrial fibrillation (treated with warfarin), hematuria (blood in the urine), and melena (blood in the stool). He also has a history of mental problems and erratic nutrition. The set of laboratory results MOST likely to be seen in this patient is:

	PT	PTT	Thrombin time
A.	shortened	shortened	shortened
B.	prolonged	prolonged	shortened
C.	prolonged	shortened	prolonged
D.	prolonged	prolonged	normal
E.	normal	normal	normal

D is correct.
Following the initiation of warfarin therapy, the PT becomes prolonged due to a rapid fall in factor VII activity. Several days later, there is prolongation of the APTT as factors II, IX and X are reduced. Thrombin time is unaffected by warfarin. Based on the history of erratic nutrition, this patient is likely to have a vitamin K deficiency, which causes a greater prolongation of PT and PTT with a normal thrombin time. Warfarin inhibits the synthesis of vitamin K-dependent proteins by the liver, which include factors II, VII, IX and X.

9.184 A 23-year-old woman presents to the obstetrics and gynecological outpatients clinic with an extreme menorrhagia (heavy periods). She has large ecchymoses which develop after light bruising. Her father showed a similar symptom and his father had died due to a hemorrhage during surgery. Her platelet count is normal. The set of laboratory results which is MOST likely to be seen in this patient is:

	PT	PTT	BT	Ristocetin
A.	prolonged	prolonged	prolonged	elevated
B.	normal	prolonged	prolonged	decreased
C.	normal	normal	normal	normal
D.	prolonged	shortened	shortened	normal
E.	shortened	prolonged	normal	elevated

B is correct.
vWD may be characterized by a predominantly mucous membrane hemorrhage such as epistaxis, gastrointestinal hemorrhage, menorrhagia, or post-surgical bleeding of variable severity in both men and women. Type I vWD, the most common type of vWD, has a test pattern of prolonged bleeding time with a normal platelet count, decreased factor VIII level (hence, prolonged APTT and normal PT), decreased vWF, and decreased ristocetin cofactor activity.

9.185 The endothelial cell receptor required for activation of protein C by thrombin is:
    A. tissue factor
    B. glycoprotein Ib/IX
    C. high-molecular-weight kininogen
    D. thrombin receptor
    E. thrombomodulin

E is correct.
The major site of protein C activation is the endothelial cell surface, where thrombin binds to the endothelial cell receptor thrombomodulin. This thrombomodulin–thrombin complex activates protein C.

9.186 The fibrinogen which binds to the surface of platelets and mediates platelet aggregation is derived from synthesis in:
- A. hepatocytes and release from platelet α granules
- B. endothelial cells and release from platelet α granules
- C. hepatocytes and release from endothelial cells
- D. hepatocytes and release from platelet dense granules
- E. hepatocytes and release from platelet lysosomes

A is correct.
Fibrinogen is a glycoprotein, weighing 340 000 daltons, synthesized in hepatocytes and megakaryocytes. Fibrinogen is present in the α granules of platelets and is released during platelet aggregation.

9.187 Which of the following combinations of clinical findings is MOST likely in a patient with 'classical' thrombotic thrombocytopenic purpura?
- A. arthritis, thrombocytopenia, purpuric skin lesions, liver failure, microangiopathic hemolytic anemia
- B. liver failure, thrombocytopenia, back pain, hemolytic anemia
- C. microangiopathic hemolytic anemia, thrombocytopenia, fever, neurologic symptoms, renal disease
- D. hemolytic anemia, thrombocytopenia, decreased LDH
- E. skin rash, hemolytic anemia, arthritis, renal failure

C is correct.
The pentad of findings in 'classical' TTP are microangiopathic hemolytic anemia, thrombocytopenia, fever, neurologic signs and symptoms, and renal disease. There are characteristic RBC changes on the peripheral blood smear, including fragmented cells, schistocytes, and microspherocytes. An increase in LDH is associated with the fragmentation of RBCs.

9.188 The two factors primarily responsible for the widespread activation of the secondary hemostatic system and microvascular thrombosis seen in disseminated intravascular coagulopathy are:
- A. spontaneous platelet aggregation and plasmin activation
- B. immune complex-mediated platelet activation and fibrinogen depletion
- C. tissue injury with tissue factor release and plasmin activation
- D. tissue injury with tissue factor release and endothelial cell injury
- E. endothelial cell injury and toxin-mediated platelet aggregation

D is correct.
The major triggering mechanisms for DIC are tissue injury with tissue factor release and endothelial cell injury.

9.189   The specific combination of factors which MOST contributes to the bleeding diathesis seen in patients with acute and chronic liver diseases is:

    A. decreased synthesis of procoagulant proteins, decreased clearance of inhibitors of fibrin polymerization (FDP and D-dimers) and thrombocytopenia

    B. decreased synthesis of procoagulant proteins, increased fibrinogen synthesis and plasmin activation

    C. decreased synthesis of procoagulant proteins, decreased synthesis of antithrombin III and plasmin activation

    D. increased factor VIII synthesis, platelet dysfunction and increased antiplasmin

    E. increased synthesis of plasminogen, fibrinogen and antiplasmin

A is correct.

The hemostatic defect in acute or chronic liver disease is due to decreased hepatic synthesis of procoagulant proteins, decreased clearance of inhibitors of fibrin polymerization (FDP and D-dimers), and thrombocytopenia (due to hypersplenism). Liver disease is associated with an increase in vWF and factor VIII activity, and a decrease in antithrombin III and protein C. Liver disease also causes platelet dysfunction with prolongation of bleeding time, and reduced hepatic synthesis of α_2-antiplasmin. A decrease in α_2-antiplasmin causes an increase in plasmin activation.

9.190   Adhesion of platelets to subendothelial collagen is mediated by the interaction of the platelet receptor glycoprotein Ib/IX complex and which of the following proteins?

    A. contact factor

    B. platelet factor 4

    C. von Willebrand's factor (vWF)

    D. fibrinogen

    E. tissue-plasminogen activator (t-PA)

C is correct.

vWF is necessary for optimal platelet adhesion to injured vessels. Initial high shear attachment of platelets to subendothelial matrix is due to vWF binding to the GP Ib/IX site on non-activated platelets and vWF binding to the subendothelial collagen.

9.191   Of the following treatments, that which is MOST commonly associated with acquired platelet dysfunction is:

    A. heparin therapy

    B. coumarin (warfarin) therapy

    C. quinidine therapy

    D. aspirin therapy

    E. cephalosporin antibiotic therapy

D is correct.

Aspirin therapy is most commonly associated with acquired platelet dysfunction. Aspirin inhibits platelet aggregation and is used for antiplatelet treatment. By blocking platelet deposition on the surface of disrupted atherosclerotic plaques, aspirin prevents acute vascular occlusion or embolization of thrombotic debris.

9.192   A 12-year-old boy presents with a history of easy bruising and recurrent bleeding into the knee joints. A blood transfusion was necessary following extraction of a tooth when he was 9 years old. Laboratory results show an activated partial thromboplastin time of 108 s (normal: < 40 s) and normal prothrombin and bleeding times. The MOST likely diagnosis for this patient is:

    A. factor II deficiency

    B. von Willebrand's disease (vWD)

    C. factor VIII deficiency

    D. factor VII deficiency

    E. factor XII deficiency

C is correct.

Hemophilia A is due to factor VIII deficiency and is associated with deep muscle and joint hemorrhage, hematoma, easy bruising, and oozing after tooth extraction. Factor VIII deficiency causes a prolonged APTT, but the PT and BT may be normal. In this case, as the bleeding time is normal, vWD is not considered. A factor VII deficiency causes a prolonged PT, and a factor XII deficiency presents as a prolonged APTT in a non-bleeding child or adult. A factor II deficiency causes a prolonged APTT and a prolonged PT. However, in this case, the PT is normal, so factor II deficiency is not the correct answer.

9.193 Which of the following combinations of pro- and anticoagulant proteins requires vitamin K-dependent γ-carboxylation for activation?
    A. factors V, VII, VIII and fibrinogen
    B. factors VI, VII, VII, IX, and X
    C. factors II, VII, IX, X, and proteins C and S
    D. factors II, V, VII, proteins C and S, and plasminogen
    E. factors II, V, X, XI, XII and protein S

C is correct.
Factors II, VII, IX, and X are the vitamin K-dependent procoagulant proteins, and protein C and protein S are the vitamin K-dependent anticoagulant proteins. Vitamin K causes a post-translational modification of specific glutamic acid residues to γ-carboxyglutamic acid which allows calcium binding to negatively charged phospholipid surfaces, resulting in the formation of critical coagulation complexes.

9.194 Which of the following proteins is required for the anticoagulant activity of heparin?
    A. protein C
    B. antiplasmin
    C. α_2-macroglobulin
    D. antithrombin III
    E. tissue factor pathway inhibitor (TFPI)

D is correct.
Heparin is anticoagulative by causing a conformational change in the structure of AT III. Heparin bound to AT III augments AT III inactivation of thrombin (factor IIa) and, to a lesser extent, factors IXa, Xa, XIa, and XIIa.

9.195 The patient presents with marked prolongation of activated partial thromboplastin time (APTT) and thrombin time (TT), and a slight prolongation of prothrombin time (PT). The MOST likely explanation for these findings is:
    A. acquired factor II deficiency
    B. congenital antithrombin III deficiency
    C. plasminogen deficiency
    D. heparin therapy
    E. congenital factor VII deficiency

D is correct.
Heparin enhances the ability of AT III to inactivate factors IIa, IXa, Xa, XIa, and XIIa. Low-dose heparin prolongs the dilute TT; heparin in larger doses prolongs TT and APTT with a slight prolongation of PT.

9.196 Type IIa von Willebrand's disease is characterized by which of the following?
    A. decrease in vWF antigen, normal multimer distribution
    B. low or normal vWF antigen, decrease in high-molecular-weight multimers
    C. decrease in vWF antigen and prolonged PT
    D. decrease in vWF antigen and normal BT
    E. low or normal vWF antigen and prolonged TT

B is correct.
Type IIa vWD is characterized by decreased HMW multimers, normal or decreased vWF antigen, decreased ristocetin cofactor, normal or decreased factor VIII, prolonged BT and APTT, and normal PT.

9.197 Of the following conditions, the MOST common cause of congenital hypercoagulability associated with episodes of recurrent vein thrombosis at a relatively young age is:
    A. antithrombin III deficiency
    B. plasminogen deficiency
    C. activated protein C resistance
    D. activated protein C deficiency
    E. fibrinogen deficiency

C is correct.
APC resistance is the most common laboratory-based cause of deep vein thrombosis. The cause of this resistance is a mutation in the factor V gene resulting in a single amino-acid substitution. There is an association between familial thrombosis and APC resistance by this mutation.

9.198   The MOST frequently encountered and clinically significant sequela of hemophilia A is:
  A. anemia secondary to chronic blood loss
  B. joint deformities and restricted motion secondary to recurrent hemarthrosis
  C. recurrent episodes of obstructive jaundice with pigmented gallstones
  D. renal failure as a result of chronic blood loss in the kidneys
  E. compromise of neurologic function secondary to hemorrhagic strokes

B is correct.

Hemophilia A is caused by a deficiency of factor VIII. The bleeding manifestations in hemophilia A include deep muscle and joint hemorrhages. The latter results in joint deformities and restricted movement secondary to recurrent hemarthrosis.

Transfusion therapy

9.199 A patient's RBCs and serum react as follows on forward and reverse grouping, respectively:

Patient RBCs with test		Patient serum with test	
anti-A	*anti-B*	*A cells*	*B cells*
positive	negative	negative	positive

The patient's ABO type is:
  A. AB
  B. O
  C. Rh-negative
  D. B
  E. A

E is correct.

On forward grouping, there is a positive reaction between the patient's RBCs and anti-A, but a negative reaction with anti-B. Therefore, the patient's RBCs have A antigen. On reverse grouping, there is a negative reaction between the patient's serum and A cells, but a positive reaction with B cells. Therefore, the patient's serum has anti-B. This combination of test results indicates group A blood.

9.200 A patient with hemophilia A presents to the emergency room of a 50-bed hospital with a history and symptoms suggestive of an acute bleeding episode in his right knee. Upon calling the blood bank, it is found that no factor VIII concentrate is available. However, the blood bank technologist tells you that another product is immediately available as a concentrated source of factor VIII. What product is this?
  A. cryoprecipitate
  B. RBCs
  C. fresh-frozen plasma
  D. platelets
  E. albumin

A is correct.

When no factor VIII concentrate is available for the treatment of hemophilia A, then cryoprecipitate may be used as a source of factor VIII. One bag of cryoprecipitate has a volume of 10–25 ml and contains at least 80 U of factor VIII. Cryoprecipitate is a more concentrated source of factor VIII than fresh-frozen plasma, which has a volume of 250 ml and contains 1 U of factor VIII/ml or 250 U in total. Cryoprecipitate is pooled such that 10 bags of cryoprecipitate constitute one pool.

9.201   A patient receiving a platelet transfusion becomes hypotensive, has respiratory collapse and is unresponsive 5 min after initiation of the transfusion. The transfusion is stopped, the patient is treated with fluids and epinephrine, and recovers without lasting sequelae. What type of transfusion reaction is this, and what is the MOST likely cause?

    A. febrile reaction due to leukocyte antibodies

    B. anaphylactic reaction due to antibody to IgA

    C. acute hemolytic transfusion reaction due to RBC antibodies

    D. allergic reaction to the blood bag

B is correct.

An anaphylactic reaction occurs when an IgA-deficient patient, who has developed antibody to IgA by sensitization from transfusion or pregnancy, is transfused with a donor blood component which has plasma containing IgA. Prevention of an anaphylactic reaction may be accomplished by: 1) removing all IgA-containing plasma from the donor blood component before transfusion by saline washing of RBCs or platelet products; or 2) transfusing blood components (FFP or cryoprecititate) from donors without IgA in their plasma. Approximately 1 in 700 Caucasians are IgA-deficient, but only 1 in 150 000 develops anti-IgA and has an anaphylactic reaction on tranfusion of donor blood components containing plasma with IgA. An anaphylactoid reaction has the same clinical presentation, with the recipient being hypersensitive to a protein in the donor plasma, but the reaction is not IgA antibody-mediated.

9.202 A patient's RBCs and serum react as follows on forward and reverse grouping, respectively:

| *Patient RBCs with test* | | *Patient serum with test* | |
anti-A	*anti-B*	*A cells*	*B cells*
positive	positive	negative	negative

The patient's ABO type is:

    A. O

    B. A

    C. B

    D. Rh-positive

    E. AB

E is correct.

On forward grouping, there is a positive reaction between the patient's RBCs and anti-A, and a positive reaction with anti-B. Therefore, the patient's RBCs have both A and B antigens. On reverse grouping, there is a negative reaction between the patient's serum and A cells, and a negative reaction with B cells. Therefore, the patient's serum has neither anti-A nor anti-B. This combination of test results indicates group AB blood.

9.203 A patient reports a history of hemophilia B (Christmas disease). He is to undergo a total knee replacement. His hematocrit is 42 (normal: 40–50) ml/dl, platelet count is 258 000 (normal: 150 000–350 000) mm^3, prothrombin time is 11.2 (normal: 10–13) s and activated partial thromboplastin time 52 (normal: 23–35) s. What is the MOST appropriate component to ensure adequate hemostasis during surgery?

    A. RBCs

    B. factor VIII concentrate

    C. cryoprecipitate

    D. platelets

    E. factor IX concentrate

E is correct.

Factor IX concentrate is the treatment for hemophilia B. There are plasma-derived factor IX concentrates which are highly purified (monoclonal or chromatographically purified) products that contain only factor IX, and are free of hepatitis and HIV viruses. Also, there is a recombinant factor IX concentrate that is free of viruses. Approximately 3% of hemophilia B patients develop a factor IX inhibitor in addition to factor IX deficiency. These patients may be treated with prothrombin-complex concentrate (PCC) products such as FEIBA (Immuno) or Autoplex-T (Baxter).

9.204 The MOST common cause of an acute hemolytic transfusion reaction is:
   A. plasma infusion
   B. clerical or patient identification error
   C. disseminated intravascular coagulation (DIC)
   D. platelet transfusion
   E. volume overload

B is correct.
Clerical or patient identification error is the most common cause of an acute hemolytic transfusion reaction. An acute hemolytic transfusion reaction occurs shortly after the transfusion of incompatible RBCs. A fatal acute hemolytic transfusion reaction occurs 1 in 100 000 transfusions. Improper patient identification is the major cause of transfusion death.

9.205 A patient with documented iron deficiency anemia who is asymptomatic is BEST treated with:
   A. transfusion of whole blood
   B. transfusion of RBCs
   C. oral iron supplementation
   D. transfusion of cryoprecipitate

C is correct.
Oral iron supplementation is the correct treatment for documented iron deficiency anemia. When there is time to use hematinics, such as iron for iron deficiency anemia, to promote erythropoiesis, this is preferable to transfusion of either whole blood or RBCs, which carry a transfusion-transmitted disease risk for hepatitis and HIV.

9.206 Blood components are irradiated:
   A. to kill intracellular viruses
   B. to inactivate coagulation-factor inhibitors
   C. to prevent graft *vs* host disease (GVHD) in immunocompromised recipients
   D. to sterilize the components

C is correct.
Only gamma irradiation with 2500 rads to cellular blood components (whole blood, RBCs, random donor platelets, plateletpheresis and leukapheresis products) prevents transfusion-associated (TA) GVHD. Neither leukocyte reduction nor saline washing of blood components is able to prevent TA-GVHD. The T lymphocytes in the cellular blood components are the cause of TA-GVHD. Leukocyte reduction or saline washing only partially removes the T lymphocytes present whereas gamma irradiation inactivates nearly all of them. Blood components from any blood relative must be gamma-irradiated to prevent TA-GVHD.

9.207 Leukocyte reduction of packed RBCs achieves all of the following EXCEPT:
   A. prevents repeated non-hemolytic febrile transfusion reactions
   B. reduces immunosuppression of recipient by donor WBCs
   C. prevents graft *vs* host disease
   D. delays HLA (human leukocyte antigen) alloimmunization
   E. renders the blood product equivalent to a cytomegalovirus seronegative blood product

C is correct.
Leukocyte reduction cannot prevent TA-GVHD, which can only be achieved by gamma irradiation. However, leukocyte reduction: 1) prevents repeated non-hemolytic febrile transfusion reactions; 2) reduces immunosuppression of recipient due to donor WBCs; 3) delays HLA alloimmunization; and 4) renders the blood product equivalent to a CMV seronegative blood product.

9.208 All of the following statements concerning Rh (D) hemolytic disease of the newborn are true EXCEPT:
  A. the father is D-positive and the mother is D-negative
  B. develops anti-D due to either blood transfusion or pregnancy
  C. maternal IgG anti-D crosses the placenta and affects the second D-positive pregnancy
  D. anti-D formation in the mother is prevented by Rh_0 (D) immune globulin (RhoGAM™) administration
  E. maternal IgM anti-D crosses the placenta and affects the D-positive pregnancy

E is correct.

In Rh (D) hemolytic disease of the newborn, the mother is D-negative and, during the first pregnancy of a D-positive fetus, the D-positive RBCs of the fetus cross the placenta and sensitize the mother. During the second pregnancy of a D-positive fetus, the D antibody in the mother, which is IgG, crosses the placenta and causes lysis of the D-positive RBCs of the fetus. RhoGAM is IgG anti-D and destroys the D-positive RBCs of the fetus in the maternal circulation before the D-negative mother becomes sensitized and produces D antibody. The D-negative mother is also able to make anti-D after being transfused with D-positive RBCs.

9.209 Cryoprecipitate can be transfused to replace all of the following EXCEPT:
  A. von Willebrand factor (vWF)
  B. factor VII
  C. factor VIII
  D. factor XIII
  E. fibrinogen

B is correct.

Cyroprecipitate is a source of vWF for the treatment of vWD, factor VIII for the treatment of hemophilia A, factor XIII for treatment of factor XIII deficiency, and fibrinogen for treatment of decreased fibrinogen. Cryoprecipitate is not a source of factor VII. Fresh-frozen plasma is a source of factor VII, with 1U/ml. The preferred product for factor VII deficiency will be recombinant factor VII concentrate as soon as it becomes available in the United States.

9.210 What is the only transfusion reaction that, once treated, the blood that is already hanging can be restarted?
  A. non-hemolytic febrile transfusion reaction
  B. septic transfusion reaction
  C. allergic (urticarial) transfusion reaction
  D. transfusion-related acute lung injury
  E. acute hemolytic transfusion reaction

C is correct.

In an allergic (urticarial) transfusion reaction, a protein (antigen) in the donor's plasma corresponds to an IgE antibody in the recipient, causing the release of histamine from the recipient's mast cells and the formation of hives. If the hives subside with either oral or intravenous diphenhydramine hydrochloride (Benadryl™) administration and there are no other presenting symptoms, then the blood component causing the allergic (urticarial) transfusion reaction can be restarted. Of the more than 20 types of transfusion reactions, this is only one in which restarting the blood which is already hanging is possible. A transfusion-reaction work-up is not required for an urticarial transfusion reaction (where hives is the only clinical symptom).

9.211   Which of the following is transfused on an emergency basis if blood is needed for a patient who is bleeding profusely and the blood type is unknown?

  A. group A, Rh-positive
  B. group O, Rh-positive
  C. group B, Rh-negative
  D. group O, Rh-negative
  E. group A, Rh-negative

D is correct.

Group O Rh-negative uncrossmatched RBCs should be transfused first in an emergency to a patient who is bleeding profusely. Around 10 min later, the recipient's ABO group and Rh type becomes known and group-specific uncrossmatched RBCs can then be transfused. Thus, if the recipient is group A Rh-positive, the recipient then receives group A Rh-positive uncrossmatched RBCs. Crossmatching means that no agglutination occurs when two drops of the recipient's serum are added to one drop of the donor's RBCs. After 30 min, crossmatching of blood can be completed, and the recipient is then able to receive group A Rh-positive crossmatched RBCs.

SECTION 10: GASTROINTESTINAL SYSTEM

10.001   Pseudomembranous colitis is associated with which one of the following organisms?
- A. toxigenic strains of *Escherichia coli*
- B. *Entamoeba histolytica*
- C. *Candida albicans*
- D. *Clostridium difficile*
- E. *Yersinia enterocolitica*

D is correct.

Psudomembranous colitis is characterized by the formation of an inflammatory pseudomembrane over areas of mucosal injury. It is usually a result of toxins of *C. difficile*, a normal gut commensal. It usually occurs after a course of broad-spectrum antibiotic therapy.

10.002   All of the following are true of carcinoid tumor EXCEPT:
- A. may be hormonally active
- B. lesions occurring in the appendix and rectum frequently show highly malignant behavior
- C. contains neurosecretory granules with affinity for silver salts
- D. arises from immature endocrine or neuroendocrine cells

B is correct.

Appendiceal and rectal carcinoids rarely metastasize, even though there may be prominent local spread. Ninety percent of carcinoids originating in the ileum, stomach and colon that have penetrated halfway through the muscle wall will have spread to lymph nodes and distant sites at the time of diagnosis.

10.003   Granulomatous inflammation is seen in which one of the following diseases?
- A. Crohn's disease
- B. ulcerative colitis
- C. pseudomembranous colitis
- D. familial polyposis

A is correct.

Non-caseating granulomas are present in around half of the patients with Crohn's disease.

10.004 Barrett's esophagus is associated with which one of the following diseases?
- A. adenocarcinoma
- B. squamous carcinoma
- C. lymphoma
- D. fibroma

A is correct.

Barrett's esophagus is a complication of long-standing gastroesophageal reflux. The distal squamous mucosa of the esophagus is replaced by metaplastic columnar epithelium. There is an associated dysplasia of this metaplastic mucosa which may progress to adenocarcinoma.

10.005   All of the following would be expected to cause symptoms of malabsorption EXCEPT:
- A. Whipple's disease
- B. Hirschsprung's disease
- C. celiac disease
- D. disaccharidase deficiency
- E. abetalipoproteinemia

B is correct.

Hirschsprung's disease (congenital aganglionic megacolon) is characterized by the absence of ganglion cells in the muscle wall and submucosa of affected segments of the colon. This leads to a functional obstruction with colonic dilation proximal to the involved segment. The small bowel, where most absorption occurs, is not affected. All of the other diseases listed are typically associated with malabsorption syndromes.

10.006 All of the following are characteristics of ulcerative colitis EXCEPT:
   A. crypt abscesses
   B. rectal involvement
   C. skip lesions
   D. increased risk of colonic adenocarcinoma
   E. increased incidence of liver disease

C is correct.
Typical findings in ulcerative colitis include an ulceroinflammatory disease extending in a continuous manner proximal from the rectum. Skip lesions are typical of Crohn's disease. There is an increased incidence of primary sclerosing cholangitis in patients with ulcerative colitis.

10.007 Which of the following polyps is a type of neoplastic polyp?
   A. tubular adenoma
   B. juvenile polyp
   C. Peutz-Jeghers polyp
   D. hyperplastic polyp
   E. inflammatory polyp

A is correct.
Tubular adenomas are polypoid neoplasms. The other polyps listed are non-neoplastic polyps.

10.008 Colonic adenocarcinoma has been found to be associated with all of the following dietary factors EXCEPT:
   A. high fat intake
   B. low intake of vegetable fiber
   C. high intake of refined carbohydrates
   D. deficiency of vitamins A and C

D is correct.
High fat intake, low intake of fiber, and high intake of refined carbohydrates are all implicated in an increased risk of colonic adenocarcinoma. No association has been found with any vitamin deficiencies.

10.009 The majority of tubular adenomas are located in the:
   A. esophagus
   B. stomach
   C. jejunum
   D. ileum
   E. colon

E is correct.
Around 90% of tubular adenomas are located in the colon.

10.010 *Helicobacter pylori* is implicated as an etiologic factor in all of the following diseases EXCEPT:
   A. chronic gastritis
   B. gastric peptic ulcer
   C. duodenal peptic ulcer
   D. hypertrophic gastritis

D is correct.
Helicobacter pylori has not been implicated in the pathogenesis of hypertrophic gastritis.

10.011 A low-fiber high-fat diet has been etiologically implicated in which one of the following diseases?
   A. carcinoid tumor
   B. colonic adenocarcinoma
   C. gastric peptic ulcer
   D. celiac sprue

B is correct.
Dietary factors which have been implicated as predisposing to carcinoma of the colon include low fiber intake, and high intake of refined carbohydrates and fat.

10.012 Which one of the following diseases is associated with macrocytic anemia?
  A. autoimmune chronic gastritis
  B. duodenal peptic ulcer
  C. pyloric stenosis
  D. ulcerative colitis
  E. Barrett's esophagus

A is correct.
In autoimmune chronic gastritis, there are autoantibodies to gastric parietal cells and intrinsic factor. The loss of production of intrinsic factor leads to pernicious anemia.

10.013 Which of the following diseases typically presents with vomiting at 2–3 weeks of age?
  A. autoimmune chronic gastritis
  B. duodenal peptic ulcer
  C. pyloric stenosis
  D. hypertrophic gastritis
  E. Barrett's esophagus

C is correct.
Congenital hypertrophic pyloric stenosis is a condition resulting from hypertrophy and hyperplasia of the muscularis propria of the pylorus. Its obstructive nature causes persistent projectile vomiting, usually starting around the second or third week of life.

10.014 Barrett's esophagus is associated with all of the following EXCEPT:
  A. occurs in the distal third of the esophagus
  B. secondary to long-standing gastroesophageal reflux
  C. histological evidence of mucosal metaplasia
  D. increased incidence of squamous carcinoma in affected areas

D is correct.
The long-standing gastroesophageal reflux stimulates a metaplastic response in the lower esophagus. Squamous epithelial cells are replaced by gastric- or intestinal-type epithelium, which is more resistant to injury by the refluxed gastric contents. These foci may be the site of adenocarcinomas of the esophagus.

10.015 Which one of the following diseases is MOST likely to respond to antibiotic therapy?
  A. ulcerative colitis
  B. Crohn's disease
  C. Whipple's disease
  D. celiac sprue
  E. ischemic colitis

C is correct.
In Whipple's disease, rod-shaped bacilli are present in distended macrophages in the lamina propria. These bacilli have been identified as the actinomycete *Tropheryma whippelii*. Appropriate antibiotic therapy produces a dramatic response.

10.016 Which one of the following diseases typically begins in the rectum?
  A. ulcerative colitis
  B. Crohn's disease
  C. Whipple's disease
  D. celiac sprue
  E. ischemic colitis

A is correct.
Ulcerative colitis is an inflammatory disease generally limited to the mucosa and submucosa. It typically begins in the rectum and extends proximally in a retrograde fashion. In severe cases, it may involve the entire colon.

10.017 Fistula formation is MOST likely to occur in which one of the following diseases?
  A. ulcerative colitis
  B. Crohn's disease
  C. Whipple's disease
  D. celiac sprue
  E. ischemic colitis

B is correct.
Crohn's disease is an inflammatory disease with transmural involvement of the bowel. This transmural involvement predisposes to the formation of fistulae.

10.018   Which one of the following diseases is MOST closely associated with advanced atherosclerosis?
   A. ulcerative colitis
   B. Crohn's disease
   C. Whipple's disease
   D. celiac sprue
   E. ischemic colitis

E is correct.
In severe atherosclerosis, involvement of the aorta and major branches, such as the arteries supplying the bowel, may result in ischemia to organs. The atherosclerotic narrowing itself may be sufficient to cause ischemic changes, or there may be superimposed thrombi which will further reduce blood flow. Emboli may also form.

10.019   Defective innervation of the bowel is a characteristic feature of which one of the following diseases?
   A. Whipple's disease
   B. Wilson's disease
   D. Hirschsprung's disease
   E. celiac sprue

D is correct.
In Hirschsprung's disease (congenital aganglionic megacolon), a segment of colon lacks both Meissner's submucosal and Auerbach's myenteric plexuses. This loss of neuronal coordination leads to a functional obstruction with dilation of the colon proximal to the affected segment.

10.020   All of the following conditions are associated with ulcerative colitis EXCEPT:
   A. toxic megacolon
   B. inflammatory pseudopolyps
   C. adenocarcinoma
   D. granulomas
   E. crypt abscesses

D is correct.
Granulomas are not a feature of ulcerative colitis. The usual picture is an ulceroinflammatory process affecting the mucosa and submucosa of the colon.

10.021   Factors important in the pathogenesis of adenocarcinoma of the colon include all of the following EXCEPT:
   A. high intake of dietary fiber
   B. activation of *ras* oncogene
   C. deletion of p53 tumor suppressor gene
   D. high intake of dietary fat

A is correct.
A diet low in indigestible fiber and high in animal fat are believed to be contributory to the development of carcinoma of the colon. A high intake of dietary fiber is believed to have some protective influence against the development of colon cancer.

10.022   The BEST treatment plan for celiac disease is:
   A. antibiotic therapy
   B. surgery
   C. dietary alteration
   D. immunosuppressive / anti-inflammatory
      agents
   E. radiation

C is correct.
Celiac sprue improves when wheat gliadins and related grain proteins are removed from the diet. The fundamental disorder is a sensitivity to gluten.

10.023 The BEST treatment plan for Hirschsprung's disease is:
   A. antibiotic therapy
   B. surgery
   C. dietary alteration
   D. immunosuppressive / anti-inflammatory
      agents
   E. radiation

B is correct.
Hirschsprung's disease or congenital aganglionic megacolon is characterized by an absence of ganglion cells in a bowel segment. The loss of enteric neuronal coordination leads to a functional obstruction. Surgical removal of the affected segment of bowel corrects the problem.

10.024   The BEST treatment plan for Whipple's disease is:
  A. antibiotic therapy
  B. surgery
  C. dietary alteration
  D. immunosuppressive / anti-inflammatory
     agents
  E. radiation

A is correct.
In Whipple's disease, rod-shaped bacilli called *Tropheryma whippelii* are found in macrophages in the lamina propria of the small intestinal mucosa. The disease responds promptly to antibiotic therapy.

10.025   The BEST treatment plan for Crohn's disease is:
  A. antibiotic therapy
  B. surgery
  C. dietary alteration
  D. immunosuppressive / anti-inflammatory
     agents
  E. radiation

D is correct.
Crohn's disease, an inflammatory bowel disease, is an idiopathic disorder. No causative organisms have been identified, and the current therapy includes immunosuppressive and/or anti-inflammatory agents.

10.026 The BEST treatment plan for hypertrophic pyloric stenosis is:
  A. antibiotic therapy
  B. surgery
  C. dietary alteration
  D. immunosuppressive / anti-inflammatory
     agents
  E. radiation

B is correct.
Congenital hypertrophic pyloric stenosis is a result of hypertrophy and hyperplasia of the muscularis propria of the pylorus. Surgical splitting of the muscle at the site of involvement is curative.

10.027   Hyperplastic gastric polyps are MOST likely to be found in association with which one of the following conditions?
  A. gastric carcinoma
  B. familial polyposis syndrome
  C. chronic gastritis
  D. Crohn's disease
  E. ulcerative colitis

C is correct.
Gastric polyps are not common. When they occur, they are usually hyperplastic polyps consisting of hyperplastic mucosal epithelium over an inflamed edematous stroma. They are most often seen in association with the chronic mucosal damage found in chronic gastritis.

10.028 Which one of the following diseases is often accompanied by severe loss of plasma proteins?
  A. autoimmune gastritis
  B. chronic idiopathic gastritis
  C. infectious gastritis
  D. hypertrophic gastropathy
  E. acute gastritis

D is correct.
Hypertrophic gastropathy, or Ménétrier's disease, is associated with marked hyperplasia of the surface mucous cells and accompanying glandular atrophy. In some patients, there is marked protein loss in the gastric secretions that produce hypoalbuminemia.

10.029 Which one of the following diseases may be caused by aspirin use?
  A. autoimmune gastritis
  B. chronic idiopathic gastritis
  C. infectious gastritis
  D. hypertrophic gastropathy
  E. acute gastritis

E is correct.
Acute gastritis is frequently associated with heavy use of non-steroidal anti-inflammatory drugs, especially aspirin.

10.030   Which one of the following is a type of hamartomatous polyp?
   A. Peutz–Jeghers polyp
   B. adenomatous polyp
   C. villous adenoma
   D. tubular adenoma

A is correct.
Peutz–Jeghers syndrome is a type of familial polyposis characterized by hamartomatous polyps.

10.031   Which one of the following types of polypoid lesion has the MOST significant malignant potential?
   A. Peutz–Jeghers polyp
   B. adenomatous polyp
   C. villous adenoma
   D. tubular adenoma

C is correct.
The risk of cancer approaches 40% in villous adenomas >4 cm in diameter.

10.032   The presence of liver metastases leads to the development of a syndrome of flushing, diarrhea, and tachycardia in which one of the following?
   A. gastrointestinal lymphoma
   B. Kaposi's sarcoma
   C. carcinoid tumor
   D. adenocarcinoma arising in familial polyposis
   E. adenocarcinoma arising in villous adenoma

C is correct.
Carcinoid tumor cells resemble the neuroendocrine cells of the gut and have the capacity to synthesize and secrete bioactive substances. Excess production of serotonin by the tumor cells is responsible for the symptomatology of flushing, diarrhea, and tachycardia. The carcinoid syndrome usually does not develop in the absence of hepatic metastases.

10.033   The MOST common cause of esophagitis is:
   A. ingestion of irritants
   B. cytotoxic anticancer therapy
   C. fungal infection in debilitated patients
   D. gastric reflux
   E. radiation

D is correct.
By far, the most frequent cause of esophagitis is reflux of gastric contents.

10.034   True statements regarding hiatal hernia include all of the following EXCEPT:
   A. paraesophageal (rolling) form is more common than the sliding form
   B. reflux esophagitis is seen commonly in association with hiatal hernia
   C. most sliding hiatal hernias are asymptomatic
   D. complications of hiatal hernia include perforation and ulceration
   E. cause of hiatal hernia is unknown

A is correct.
There are two types of hiatal hernias: sliding; and paraesophageal. The sliding hernia constitutes 95% of cases of hiatal hernia.

10.035 A 62-year-old woman presents with weight loss, abdominal pain, and anorexia. Based on endoscopic biopsy, you make the diagnosis of gastric carcinoma. True statements regarding this disease process include each of the following EXCEPT:
  A. prognosis depends more on depth of invasion than histologic type
  B. dietary carcinogens are suspected to be prime offenders
  C. partial gastrectomy patients are at increased risk for development of gastric carcinoma
  D. *Helicobacter pylori* appears to serve as a cofactor in gastric carcinogenesis of the intestinal type
  E. frequency of the diffuse-type gastric carcinoma has decreased in the last 60 years

E is correct.
The frequency of diffuse gastric carcinoma has not significantly changed over the past 60 years.

10.036 True statements regarding colorectal carcinoma include each of the following EXCEPT:
  A. cancers in the large intestine are almost always adenocarcinomas
  B. tumors in the proximal colon tend to be annular, inducing 'napkin-ring' constrictions
  C. high dietary fat intake is a risk factor
  D. the most important prognostic indicator is the stage at the time of diagnosis
  E. when diagnosed in a young person, preexisting ulcerative colitis or a polyposis syndrome is to be suspected

B is correct.
Carcinomas of the ascending colon and cecum tend to be polypoid masses whereas those of the distal colon are more likely to be annular, encircling lesions.

10.037 Variants of hypertrophic gastritis are associated with all of the following features EXCEPT:
  A. hyperplasia of parietal and chief cells in gastric glands
  B. hyperplasia of surface mucous cells with glandular atrophy
  C. gastrinomas
  D. megaloblastic anemia
  E. hypoalbuminemia

D is correct.
Megaloblastic anemia is a feature of autoimmune gastritis, wherein autoantibodies to gastric gland parietal cells and intrinsic factor are present.

10.038 Each of the following statements correctly characterizes acute appendicitis EXCEPT:
  A. mainly a disease of adolescents and young adults
  B. clinically mimicked by mesenteric lymphadenitis
  C. accompanied by luminal obstruction in most cases
  D. diagnosed histologically by the presence of neutrophils in the lumen
  E. presents typically with right lower-quadrant pain and tenderness

D is correct.
The histologic diagnosis of acute appendicitis is made by identifying neutrophil infiltration of the muscularis of the appendix. The inflammatory exudate may extend to the serosal surface as well.

10.039 A 57-year-old woman presents with vaso-motor disturbances, intestinal hypermotility and asthmatic bronchoconstrictive attacks. Biopsy of an ileal mass shows a tumor composed of nests and cords of uniform cells. True statements regarding this disease process include each of the following EXCEPT:

    A. the overall 5-year survival rate is approximately 10%

    B. elevated levels of 5-hydroxyindoleacetic acid (5-HIAA) are typical in urine

    C. within the gut, the appendix is the most common site of this tumor

    D. this tumor type, when present in the appendix and rectum, rarely metastasizes

    E. this patient probably has hepatic metastases

A is correct.

The 5-year survival rate for patients with carcinoid tumors is about 90%. Even in patients with carcinoids originating in the small intestine with hepatic metastases, the 5-year survival rate is > 50%.

10.040 A 47-year-old executive presents with acute hematemesis. After you have stabilized the patient, you perform gastroduodenal endoscopy and observe a 2 cm-diameter ulcer with non-raised margins on the greater curvature of the stomach. Which of the following is the BEST applicable statement?

    A. location, size, and morphology rule out a malignant tumor

    B. the patient is unlikely to be infected with *Helicobacter pylori*

    C. heaped-up margins around a gastric ulcer are characteristic of benign lesions

    D. biopsy of the gastric antrum along its lesser curvature would probably show chronic gastritis

    E. balance between mucosal defense mechanisms and gastric acid/peptic activity is probably normal

D is correct.

Chronic gastritis occurs in almost all patients with peptic ulcer disease.

10.041 A 72-year-old man presents with lower GI bleeding. Endoscopic examination reveals a single pedunculated polyp, which is removed. Histologic examination reveals an adenomatous polyp with early carcinomatous change limited to the mucosa. What is the most likely probability for a 5-year survival for this patient?

    A. 0%

    B. 10%

    C. 25%

    D. 50%

    E. 100%

E is correct.

Patients with carcinoma of the colon limited to the mucosa have a virtually 100% probability for a 5-year survival after resection.

10.042 Which one of the following organisms has been implicated as a factor in the development of peptic ulcer disease?
  A. *Streptococcus bovis*
  B. *Helicobacter pylori*
  C. *Streptococcus pyogenes*
  D. *Clostridium difficile*

B is correct.
Helicobacter pylori infection of the gastric mucosa is present in 90–100% of patients with duodenal ulcer and in 70% of patients with gastric ulcer.

10.043 Barrett's esophagus is associated with:
  A. an increased risk of squamous cell carcinoma
  B. Crohn's disease
  C. Mallory–Weiss syndrome
  D. a long history of reflux
  E. tracheoesophageal fistula

D is correct.
Chronic reflux of gastric contents into the esophagus results in a metaplastic transformation of the lower esophageal mucosa into columnar epithelium. This epithelium differentiates into either gastric or intestinal types. Dysplasia and even adenocarcinoma may occur in these metaplastic foci.

10.044 A 50-year-old woman presents with pernicious anemia. Gastric endoscopy with biopsy shows thinning of the fundic mucosa. An additional likely finding in the work-up of this patient is:
  A. autoantibodies to gastrin-producing cells (G cells)
  B. hypochlorhydria
  C. marked acute inflammation of the fundic lamina propria
  D. duodenal ulcers
  E. aphthous ulcers of the esophagus

B is correct.
In pernicious anemia, there are antibodies to parietal cells and intrinsic factor. The antibodies to parietal cells include one directed against an acid-producing enzyme. A result is hypochlorhydria, or a reduction of gastric acid.

10.045 Meckel's diverticulum results from:
  A. a congenital defect in the muscular wall of the ileum
  B. excessive intraluminal pressure during vomiting
  C. hiatal herniation with gastric obstruction
  D. incomplete closure of the vitelline duct
  E. acid production by hypertrophic gastric mucosa

D is correct.
The vitelline duct connects the lumen of the gut to the yolk sac during embryogenesis. It usually evolves *in utero*, resulting in a ligamentous cord. Persistence of this duct may give rise to a diverticulum, which is usually within 30 cm of the ileocecal valve.

10.046 The term 'linitis plastica' refers to:
  A. a pipe-like esophagus in scleroderma
  B. a firm gastric wall infiltrated by tumor
  C. mucosal 'puckering' seen around benign peptic ulcers
  D. a dense purulent exudate at a site of appendiceal rupture
  E. linear colonic fissures in Crohn's disease

B is correct.
Linitis plastica or 'leather bottle stomach' is a term used to describe the diffuse thickening of the gastric wall due to infiltration by adenocarcinoma cells. The tumor is usually of the 'signet-ring' type.

10.047 The features of familial adenomatous polyposis include all of the following EXCEPT:
   A. autosomal-dominant inheritance
   B. genetic defect localized to chromosome 5q21
   C. adenomas found in areas of the gastrointestinal tract other than the colon
   D. 25% risk of colonic cancer in patients without prophylactic colectomy
   E. most of the polyps are tubular adenomas

E is correct.
Villous adenomas are large sessile masses. The risk of cancer is around 40% in sessile villous adenomas >4 cm in diameter.

10.048 The MOST important prognostic factor in colon carcinomas is:
   A. Dukes stage
   B. histologic grade
   C. histologic type
   D. pattern of oncogene activation
   E. polypoid *vs* infiltrative growth pattern

A is correct.
The most important factor in determining the prognosis in a patient with colon cancer is the clinical stage, or extent of the tumor. A patient with stage A lesions, which are limited to the mucosa, has essentially a 100% chance for 5-year survival. A patient with C2 lesions (penetrating through the muscularis propria and involving nodes) has only a 23% chance of 5-year survival.

10.049 Exsanguinating hematemesis is MOST commonly associated with:
   A. pyloric stenosis
   B. hepatic cirrhosis
   C. paraesophageal (rolling) hiatal hernia
   D. Schatzki's ring
   E. squamous cell carcinoma

B is correct.
Hepatic cirrhosis is associated with portal hypertension and esophageal varices, which are prone to produce massive hemorrhages. Also, in cirrhosis, the liver fails to manufacture sufficient quantities of many coagulation factors. There may also be a thrombocytopenia secondary to hypersplenism.

10.050 Which one of the following statements is TRUE concerning *Helicobacter pylori* infection?
   A. is associated with gastric, but not duodenal, peptic ulcer disease
   B. does not appear to be a significant risk factor for gastric carcinoma
   C. is commonly asymptomatic
   D. increases gastric acidity
   E. is often transmural in the antral region

C is correct.
Most patients infected with *H. pylori* are asymptomatic.

10.051 The variant of hypertrophic gastropathy termed Ménétrier's disease is characterized by:
   A. abnormal autonomic innervation of the gastric cardia
   B. hypertrophy of gastric muscularis
   C. increased gastric mucus secretion
   D. inflammation of gastric crypts
   E. pyloric outlet obstruction

C is correct.
This form of hypertrophic gastritis is characterized by a marked hyperplasia of the surface mucous cells along with glandular atrophy.

10.052 A 60-year-old woman at 1 year postmyocardial infarction presents with severe abdominal pain, nausea, and vomiting. Exploratory laparoscopy reveals a sharply defined segment of colonic serosal hemorrhage at the splenic flexure. The MOST likely etiology is:
  A. embolic occlusion of the superior mesenteric artery
  B. use of vasoactive drugs (such as propranolol)
  C. ulcerative colitis
  D. angiodysplasia
  E. hypoperfusion due to cardiac failure

A is correct.
The sharp demarcation of the affected segment of bowel suggests an ischemic infarct. A mural thrombus in the left ventricle may have developed, resulting in embolization.

10.053 A distinctive feature of ulcerative colitis is:
  A. granuloma formation
  B. deep linear ulcers
  C. pseudopolyps
  D. fistulas
  E. skip lesions

C is correct.
Areas of regenerating mucosa adjacent to ulcerous areas bulge upwards, creating pseudopolyps.

10.054 The pathogenesis of celiac sprue involves:
  A. a rod-shaped organism recently identified as *Tropheryma* species
  B. acquisition of infection in tropical climes
  C. antibodies against a normal food component
  D. deficiency of a specific disaccharidase enzyme
  E. loss of ganglion cells

C is correct.
Celiac sprue is due to a sensitivity to gluten in the diet. It is thought that genetic susceptibility and immune-mediated intestinal injury play a role in the pathogenesis of this disease.

10.055 Signet-ring cells are characteristic of:
  A. esophageal squamous cell carcinoma
  B. diffuse infiltrating gastric adenocarcinoma
  C. intestinal lymphoma
  D. carcinoid tumor
  E. colonic adenocarcinoma

B is correct.
Although signet-ring cells may occasionally be seen in any mucin-secreting adenocarcinoma, diffuse infiltrating gastric adenocarcinomas are characteristically composed of large numbers of signet-ring cells.

10.056 Gastrointestinal carcinoid tumors produce the 'carcinoid syndrome' only in the presence of:
  A. a host antitumor humoral response
  B. hepatic metastases
  C. intestinal obstruction
  D. tumor necrosis
  E. tumor insulin secretion

B is correct.
This syndrome is thought to arise from excess secretion of serotonin. The liver normally degrades serotonin into a functionally inactive compound. The serotonin secreted by intestinal carcinoids which have not metastasized is carried to the liver, via the portal vein, where it is metabolized. Metastases to the liver may secrete serotonin, which then has gained access to the hepatic venous outflow and may then reach the systemic circulation.

10.057 A 20-year-old man presents with multiple osteomas of the skull and epidermal cysts. Colonoscopy reveals approximately 200 adenomatous polyps. Features consistent with the diagnosis for this patient include:
  A. almost certain colonic carcinoma within 15 years without colectomy
  B. autosomal-recessive inheritance
  C. polyps which have predominantly villous features
  D. coexistent gastric hamartomas
  E. increased incidence of XXY karyotype

A is correct.
Gardner's syndrome consists of familial adenomatous polyposis, which is an autosomal-dominant condition, together with multiple osteomas, epidermal cysts, and fibromatosis. The frequency of developing adenocarcinoma of the colon approaches 100% with this syndrome.

10.058 Loss of myenteric ganglion cells may result in:
  A. esophageal dilation
  B. gastric sclerosis and atrophy
  C. hiatal hernia
  D. colonic polyps
  E. rectal incontinence

A is correct.
Secondary achalasia may occur in Chagas' disease. The disease process, caused by *Trypanosoma cruzi*, may result in injury to the myenteric plexus of the esophagus with resultant esophageal dilation.

10.059 Infectious enterocolitis is MOST commonly caused by rotavirus, Norwalk virus and:
  A. *Entamoeba histolytica*
  B. *Yersinia enterocolitica*
  C. enterotoxigenic *Escherichia coli*
  D. *Vibrio cholerae*

C is correct.
Infectious enterocolitis is a serious world problem significantly contributing to child death in developing countries. The most common etiologic agents are rotavirus, Norwalk virus and enterotoxigenic *E. coli*.

10.060 All of the following are true of squamous cell carcinoma of the oral cavity EXCEPT:
  A. most common malignancy in this location
  B. male predominance
  C. associated with tobacco use
  D. leukoplakia is a precursor lesion
  E. floor-of-mouth lesions have better prognosis than lip lesions

E is correct.
Squamous cell carcinomas of the lip have the best prognosis. Tumors of the floor of the mouth and at the base of the tongue have a much poorer prognosis, with approximately 75% of these tumors recurring during a 5-year period postoperatively.

10.061 Which one of the following salivary gland tumors consists of a benign epithelial proliferation with a prominent benign lymphoid infiltrate?
  A. Warthin's tumor
  B. lymphoepithelioma
  C. oncocytoma
  D. pleomorphic adenoma

A is correct.
Warthin's tumor (papillary cystadenoma lymphomatosum) is the second most common salivary gland neoplasm. It usually occurs in the parotid gland. Histologically, it is composed of spaces lined by a double layer of epithelial cells along with a dense lymphoid stroma. Often, prominent germinal centers are present.

10.062 Leukoplakia is associated with which one of the following conditions?
A. Wegener's granulomatosis
B. herpetic stomatitis
C. aphthous ulcers
D. cholesteatoma
E. squamous cell carcinoma

E is correct.
Histologically, leukoplakia ranges from hyperkeratosis overlying an orderly acanthotic mucosal epithelium to lesions showing dysplastic changes with some also showing squamous cell carcinoma.

10.063 Which one of the following is the MOST frequent tumor of the parotid gland?
A. pleomorphic adenoma
B. adenolymphoma
C. mucoepidermoid tumor
D. adenoid cystic carcinoma
E. acinar cell tumor

A is correct.
The pleomorphic adenoma, or mixed tumor, represents around 60% of parotid tumors.

10.064 Which one of the following salivary gland tumors demonstrates a behavior which ranges from benign to overtly malignant?
A. pleomorphic adenoma
B. adenolymphoma
C. mucoepidermoid tumor
D. adenoid cystic carcinoma
E. acinar cell tumor

C is correct.
These range from low-grade tumors with a 5-year survival rate of 90% to high-grade tumors with a 5-year survival rate of around 50%. These tumors represent only 10–15% of all salivary gland tumors.

10.065 Inflammation of the salivary gland mediated by autoantibodies eventually produces the clinical picture of:
A. dysphagia
B. induration and pain
C. perioral muscular spasm
D. excessive salivation
E. xerostomia

E is correct.
Xerostomia refers to dry mouth. This is a prominent clinical feature of the autoimmune disorder Sjögren's syndrome. Dry eyes are also a typical feature.

10.066 All of the following are true of squamous cell carcinoma of the esophagus EXCEPT:
A. most common type of esophageal cancer
B. tobacco and alcohol use are important predisposing factors
C. lesions occur most commonly in the middle one-third of the esophagus
D. occurs most commonly in adults over 50 years of age
E. patients present with difficulty in swallowing early in the course of the disease

E is correct.
Esophageal carcinoma is typically insidious in onset, producing symptoms of dysphagia and obstruction late in the course of the disease.

SECTION 11: LIVER, BILIARY TRACT, AND EXOCRINE PANCREAS

11.001 Which of the following two hepatitis viruses are MOST likely to be associated with the development of chronic liver disease?
  A. HBV and HCV
  B. HAV and HBV
  C. HAV and HCV
  D. HBV and HEV
  E. HEV and HCV

A is correct.
Chronic liver disease, such as chronic-persistent or chronic-active hepatitis, is associated with hepatitis viruses B and C. Hepatitis viruses A and E are not associated with chronic disease.

11.002 Which of the following primary liver neoplasms tend to occur in young women taking oral contraceptives?
  A. bile duct adenoma
  B. liver cell adenoma
  C. hepatocellular carcinoma
  D. cholangiocarcinoma
  E. angiosarcoma

B is correct.
Oral contraceptives have been implicated in the development of liver cell adenomas. These neoplasms have a tendency to bleed and may precipitate an acute surgical emergency.

11.003 On histologic examination of a liver biopsy, the finding of 'ground-glass' hepatocytes (a granular eosinophilic cytoplasm) is characteristic of hepatic disease secondary to which one of the following etiologic agents?
  A. HAV
  B. HBV
  C. HCV
  D. HEV
  E. alcohol

B is correct.
Most of the hepatotropic viruses do not cause specific cytopathic changes in hepatocytes. However, the hepatitis B virus may cause a finely granular, eosinophilic, cytoplasmic alteration in hepatocytes, described as a 'ground-glass' appearance. Electron microscopy shows that these hepatocytes contain spheres and tubules of HBsAg.

11.004 Which one of the following pairs of hepatitis viruses are transmitted by means of the enteric (fecal–oral) route?
  A. HBV and HAV
  B. HAV and HEV
  C. HAV and HCV
  D. HAV and HDV
  E. HBV and HEV

B is correct.
Both HAV and HEV are classically transmitted via the fecal–oral route. HBV, HCV, and HDV are typically transmitted via blood and body fluids.

11.005 The histologic finding of eosinophilic cytoplasmic inclusions in degenerating liver cells is a characteristic feature of which one of the following conditions?
  A. acute alcoholic hepatitis
  B. acute HAV hepatitis
  C. acute HBV hepatitis
  D. chronic HBV hepatitis
  E. tetracycline toxicity to hepatocytes

A is correct.
A typical histologic feature of acute alcoholic hepatitis is the finding of eosinophilic cytoplasmic inclusions in scattered hepatocytes. These inclusions contain tangled cytokeratin intermediate filaments and are termed 'Mallory bodies'. These inclusions are characteristic of acute alcoholic hepatitis, but may also be seen in other hepatic diseases.

11.006   All of the following are true concerning primary biliary cirrhosis EXCEPT:
    A. presence of antimitochondrial antibodies
    B. prominent cholestasis
    C. granulomas are seen microscopically
    D. increased incidence of hepatocellular carcinoma
    E. occurs predominantly in men

E is correct.
Primary biliary cirrhosis has a female : male predominance in excess of 6 : 1. All of the other features are typical of primary biliary cirrhosis.

11.007   Which one of the following lesions has a close link with the hepatitis B virus?
    A. bile duct adenoma
    B. liver cell adenoma
    C. hepatocellular carcinoma
    D. cholangiocarcinoma
    E. angiosarcoma

C is correct.
There is a recognized association between the hepatitis B and C viruses, and the development of hepatocellular carcinoma. Angiosarcomas are associated with vinyl chloride exposure. Cholangiocarcinomas are associated with 'Thorotrast' and liver-fluke infestation. Liver cell adenomas occur in increased frequency in young women taking oral contraceptives.

11.008   Unconjugated hyperbilirubinemia is often found in each of the following conditions EXCEPT:
    A. hemolytic anemia
    B. posthepatic biliary obstruction
    C. jaundice during the neonatal period
    D. Gilbert's disease
    E. Crigler–Najjar syndrome

B is correct.
Hemolytic anemia, neonatal jaundice, Gilbert's disease and Crigler–Najjar syndrome are all characteristically associated with unconjugated (indirect) hyperbilirubinemia. Gilbert's disease and Crigler–Najjar syndrome are both genetic deficiencies involving failure of adequate conjugation of bilirubin. In posthepatic biliary obstruction, bilirubin has already been conjugated by the liver.

11.009   Alkaline phosphatase is abundant in the liver, intestine, placenta and bone. In a patient with elevated serum alkaline phosphatase activity, measurement of which of the following is MOST useful in determining whether the source of the elevated enzyme activity was the liver or some other organ?
    A. serum creatine kinase (CK)
    B. prothrombin time (PT)
    C. serum calcium and parathyroid hormone
    D. human placental lactogen
    E. serum γ-glutamyltransferase (γ-GT) activity

E is correct.
γ–Glutamyltransferase is a sensitive screen for liver disease. It is elevated in many hepatic diseases.

11.010   All of the following are implicated in chronic hepatitis EXCEPT:
    A. hepatitis B virus
    B. hepatitis C virus
    C. hepatitis E virus
    D. Wilson's disease
    E. α_1-antitrypsin deficiency

C is correct.
There has as yet been no correlation between the hepatitis E virus and chronic hepatic disease.

11.011 Complications or well-established associations with gallstones include all of the following EXCEPT:
  A. biliary obstruction
  B. primary biliary cirrhosis
  C. pancreatitis
  D. intestinal obstruction

B is correct.
Primary biliary cirrhosis is a chronic, progressive cholestatic hepatic disease with destruction of intrahepatic bile ducts. There is a strong suggestion of an autoimmune etiology. There is no known association with cholelithiasis.

11.012 Hemolytic anemia is associated with which type of gallstones?
  A. pigment
  B. cholesterol
  C. mixed
  D. calcium carbonate

A is correct.
Pigment stones in the gallbladder are composed of oxidized polymers of the calcium salts of unconjugated bilirubin along with small amounts of calcium carbonate and calcium phosphate. Chronic hemolytic syndromes increase the likelihood of developing this type of gallstone.

11.013 A patient with which one of the following diseases is at GREATEST risk of developing chronic active hepatitis?
  A. hepatitis A
  B. hepatitis B
  C. hepatitis C
  D. hepatitis E

C is correct.
Over 50% of patients with hepatitis C progress to chronic disease and eventual cirrhosis.

11.014 Which one of the following diseases is MOST likely to be associated with primary sclerosing cholangitis?
  A. α_1-antitrypsin deficiency
  B. Wilson's disease
  C. ulcerative colitis
  D. chronic persistent hepatitis
  E. cholelithiasis

C is correct.
Approximately 70% of patients with primary sclerosing cholangitis have a coexisting ulcerative colitis.

11.015 A unique histologic feature of primary biliary cirrhosis which is NOT characteristically seen in other types of cirrhosis is:
  A. bile stasis
  B. 'piecemeal necrosis' of hepatocytes
  C. perivenular fibrosis in zone 3
  D. granulomas
  E. chronic inflammatory cells

D is correct.
In the florid duct lesion phase of the disease, granulomatous destruction of interlobular bile ducts is characteristically seen.

11.016 An 18-year-old boy has the following test results: total bilirubin = 3.5 mg/dl (normal = 1.2 mg/dl); direct bilirubin = 2.8 mg/dl (normal = < 1.0 mg/dl). Possible etiologies for these results include:
  A. glucose-6-phosphatase deficiency (G6PD)
  B. Gilbert's disease
  C. sickle cell anemia
  D. hepatitis

D is correct.
As most of the bilirubin is in the conjugated or direct form, hepatitis is the most likely cause among those listed. In hepatitis, the hepatocytes can still conjugate bilirubin. The other diseases listed either involve a deficiency in conjugation of bilirubin or excess production of unconjugated bilirubin.

11.017 Abnormal copper metabolism is a characteristic of which one of the following diseases?
 A. α_1-antitrypsin deficiency
 B. hemochromatosis
 C. hepatitis B
 D. Wilson's disease
 E. chronic alcohol abuse

D is correct.
In Wilson's disease, there is a deficiency of ceruloplasmin, the copper-transport protein. As a consequence, there is deposition of copper in various organs, including the liver. In the liver, there may be fatty change, with the histologic picture of acute or chronic hepatitis or cirrhosis.

11.018 PAS-positive globules in hepatocytes are seen in which one of the following diseases?
 A. α_1-antitrypsin deficiency
 B. hemochromatosis
 C. hepatitis B
 D. Wilson's disease
 E. chronic alcohol abuse

A is correct.
In α_1-antitrypsin deficiency, this enzyme, synthesized by hepatocytes, is not able to be secreted by the hepatocyte and collects in large quantities in the hepatocyte, appearing as PAS-positive globules. As the enzyme cannot be secreted, there is a relative deficiency of the enzyme. There may be an associated pulmonary emphysema due to the lack of enzyme activity in inhibiting proteases, especially neutrophil elastase, which is released at sites of inflammation.

11.019 Which hepatic disease is MOST likely to have the following laboratory data: total anti-HAV negative; anti-HBe positive; anti-HBs positive; anti-HCV negative?
 A. acute HAV infection
 B. acute HBV infection
 C. chronic HDV infection
 D. remote HBV infection
 E. acute or chronic HCV infection

D is correct.
The negative anti-HAV rules out recent or remote HAV infection. The anti-HCV negativity rules out HCV infection. Positive antibodies to e and s antigens of HBV indicate a remote infection with HBV. An acute HBV infection would have negative antibodies to e and s antigens, but positive results for these antigens.

11.020 Which hepatic disease is MOST likely to have the following laboratory data: total anti-HAV positive; IgM anti-HAV negative; IgM anti-HBc positive; HBsAg positive; anti-HCV negative?
 A. acute HAV infection
 B. acute HBV infection
 C. chronic HDV infection
 D. remote HBV infection
 E. chronic HCV infection

B is correct.
The negative IgM anti-HAV and positive total anti-HAV indicate a remote infection with HAV. If there were an acute infection, the IgM antibody would be positive. The negative results for anti-HCV rule out an HCV infection. In the acute phase of HBV infection, there is the presence in the serum of HBV surface antigen as well as IgM antibody to core antigen.

11.021 Which hepatic disease is MOST likely to have the following laboratory data: IgM anti-HAV positive; anti-HBe negative; anti-HBs negative; anti-HCV negative?
 A. acute HAV infection
 B. acute HBV infection
 C. chronic HDV infection
 D. remote HBV infection
 E. chronic HCV infection

A is correct.
A positive IgM anti-HAV indicates a current or recent infection with HAV.

11.022   Which one of the following conditions does NOT have a known causal influence on the development of cholangiocarcinoma?
    A. HBV infection
    B. *Opisthorchis sinensis* infestation
    C. primary sclerosing cholangitis
    D. Thorotrast exposure

A is correct.
Hepatitis B virus has a strong association with the development of hepatocellular carcinoma. Chronic carriers of HBV may have a 200-fold increased risk for hepatocellular carcinoma. No association has been identified between HBV and cholangiocarcinoma.

11.023   Which one of the following conditions demonstrates a central stellate scar surrounded by normal hepatocytes?
    A. bile duct adenoma
    B. focal nodular hyperplasia
    C. liver cell adenoma
    D. hepatoblastoma
    E. hepatocellular carcinoma

B is correct.
Focal nodular hyperplasia in the liver appears as a well-demarcated lesion. Typically, there is a central gray-white stellate scar. Between the fibrous extensions of the scar are found apparently normal hepatocytes.

11.024   All of the following are typical morphologic features of acute viral hepatitis EXCEPT:
    A. hepatocyte regeneration
    B. Kupffer's cell hyperplasia
    C. acidophilic bodies
    D. polymorphonuclear leukocyte infiltrates
    E. ballooning degeneration of hepatocytes

D is correct.
The inflammatory infiltrate in acute viral hepatitis is typically composed of mononuclear cells, predominantly lymphocytes.

11.025   A tissue reaction consistent with chronic active hepatitis has been reported in each of the following EXCEPT:
    A. hepatitis B
    B. hepatitis C
    C. hepatitis E
    D. autoimmune hepatitis
    E. drug-induced hepatic injury

C is correct.
The hepatitis E virus has not been implicated in chronic liver disease.

11.026   All of the following contribute to the formation of portal hypertension in patients with cirrhosis EXCEPT:
    A. regenerative nodules impinging on central veins
    B. compression of the portal vein
    C. sinusoidal fibrosis
    D. opening of arteriovenous communications

B is correct.
Portal hypertension secondary to cirrhosis is an intrahepatic type of portal hypertension. Compression of the portal vein is not a component of cirrhosis, but may occur with enlarged lymph nodes in the porta hepatis.

11.027 Of the following serum results, which is the MOST indicative of biliary tract involvement (as opposed to liver parenchymal cell damage)?
    A. alanine aminotransferase (ALT) = 1500 U/l (normal 5–40)
    B. aspartate aminotransferase (AST) = 3000 U/l (normal 5–40), ALT = 500 U/l
    C. lactate dehydrogenase $(LDH)_5$ isoenzyme = 20% of total LDH (normal 6–16%)
    D. alkaline phosphatase = 650 U/l (normal 30–100), γ–glutamyltransferase (GGT) = 130 U/l (normal 10–50)
    E. total bilirubin 4.0 mg/dl (normal 0.2–1.0), direct bilirubin 1.0 mg/dl (normal 0.0–0.2)

D is correct.
In the presence of known liver disease, alkaline phosphatase serum levels are useful in distinguishing biliary tract obstruction from hepatocellular injury. GGT serum elevation also reflects biliary tract disease. Elevated AST and ALT are seen in hepatocellular damage.

11.028 In acute viral hepatitis, which of the following clinical laboratory findings would NOT be expected?
    A. aspartate aminotransferase (AST) increases of 10–100 times higher than normal
    B. total lactate dehydrogenase (LDH) elevations between 10 and 40 times higher than normal
    C. an AST : ALT ratio of < 1
    D. an elevation in total bilirubin beyond the normal range
    E. an elevation in alkaline phosphatase that is < 3 times the normal range

B is correct.
In acute viral hepatitis, the serum LDH is usually elevated no more than twice the normal concentration. High elevations of LDH in the range of 10–40 times normal are more likely to be seen in toxic or ischemic hepatocellular disease.

11.029 Which of the following statements is NOT true concerning bilirubin?
    A. synthesized primarily within hepatic parenchymal cells
    B. the unconjugated form is normally > 50% of the total bilirubin in plasma
    C. elevations of the unconjugated form of bilirubin are toxic to the nervous system
    D. soluble in water when in the conjugated form
    E. conjugated in the liver to glucuronic acid

A is correct.
Bilirubin is the final breakdown product of hemoglobin and is produced by the reticuloendothelial system.

11.030 Elevations of unconjugated (indirect) bilirubin are MOST commonly seen in which one of the following?
    A. biliary obstruction
    B. Crigler–Najjar syndrome
    C. cholestasis
    D. hepatitis
    E. Dubin–Johnson syndrome

B is correct.
Crigler–Najjar syndrome is a form of unconjugated hyperbilirubinemia with a deficiency of uridine diphosphate-glucuronosyltransferase, an enzyme responsible for the conjugation of bilirubin in the liver. The other diseases listed all present predominantly with a conjugated hyperbilirubinemia.

11.031   Cirrhosis is associated with which type of gallstones?

    A. bilirubin pigment
    B. cholesterol
    C. mixed
    D. brown
    E. calcium carbonate

A is correct.

Cirrhosis, either because of an associated increased hemolysis or because of damage to hepatocytes, may be associated with an increased incidence of bilirubin pigment gallstones.

11.032   At a community hospital, all employees who are exposed to blood routinely are offered hepatitis B vaccine. Prior to receiving the vaccine, all employees are screened for HBsAg and anti-HBs. One employee is found to be HBsAg-positive. This employee is then tested for IgM anti-HBc. The reason for testing for IgM anti-HBc is to:

    A. rule out a concurrent C virus infection
    B. rule out a concurrent D virus infection
    C. determine the amount of liver damage present
    D. determine if the infection is recent
    E. determine if the employee is infectious

D is correct.

A patient may be HBsAg positive because of either an acute HBV infection, chronic disease, or as a carrier. The presence of IgM anti-HBc indicates an acute or recent infection.

11.033   Hepatitis A virus is MORE likely than hepatitis B virus to produce:

    A. chronic liver disease
    B. hepatocellular carcinoma
    C. acute fulminant hepatitis
    D. carrier state
    E. epidemic disease

E is correct.

Hepatitis A virus is implicated in epidemics of hepatitis. It is not associated with chronic liver disease and very rarely causes acute fulminant hepatitis.

11.034   A 35-year-old woman who is HBsAg-positive becomes pregnant. Soon after delivery of a term male infant, serologic studies are performed on the newborn. The infant is found to be infected with the hepatitis B virus. What percent of newborns contracting hepatitis B from their mothers are likely to become carriers?

    A. 90%
    B. 50%
    C. 25%
    D. 5%
    E. < 1%

A is correct.

Vertical transmission of HBV has a probability of at least 90% of those infants developing the carrier state.

11.035   Chronic alcohol ingestion may increase toxicity and carcinogenic potential in certain compounds because of:
A. injury to plasma membranes with resultant increased permeability
B. injury to mitochondria with damage of mitochondrial enzyme systems
C. formation of haptenes with sensitization of cell matrix
D. stimulation of smooth endoplasmic reticulum mixed-function oxidases
E. inhibition of excretion of these compounds in the bile

D is correct.
Chronic alcohol ingestion causes stimulation of hepatic mixed-function oxidases. Certain toxins and carcinogens are metabolized by these enzymes and converted into a more toxic or active carcinogen.

11.036   Hemochromatosis and α_1-antitrypsin deficiency place the patient at an increased risk for the development of:
A. hepatic adenoma
B. focal nodular hyperplasia
C. hepatocellular carcinoma
D. cholangiocarcinoma
E. hepatic hemangiosarcoma

C is correct.
There is a significant increase in the incidence of hepatocellular carcinoma in livers of patients with hemochromatosis as well as with α_1-antitrypsin deficiency.

11.037   Which one of the following diseases has an increased incidence in patients using oral contraceptives?
A. hepatic adenoma
B. focal nodular hyperplasia
C. hepatocellular carcinoma
D. cholangiocarcinoma
E. hepatic hemangiosarcoma

A is correct.
Increased incidence of hepatic adenomas are associated with long-term oral contraceptive use. On occasions, these benign neoplasms hemorrhage into the peritoneal cavity.

11.038   Which one of the following diseases is etiologically linked to vinyl chloride and arsenic?
A. hepatic adenoma
B. focal nodular hyperplasia
C. hepatocellular carcinoma
D. cholangiocarcinoma
E. hepatic hemangiosarcoma

E is correct.
Hemangiosarcomas of the liver have an association with vinyl chloride, arsenic and Thorotrast.

11.039   Chronic hepatitis has been attributed to all of the following conditions EXCEPT:
A. Wilson's disease
B. α_1-antitrypsin deficiency
C. isoniazid therapy
D diabetes mellitus
E. autoimmunity

D is correct.
Diabetes mellitus has not been implicated in chronic hepatitis. Renal disease is a major manifestation of diabetes mellitus.

11.040 Complications of gallstones include all of the following EXCEPT:
  A. adenocarcinoma of the ampulla of Vater
  B. acute intrahepatic cholangitis
  C. acute pancreatitis
  D. gangrenous cholecystitis
  E. intestinal obstruction

A is correct.
Gallstones may have an association with carcinoma of the gallbladder, but not with carcinoma of the ampulla.

11.041 Large increases in conjugated (direct) bilirubin is MOST commonly seen in which of the following?
  A. Dubin–Johnson syndrome
  B. hemolytic anemia
  C. Gilbert's disease
  D. physiologic jaundice of the newborn
  E. Crigler–Najjar disease

A is correct.
Dubin–Johnson syndrome is an autosomal-recessive hereditary hyperbilirubinemia. There is no defect in the conjugation of bilirubin, but in the excretion of the conjugated bilirubin across the hepatocyte canalicular membrane.

11.042 The clinical picture which is MOST likely to result in a 70–90% probability of developing the carrier state for hepatitis B is:
  A. occurrence in elderly populations
  B. vertical transmission
  C. previous history of hepatitis A
  D. production of large amounts of surface antigen during the acute infection
  E. consumption of alcohol during the acute phase of the infection

B is correct.
The transmission of hepatitis B virus from mother to child *in utero* (vertical transmission) results in a very high probability that the child will become a carrier.

11.043 Increased resistance to blood flow at the level of the hepatic sinusoid along with abnormal arteriovenous anastomoses in the liver are MOST likely to be associated with which one of the following conditions?
  A. high-output cardiac failure
  B. hypersplenism
  C. restrictive pulmonary disease
  D. acute hepatic steatosis
  E. acute hepatitis A viral infection

B is correct.
Increased resistance to blood flow and abnormal arteriovenous anastomoses are features in cirrhosis which contribute to portal venous hypertension. The splenic vein empties into the portal venous system, hence the increased pressure reflected in the spleen. An enlarged congested spleen more actively removes red cells, white cells, and platelets from the blood (hypersplenism).

11.044 All of the following predispose to cholesterol gallstones EXCEPT:
  A. obesity
  B. Crohn's disease
  C. diabetes mellitus
  D. chronic hemolytic anemia
  E. estrogen therapy

D is correct.
Chronic hemolytic anemia predisposes to black pigment stones.

11.045 The following results were obtained on a serum specimen: alkaline phosphatase normal; γ-glutamyltransferase (GGT) normal; alanine aminotransferase (ALT) 3000 U/l (normal 5–50); aspartate aminotransferase (AST) 2000 U/l (normal 5–50); lactate dehydrogenase (LDH) 300 U/l (normal 100–200); total bilirubin 4.0 mg/dl (normal 0.2–1.0) with 70% in the conjugated form. These results are MOST consistent with:

   A. biliary tract obstruction
   B. acute viral hepatitis
   C. alcoholic hepatitis
   D. lytic bone lesions
   E. hemolytic anemia

B is correct.
The elevation of both AST and ALT of > 10 times normal is virtually diagnostic of severe hepatocyte damage. In viral hepatitis, the AST : ALT ratio is < 1 whereas, in alcoholic hepatitis, the ratio is > 2.

11.046 These characteristics best describe which one of the following hepatitis viruses: small, enveloped, single-stranded complete RNA virus; major route of transmission parenteral; transmission by sexual contact apparently low; and > 50% of patients develop chronic liver disease?

   A. HAV
   B. HBV
   C. HCV
   D. HDV
   E. HEV

C is correct.
The virus with which you might confuse these characteristics is the B virus. However, the B virus is a DNA virus with significant transmission by sexual contact. A much smaller percentage of patients develop chronic liver disease with hepatitis B.

11.047 This following characteristic BEST describes which one of the following hepatitis viruses: Infection can only occur in conjunction with another hepatitis virus:

   A. HAV
   B. HBV
   C. HCV
   D. HDV
   E. HEV

D is correct.
HDV is an incomplete RNA virus which can only cause infection when it is encapsulated by HBsAg. Therefore, it can only cause disease in the presence of HBV.

11.048 Well-documented e antigen in serum indicates infectivity with which one of the following?

   A. HAV
   B. HBV
   C. HCV
   D. HDV
   E. HEV

B is correct.
In hepatitis secondary to HBV, the HBeAg peaks during the acute phase. During normal convalescence, anti-HBeAg appears and HBeAg disappears. HBeAg continues to be detected in some patients who become chronic carriers. Its presence signifies continued infectivity.

11.049   A 42-year-old man with a long history of ulcerative colitis presents with progressive fatigue, pruritus, and jaundice. He has elevated serum alkaline phosphatase, elevated direct bilirubin, and normal AST and ALT. Which one of the following is the MOST likely diagnosis?

    A. alcoholic cirrhosis
    B. hemochromatosis
    C. Wilson's disease
    D. α_1-antitrypsin deficiency
    E. Reye's syndrome
    F. primary biliary cirrhosis
    G. primary sclerosing cholangitis
    H. hepatic adenoma
    I. hepatocellular carcinoma
    J. cholangiocarcinoma

G is correct.

The normal AST and ALT indicate that there is no significant component of acute hepatocellular damage present. Elevated serum alkaline phosphatase in the presence of hepatic disease suggests biliary obstruction. The pruritus is also suggestive of biliary obstruction. The clinical setting of a 42-year-old man with ulcerative colitis with these hepatic findings suggests primary sclerosing cholangitis.

11.050   A 54-year-old woman presents with pruritus, fatigue, and xanthomas. Laboratory data indicate hypercholesterolemia and the presence of antimitochondrial antibodies. Which one of the following is the MOST likely diagnosis?

    A. alcoholic cirrhosis
    B. hemochromatosis
    C. Wilson's disease
    D. α_1-antitrypsin deficiency
    E. Reye's syndrome
    F. primary biliary cirrhosis
    G. primary sclerosing cholangitis
    H. hepatic adenoma
    I. hepatocellular carcinoma
    J. cholangiocarcinoma

F is correct.

Primary biliary cirrhosis is a disease of middle-aged women presenting with pruritus. Cholesterol retention may produce xanthomas. Autoantibodies, especially antimitochondrial antibodies, are present in 90% of patients.

11.051   A 23-year-old woman taking oral contraceptives presents with an acute abdomen. Examination reveals intraperitoneal hemorrhage. Which one of the following is the MOST likely diagnosis?

    A. alcoholic cirrhosis
    B. hemochromatosis
    C. Wilson's disease
    D. α_1-antitrypsin deficiency
    E. Reye's syndrome
    F. primary biliary cirrhosis
    G. primary sclerosing cholangitis
    H. hepatic adenoma
    I. hepatocellular carcinoma
    J. cholangiocarcinoma

H is correct.

Women taking long-term oral contraceptives have an increased incidence of hepatic adenoma. These tumors are benign, but have the potential to bleed with the possibility of massive intraperitoneal hemorrhage.

11.052 A 58-year-old man presents with an enlarged nodular liver. He has been diagnosed to be an HBV carrier for the past 10 years. Which one of the following is the MOST likely diagnosis?
    A. alcoholic cirrhosis
    B. hemochromatosis
    C. Wilson's disease
    D. α_1-antitrypsin deficiency
    E. Reye's syndrome
    F. primary biliary cirrhosis
    G. primary sclerosing cholangitis
    H. hepatic adenoma
    I. hepatocellular carcinoma
    J. cholangiocarcinoma

I is correct.
There is a significant increased risk for hepatocellular carcinoma in patients with chronic liver disease associated with HBV. The enlarged nodular liver suggests the possibility of neoplasm in this patient.

11.053 A 48-year-old woman presents with malaise, weakness, and jaundice. Liver biopsy reveals fatty liver, and perivenular and pericellular fibrosis. Which one of the following is the MOST likely diagnosis?
    A. alcoholic cirrhosis
    B. hemochromatosis
    C. Wilson's disease
    D. α_1-antitrypsin deficiency
    E. Reye's syndrome
    F. primary biliary cirrhosis
    G. primary sclerosing cholangitis
    H. hepatic adenoma
    I. hepatocellular carcinoma
    J. cholangiocarcinoma

A is correct.
Alcoholic cirrhosis is characterized by fatty change in the hepatocytes and fibrosis. In the early stages of this disease, the fibrosis begins in the perivenular areas.

11.054 Which one of the following etiologic agents has NOT been implicated in the development of hepatocellular carcinoma?
    A. alcohol
    B. *Aspergillus flavus* toxins
    C. HBV
    D. HCV
    E. vinyl chloride

E is correct.
Vinyl chloride has been implicated as a causative factor in the development of primary hepatic angiosarcomas. No association has been identified between vinyl chloride and the development of hepatocellular carcinoma.

11.055 Two of the main factors in the pathogenesis of portal hypertension in cirrhosis are an increased intrahepatic resistance to blood flow and:
    A. increased renal excretion of sodium
    B. right heart failure
    C. hepatic vein thrombosis
    D. veno-occlusive disease
    E. hepatic arteriovenous anastomoses

E is correct.
In the fibrotic reaction in the cirrhotic liver, numerous arteriovenous anastomoses are formed, causing shunting of blood into the venous system. This results in an increased hepatic venous pressure which is reflected in the portal system.

11.056   Hepatitis D virus can only cause hepatitis in the presence of which one of the following viruses?
- A. AIDS virus
- B. HBV
- C. HCV
- D. HEV
- E. Epstein–Barr virus

B is correct.
HDV is an incomplete RNA virus which must be encapsulated with HBsAg in order to replicate and cause disease.

11.057   A 45-year-old man presents with chronic hepatitis. Which one of the following is LEAST likely to be the cause of the chronic hepatitis?
- A. HAV
- B. HBV
- C. HCV
- D. prescribed drugs

A is correct.
HAV is not associated with chronic liver disease.

11.058   Which of the following pairs of hepatitis viruses are MOST similar in clinical presentation?
- A. HAV & HBV
- B. HBV & HEV
- C. HCV & HAV
- D. HEV & HAV

D is correct.
Both HEV and HAV are primarily transmitted by the fecal–oral route. Clinical disease has a similar onset, and full recovery without chronic disease is typical.

11.059   Mural calcification and fibrosis are typically seen in:
- A. Rokitansky–Aschoff sinus
- B. porcelain gallbladder
- C. hydrops of the gallbladder
- D. cholesterol polyps
- E. primary sclerosing cholangitis

B is correct.
'Porcelain gallbladder' is a term used to describe extensive dystrophic calcification in the gallbladder wall. There is an increased incidence of carcinoma of the gallbladder associated with this condition.

11.060   A distended viscus containing mucoid fluid is seen in:
- A. Rokitansky–Aschoff sinus
- B. porcelain gallbladder
- C. hydrops of the gallbladder
- D. cholesterol polyps
- E. primary sclerosing cholangitis

C is correct.
On occasions, progressive removal of lipids in an obstructed gallbladder may lead to the presence of a clear mucinous secretion in the distended gallbladder. This condition is called hydrops or mucocele of the gallbladder.

11.061   Diverticulum-like invaginations of the epithelium into and beyond the smooth muscle layer describes:
- A. Rokitansky–Aschoff sinus
- B. porcelain gallbladder
- C. hydrops of the gallbladder
- D. cholesterol polyps
- E. primary sclerosing cholangitis

A is correct.
Small outpouchings of gallbladder mucosa which penetrate into the muscle wall are called Rokitansky–Aschoff sinuses. They may be acquired herniations.

11.062 Which of the following is NOT a test that can be used to assess the functional capacity of the liver? Measurement of:
    A. coagulation factors
    B. serum albumin concentration
    C. caffeine metabolism
    D. serum bile acid concentrations
    E. serum aspartate aminotransferase (AST) activity

E is correct.
Increased AST levels in the serum reflect hepatocyte injury with increased permeability. It has no relationship to the functional capacity of the liver.

11.063 Large increases in which of the following in serum is MOST commonly associated with cholestatic liver disease?
    A. alkaline phosphatase
    B. alanine aminotransferase
    C. aspartate aminotransferase
    D. lactate dehydrogenase
    E. unconjugated bilirubin

A is correct.
Alkaline phosphatase elevations in the serum may be indicative of obstructive or cholestatic biliary disease. Alkaline phosphatase in the serum may be derived from non-hepatic sources but, in cases of known liver disease, elevated alkaline phosphatase is indicative of obstructive hepatic disease. Alkaline phosphatase is secreted by bile duct epithelium.

11.064 Large increases in unconjugated (indirect) bilirubin is MOST commonly seen in which of the following?
    A. liver cancer
    B. hemolysis
    C. gallstones
    D. viral hepatitis
    E. alcoholic hepatitis

B is correct.
Massive hemolysis releases large quantities of unconjugated bilirubin into the serum which may temporarily overload the capacity of the liver to conjugate it. The result is a hyperbilirubinemia of the indirect type.

11.065 Wilson's disease (hepatolenticular degeneration) has all of the following features EXCEPT:
    A. decreased serum ceruloplasmin
    B. increased urinary excretion of copper
    C. hepatic fatty change
    D. chronic hepatitis
    E. decreased α_1-antitrypsin

E is correct.
In Wilson's disease, there is a defect in copper metabolism. The serum binding protein ceruloplasmin is deficient, resulting in increased copper which settles in various organs. In the liver, changes include fatty liver, acute hepatitis, chronic hepatitis and cirrhosis. α_1-Antitrypsin synthesis and secretion are not affected.

11.066 Which of the following is TRUE regarding bilirubin?
    A. most is produced as a by-product of hemoglobin synthesis
    B. normally found in plasma predominantly as the conjugated form (direct)
    C. soluble in water when in the unconjugated form (indirect)
    D. conjugated with glucuronic acid in the liver
    E. conjugated form is toxic to the central nervous system

D is correct.
Bilirubin is mainly a product of hemoglobin breakdown and is primarily in the unconjugated form in the serum. It is taken up by the hepatocyte, where it is conjugated with glucuronic acid to a soluble bilirubin diglucuronide.

11.067   Elevations of conjugated (direct) bilirubin are MOST commonly seen in which of the following?
   A. hemolysis
   B. physiologic jaundice of the newborn
   C. acute hepatitis
   D. Gilbert's disease
   E. Crigler–Najjar disease

11.068   The following results were obtained on a serum specimen: alkaline phosphatase and 5'-nucleotidase normal; LDH (lactate dehydrogenase) 300 U/l (normal 100–200); total bilirubin 8 mg/dl (normal 0.2–1.4); ALT 200 U/l (normal 5–50); AST 500 U/l (normal 5–50). These results are MOST consistent with:
   A. acute viral hepatitis
   B. alcoholic hepatitis
   C. biliary tract obstruction
   D. hemolytic anemia
   E. lytic bone lesions

11.069   Which one of the following factors has the MOST effect in determining whether or not a carrier state will develop for patients with HBV?
   A. age at time of infection
   B. extent of hepatocellular necrosis during the acute phase
   C. size of the initial viral inoculum
   D. absence of jaundice during the acute phase
   E. serum level of alanine aminotransferase (ALT) during the acute phase

11.070   A 64-year-old man presents with pigment cirrhosis. Six months later, he returns with a palpable mass in the liver and bloody ascites. Measurement of which one of the following substances in serum is MOST likely to aid in the diagnosis of this recent development?
   A. bilirubin
   B. alanine aminotransferase (ALT)
   C. HBsAg
   D. α-fetoprotein
   E. chorioembryonic antigen

C is correct.

In acute hepatitis, bilirubin is conjugated by the hepatocytes, but there is a problem with secretion of the conjugated bilirubin. The jaundice which occurs is therefore predominantly due to conjugated or direct bilirubin. In all of the other diseases listed, the hyperbilirubinemia is of the unconjugated, or indirect, type.

B is correct.

In alcoholic hepatitis, the AST:ALT ratio is usually >2, AST is usually 1–10 times greater than normal, LDH is 1–2 times greater than normal, and the peak bilirubin concentration is 3–20 mg/dl.

A is correct.

Vertical transmission (transmission to an infant *in utero*) has a 90% probability that the infant will become a carrier.

D is correct.

Bloody ascites should alert the physician to the possibility of malignancy. Also, pigment cirrhosis has an increased incidence for the development of hepatocellular carcinoma. Elevated serum levels of α-fetoprotein are found in 60–75% of patients with hepatocellular carcinoma. Therefore, in the clinical setting which is suspicious for hepatocellular carcinoma, measurement of α-fetoprotein may provide helpful information.

11.071   A 45-year-old man with a long history of chronic ulcerative colitis presents with biliary obstruction. Liver biopsy reveals inflammation, obliterative fibrosis, and segmental dilation of the intrahepatic and extrahepatic bile ducts. This patient is MOST likely to have:
 A. primary biliary cirrhosis
 B. congenital hepatic fibrosis
 C. primary sclerosing cholangitis
 D. veno-occlusive disease
 E. Wilson's disease (hepatolenticular
    degeneration)

C is correct.
Primary sclerosing cholangitis is a cholestatic hepatic disease which affects men more than women. It is of unknown etiology, but around 70% of patients with this disease have an associated ulcerative colitis.

11.072   Which of the following pairs of hepatitis viruses are MOST closely linked etiologically to hepatocellular carcinoma?
 A. HAV and HBV
 B. HBV and HEV
 C. HBV and HCV
 D. HEV and HAV

C is correct.
HBV and HCV are both associated with an increased incidence of hepatocellular carcinoma. No such association has been seen with HAV or HEV.

11.073   Renal failure in the hepatorenal syndrome is believed to be primarily due to:
 A. acute renal tubular necrosis
 B. fibrinoid necrosis of glomeruli
 C. glomerular amyloid deposition
 D. obstruction of the renal tubules by bile
    casts
 E. reduction of renal cortical blood flow

E is correct.
The hepatorenal syndrome refers to the development of renal failure in patients with severe hepatic disease, without renal morphologic abnormalities. Although the cause of this syndrome has not been conclusively determined, most evidence suggests that the renal failure is pathogenetically related to vasoconstriction and reduction of renal blood flow to the cortex.

11.074   The major source of excess collagen in cirrhosis appears to be which one of the following cells?
 A. portal fibroblasts
 B. transformed Kupffer's cells
 C. Disse's space Ito cells
 D. metaplastic smooth muscle cells of arteriolar
    walls
 E. injured hepatocytes

C is correct.
One of the major pathogenetic processes in the development of cirrhosis is progressive fibrosis. The primary source of this excess collagen appears to be the Ito cells which are found in the space of Disse. These cells normally function as vitamin A fat-storage cells. In cirrhosis, they transform into myofibroblast-like cells and are capable of collagen synthesis.

11.075   Fibrosis and ductal calcifications are features of which one of the following diseases?
 A. annular pancreas
 B. pancreatic pseudocyst
 C. acute pancreatitis
 D. chronic pancreatitis
 E. pancreatic carcinoma

D is correct.
Chronic pancreatitis may be associated with pancreatic ductal concretions causing ductal obstruction. There is an irregular diffuse fibrosis in the pancreatic tissue along with reduced number and size of acini. There is relative sparing of the islets of Langerhans.

11.076   All of the following may be features of acute pancreatitis EXCEPT:
   A. fat necrosis
   B. hemorrhage
   C. hypocalcemia
   D. reactive islet-cell hyperplasia

D is correct.
Islet-cell hyperplasia has no association with acute pancreatitis.

11.077   Migratory thrombophlebitis is associated with which one of the following diseases?
   A. diabetes mellitus
   B. cystic fibrosis
   C. acute pancreatitis
   D. chronic relapsing pancreatitis
   E. pancreatic carcinoma

E is correct.
Migratory thrombophlebitis (Trousseau's syndrome) occurs in approximately 10% of patients with adenocarcinoma of the pancreas. It is believed to be due to platelet-aggregating factors and procoagulants derived from the tumor cells. This syndrome may also be seen in other types of malignancies.

11.078   Adenocarcinoma of the pancreas originates from:
   A. acinar cells
   B. islet beta cells
   C. islet delta cells
   D. ductal epithelium
   E. hamartomas

D is correct.
Virtually all adenocarcinomas of the pancreas originate in the epithelial lining of the pancreatic ducts.

11.079   All of the following are features of pancreatic carcinoma EXCEPT:
   A. most of the neoplasms are derived from duct epithelium
   B. most cases develop in the head of the pancreas
   C. obstructive jaundice may be a presenting sign
   D. tumor cells secrete amylase and lipase
   E. associated with migratory thrombophlebitis

D is correct.
Pancreatic carcinomas are derived from ductal epithelial cells. It is not the duct cells which have the capability of secreting amylase and lipase, but the acinar cells.

11.080   Typical laboratory findings in acute hemorrhagic pancreatitis include all of the following EXCEPT:
   A. decreased serum calcium
   B. increased serum amylase
   C. increased serum ammonia
   D. hyperglycemia
   E. increased serum lipase

C is correct.
Increased serum ammonia does not occur with acute hemorrhagic pancreatitis. Hypocalcemia may occur due to the extensive fat necrosis and binding of calcium to free fatty acids.

11.081   A common sequela of acute pancreatitis is:
   A. diabetes mellitus
   B. islet cell hyperplasia
   C. pancreatic carcinoma
   D. pancreatic pseudocyst
   E. Zollinger–Ellison syndrome

D is correct.
In acute pancreatitis, there is proteolytic destruction of pancreatic tissue. These areas of necrotic pancreatic tissue may be walled off by fibrous tissue, forming a cystic space. The space does not contain an epithelial lining and is, therefore, a pseudocyst and not a true cyst.

11.082 Hemorrhage, fat, and parenchymal necrosis may be seen in association with:
    A. annular pancreas
    B. pancreatic pseudocyst
    C. acute pancreatitis
    D. chronic pancreatitis
    E. pancreatic carcinoma

C is correct.
In acute hemorrhagic pancreatitis, there is widespread pancreatic necrosis and hemorrhage.

SECTION 12: KIDNEY AND LOWER URINARY TRACT

12.001 By definition, the nephritic syndrome is associated with each of the following EXCEPT:
- A. red blood cell casts
- B. hematuria
- C. mild proteinuria
- D. rapid progression to renal failure in weeks
- E. elevated BUN and creatinine

D is correct.

Red cell casts, hematuria, mild proteinuria, and elevated BUN and creatinine are classical findings in the typical nephritic syndrome. Patients usually recover within a few weeks. Rapid progression to renal failure is not typical of the nephritic syndrome, but is associated with glomerular crescent formation in rapidly progressive glomerulonephritis.

12.002 The nephrotic syndrome is associated with each of the following EXCEPT:
- A. red blood cell casts
- B. moderate-to-severe proteinuria
- C. membranous nephropathy
- D. minimal-change disease
- E. normal BUN and creatinine

A is correct.

The nephrotic syndrome consists of proteinuria ($\geq 3.5\,g$ over a 24-hour period). Hypoproteinemia and hyperlipidemia also occur. Unless there are other underlying causes, the BUN and creatinine are not elevated in the typical nephrotic syndrome. There are many causes of the nephrotic syndrome, including membranous nephropathy and minimal-change disease.

12.003 Each of the following cell types is normally found in the glomerulus EXCEPT:
- A. endothelial
- B. mesangial
- C. parietal epithelial
- D. visceral epithelial
- E. fibroblast

E is correct.

Fibroblasts are not components of a normal glomerulus. Fibroblastic proliferation in the glomerulus is indicative of disease.

12.004 The histologic hallmark of crescentic glomerulonephritis is:
- A. endothelial cell proliferation
- B. epithelial cell proliferation
- C. the 'wireloop'
- D. 'apple-green' birefringence
- E. basement membrane 'spike' formation

B is correct.

Histology shows the formation of epithelial crescents in the glomeruli as a result of proliferation of parietal epithelial cells and migration of monocytes and macrophages into Bowman's space. The 'wireloop' lesion is classic for glomerulonephritis associated with lupus. Basement membrane 'spike' formation is seen in membranous glomerulopathy. 'Apple-green' birefringence is seen in histologic sections of amyloid stained with Congo red.

12.005 Postrenal acute renal failure is characteristic of which one of the following conditions?
- A. minimal-change nephrotic syndrome
- B. cystitis
- C. congestive heart failure
- D. obstructive prostatic hyperplasia
- E. polyarteritis nodosa

D is correct.

Postrenal acute renal failure describes renal failure due to a process occurring in the urinary tract beyond the kidneys. The most common process causing this type of acute renal failure is obstructive prostatic hyperplasia. There is usually a history of chronic prostatic urinary obstruction, but infection, edema or some other local occurrence may totally occlude the urethra, leading to acute renal failure.

12.006   Each of the following statements about Goodpasture's syndrome is true EXCEPT:
   A. clinical presentation usually includes hemoptysis
   B. RBC casts in urine are an important diagnostic feature
   C. linear IgG-staining by immunofluorescence is characteristic
   D. long-term prognosis is usually complete recovery of renal function
   E. histologic hallmark is renal glomerular 'crescent' formation.

D is correct.
Goodpasture's syndrome is characterized by pulmonary hemorrhages, linear deposits of IgG in glomeruli, and rapidly progressive renal failure with glomerular crescent formation. Despite therapy, patients generally require chronic dialysis or renal transplantation.

12.007   Each of the following may play a pathogenetic role in glomerular injury EXCEPT:
   A. complement components
   B. immune-complex deposition into the glomerular basement membrane
   C. neutrophil infiltration into the glomerulus
   D. monocyte, macrophage and/or platelet infiltration into the glomerulus
   E. creatinine infiltration into the mesangial region

E is correct.
There is no recognized role of creatinine in causing glomerular injury.

12.008   To determine creatinine clearance, all of the following measurements are needed EXCEPT:
   A. urine creatinine concentration
   B. plasma (or serum) creatinine concentration
   C. sample blood volume
   D. volume of urine collected
   E. total time of urine collection

C is correct.
Measurement of creatinine clearance requires a 24-hour urine sample. Urine creatinine concentration, plasma creatinine concentration, and volume of urine collected are also necessary to calculate creatinine clearance. The volume of the blood sample is not necessary for the calculation.

12.009   When examining urinary sediment, the finding which is MOST indicative (highest positive predictive value) of intrinsic renal disease is:
   A. squamous epithelial cells
   B. cysteine crystals
   C. *Trichomonas vaginalis* organisms
   D. cellular casts
   E. starch granules

D is correct.
Cellular casts are formed within the renal tubules. The cells form a 'cast' of the tubule lumen. The finding of cellular casts in the urine indicates intrinsic disease in the kidney.

12.010 Which one of the following statements about renal cell carcinoma is TRUE?
   A. frequently presents with nephrotic syndrome
   B. arises from the glomerular mesangial cell
   C. primarily a neoplasm found in adults (peak incidence in sixth decade)
   D. only rarely metastasizes to lung
   E. derived from parietal squamous epithelial cells

C is correct.
Renal cell carcinoma is a neoplasm arising from tubular epithelial cells. It may metastasize widely. Presentation is typically with painless hematuria. Peak incidence is in the sixth decade of life.

12.011   A positive chemical test for blood (as measured by the pseudoperoxidase activity of heme-containing proteins) on a routine dipstick urinalysis is consistent with all of the following conditions EXCEPT:
  A. myoglobinuria
  B. hemoglobinuria
  C. bilirubinuria
  D. microscopic hematuria (RBC in urine)
  E. menstrual bleeding contaminating the urine specimen

C is correct.
Bilirubin does not contain heme.

12.012   Which one of the following statements about malignant hypertension is TRUE?
  A. this condition is the result of a malignant neoplasm, usually primary, in the kidney
  B. morbidity and mortality are very low
  C. most often arises *de novo* in a previously normotensive patient
  D. histologically characterized by atherosclerosis
  E. characterized by renal failure

E is correct.
Malignant hypertension usually arises in a patient with essential hypertension. The full-blown syndrome is characterized by a diastolic pressure > 130 mmHg, papilledema, encephalopathy, cardiovascular abnormalities, and renal failure.

12.013   Severe proteinuria (also called 'massive' proteinuria or nephrotic-range proteinuria) is defined as a urinary total protein excretion rate of:
  A. $< 500\,mg/day$
  B. $> 30\,g/day$
  C. $< 10\,\mu g/day$
  D. $> 3\text{-}4\,g/day$
  E. $< 1\,ng/min$

D is correct.
The typical definition of nephrotic-range proteinuria is 24-hour excretion of $\geq 3.5\,g$ of protein.

12.014   Each of the following statements about acute tubular necrosis is true EXCEPT:
  A. proximal tubule and thick ascending limb of Henle's loop are most frequently affected
  B. almost always irreversible
  C. may follow myoglobinuria due to crush injury
  D. nephrotoxic-induced acute tubular necrosis may result from certain antibiotics (e.g. aminoglycosides)
  E. pathogenesis may be related to tubular obstruction

B is correct.
Acute tubular necrosis which results in the necrosis of tubular epithelial cells with preservation of the underlying basement membrane is a potentially reversible process. If the cause of the necrosis is corrected, the tubular epithelial cells may regenerate.

12.015   The nephrotic syndrome is LEAST likely to occur in which one of the following diseases?
  A. diabetic nephropathy
  B. minimal-change disease
  C. poststreptococcal glomerulonephritis
  D. membranous glomerulopathy
  E. systemic lupus erythematosus

C is correct.
The nephrotic syndrome may be a clinical manifestation of all of the diseases listed except poststreptococcal glomerulonephritis. The clinical syndrome typically associated with that disease is the nephritic syndrome.

12.016 Which one of the following statements about membranous nephropathy is TRUE?
  A. mesangial deposits of IgA are prominent
  B. polymorphonuclear leukocytes are prominent in the mesangium
  C. glomerular epithelial crescents are prominent
  D. glomerular basement membrane 'spikes' are a histologic feature

D is correct.

In membranous nephropathy, there are numerous deposits of antigen–antibody complexes between the glomerular basement membrane and the overlying epithelial cells. Basement membrane material is deposited between these antigen–antibody complexes, appearing as irregular spikes protruding from the glomerular basement membrane.

12.017 Which one of the following statements about Berger's disease is TRUE?
  A. glomerular epithelial crescents are a common feature
  B. characterized by IgA deposits in the mesangium
  C. polymorphonuclear leukocytes are prominent in the glomerulus
  D. glomerular deposits of antinuclear antibody are often seen

B is correct.

Berger's disease, also known as IgA nephropathy, has mesangial deposition of IgA. The etiology may be related to increased mucosal IgA synthesis secondary to respiratory or gastrointestinal exposure to certain bacteria or viruses. IgA complexes may then be trapped in the glomerulus.

12.018 Which one of the following statements about diabetic nephropathy is TRUE?
  A. characterized by amyloid deposition in mesangial nodules
  B. prominent glomerular deposits of IgA
  C. glomerular basement membrane thickening is a prominent feature
  D. antigen–antibody complexes are deposited on the epithelial side of the glomerular basement membrane

C is correct.

In diabetic nephropathy, there is a widespread thickening of the glomerular basement membrane. There is also an associated increase in mesangial matrix and a mild proliferation of mesangial cells. There are no deposits of antigen–antibody complexes, IgA or amyloid associated with diabetic nephropathy.

12.019 Each of the following statements about post-streptococcal glomerulonephritis is true EXCEPT:
  A. IgA is usually seen in the mesangium using immunofluorescence
  B. RBC casts in urine are an important diagnostic feature
  C. clinical presentation usually includes hematuria
  D. most children with this disease completely recover with no sequelae
  E. the antistreptolysin O titer (ASO) is usually elevated

A is correct.

In poststreptococcal glomerulonephritis, there are granular deposits of IgG, IgM, and C3 in the mesangium. IgA is typically found in the mesangium in cases of Berger's disease (IgA nephropathy).

12.020 Each of the following is part of the definition of nephrotic syndrome EXCEPT:
  A. proteinuria
  B. edema
  C. elevated serum creatinine
  D. hypoalbuminemia
  E. hyperlipidemia

C is correct.

Nephrotic syndrome basically involves damage to the selective filtration barrier of the glomerulus and loss of protein in the urine. The etiology of the hyperlipidemia is complex but, in part, involves increased hepatic synthesis. There is no elevation of serum creatinine or BUN in uncomplicated nephrotic syndrome.

12.021 Typical histologic alterations seen in glomerular disease include each of the following EXCEPT:
A. cellular proliferation of mesangial cells
B. leukocyte infiltration
C. malignant transformation of endothelial cells
D. hyalinization and sclerosis
E. glomerular basement membrane-thickening

C is correct.
Malignant transformation of glomerular endothelial cells is not a feature of glomerular disease.

12.022 Each of the following statements about membranoproliferative glomerulonephritis is true EXCEPT:
A. high recurrence rate in transplantation
B. light microscopy reveals alterations in the glomerular basement membrane
C. light microscopy reveals cellular proliferation in the glomeruli
D. may present as nephrotic syndrome with RBC casts
E. the classic pattern of glomerular disease in diabetic nephropathy

E is correct.
The classic pattern of glomerular disease in diabetic nephropathy is either diffuse glomerulosclerosis, nodular glomerulosclerosis, or exudative lesions.

12.023 Acute tubular necrosis (ATN) is typically associated with each of the following EXCEPT:
A. ischemic renal injury
B. rhabdomyolysis
C. IgA nephropathy
D. nephrotoxic renal injury
E. shock

C is correct.
IgA nephropathy characteristically is associated with recurrent gross or microscopic hematuria, mild proteinuria and, occasionally, the nephrotic syndrome. ATN is not a feature of this disease.

12.024 Which of the following is typically associated with the development of acute renal failure?
A. unilateral renal stone
B. renal ischemia
C. renal cell carcinoma
D. cystitis
E. proteinuria

B is correct.
Renal ischemia, if severe, can cause acute tubular necrosis and subsequent acute renal failure. If the ischemia is due to hypotension, there may also be a decrease or cessation of glomerular filtration.

12.025 Three key features of the nephrotic syndrome are:
A. azotemia, hypertension and RBC casts
B. cellular 'crescents', linear IgG deposition, and pulmonary hemorrhage
C. pericarditis, cerebritis, and elevated antinuclear antibodies
D. proteinuria, hypoalbuminemia, and edema
E. hyperkalemia, hypokaluria, and nephrolithiasis

D is correct.
The nephrotic syndrome is associated with proteinuria of $\geq 3.5\,g$ over a 24-hour period. This results in hypoalbuminemia, and a subsequent decrease in plasma osmotic pressure leading to edema.

12.026   Which of the following statements about minimal-change disease is TRUE?
- A. typically fails to respond to corticosteroid therapy
- B. most common cause of idiopathic nephrotic syndrome in children
- C. typically secondary to systemic lupus erythematosus
- D. glomeruli normal except for mild 'spike' formation
- E. immunofluorescence positive for complement deposition

B is correct.
Minimal-change disease is the most frequent cause of nephrotic syndrome in children. There is diffuse loss of the foot processes of epithelial cells, seen by electron microscopy. By light microscopy, the glomeruli appear entirely normal.

12.027   A 65-year-old man presents with flank pain, hematuria, hypercalcemia, polycythemia and weight loss. This patient is MOST likely to have which one of the following diseases?
- A. renal cell carcinoma
- B. Kimmelstiel–Wilson lesion
- C. malignant hypertension
- D. autosomal-recessive polycystic kidney disease
- E. Wilms' tumor

A is correct.
The classic diagnostic features of renal cell carcinoma are flank pain, mass, and hematuria. This occurs most frequently in the sixth and seventh decades with a male preponderance of $3:1$. Paraneoplastic syndromes associated with renal cell carcinoma include polycythemia and hypercalcemia.

12.028   Rapidly progressive glomerulonephritis is characterized by each of the following EXCEPT:
- A. renal colic
- B. crescent formation in glomeruli
- C. RBC casts
- D. renal failure developing over weeks to months

A is correct.
Renal colic is a term used to describe the intense pain caused by renal stones which have passed into the ureters.

12.029   Which one of the following diseases is LEAST likely to present with the nephrotic syndrome?
- A. minimal-change disease
- B. membranous nephropathy
- C. focal-segmental glomerulosclerosis
- D. IgA nephropathy

D is correct.
IgA nephropathy most often presents with recurrent gross or microscopic hematuria. Mild proteinuria is usually present, but the nephrotic syndrome only occurs occasionally. The nephrotic syndrome is a prominent feature in each of the other diseases listed.

12.030   Focal-segmental glomerulosclerosis progresses to end-stage renal disease within 10 years in approximately what percent of cases?
- A. 0%
- B. 2%
- C. 10%
- D. 50%
- E. 90%

D is correct.
A little more than 50% of patients with focal-segmental glomerulonephritis develop end-stage renal disease within 10 years.

12.031 White blood cell (WBC) casts in the urine suggest:
  A. leukemia
  B. pyelonephritis
  C. cystitis
  D. decreased urine pH

B is correct.
White cell casts indicate the presence of WBC within the renal tubules. These cells form a mold or 'cast' of the tubular lumen. The finding of WBC casts in the urine therefore suggests acute infection within the kidney, or pyelonephritis.

12.032 Glomerular disease is suggested by each of the following EXCEPT:
  A. nephrotic range proteinuria ($>3.5\,g/24\,h$)
  B. RBC casts in the urine
  C. loss of foot processes of podocytes
  D. urine with low specific gravity

D is correct.
The specific gravity of the urine is largely a result of tubular epithelial function.

12.033 Acute poststreptococcal glomerulonephritis is typically associated with:
  A. glomerular microabscesses
  B. granular immune-complex deposits on the glomerular basement membrane
  C. diffuse glomerular crescent formation
  D. IgA deposits in the glomerular mesangium

B is correct.
In acute poststreptococcal glomerulonephritis, granular deposits of immune complexes are seen along the glomerular basement membrane.

12.034 Clinical features of cystitis include each of the following EXCEPT:
  A. dysuria
  B. white blood cell casts
  C. hematuria
  D. urinary frequency

B is correct.
White cell casts indicate the presence of WBC within the renal tubules. These cells form a mold or 'cast' of the tubular lumen. The finding of WBC casts in the urine therefore suggests acute infection within the kidney, or pyelonephritis. These casts are not found in cystitis alone.

12.035 Each of the following features is usually associated with the nephritic syndrome EXCEPT:
  A. edema
  B. acute renal failure
  C. proteinuria
  D. RBC casts
  E. hypertension

B is correct.
Acute renal failure refers to a rapid deterioration of renal function. This is not a feature of uncomplicated nephritic syndrome.

12.036 Rapidly progressive glomerulonephritis associated with Goodpasture's syndrome is a classic example of which one of the following mechanisms of glomerular injury?
  A. nephritis caused by antibodies against 'planted' non-glomerular antigens
  B. circulating immune-complex nephritis
  C. antiglomerular basement-membrane antibody nephritis
  D. nephritis associated with activation of the alternative complement pathway

C is correct.
In Goodpasture's syndrome, antibodies which are directed against intrinsic fixed antigens in the glomerular basement membrane (GBM) are found. They bind along the GBM, inducing a linear immunofluorescent pattern. These antibodies crossreact with pulmonary alveolar basement membrane, producing pulmonary hemorrhage.

12.037 Each of the following may play a role in the pathogenesis of glomerular injury EXCEPT:
   A. immune-complex formation *in situ*
   B. circulating immune-complex deposition
   C. cytotoxic antibodies
   D. amyloid deposition
   E. blood urea nitrogen (BUN)

E is correct.
There is no known association between BUN and the pathogenesis of glomerular injury.

12.038 Each of the following statements is typical of renal cell carcinoma EXCEPT:
   A. flank pain
   B. abdominal mass in a child
   C. hematuria
   D. weight loss
   E. may recur many years after the initial presentation

B is correct.
Renal cell carcinoma is most prevalent in the sixth and seventh decades of life. It is extremely uncommon in children. Renal neoplasms in children are most likely to be Wilms' tumor.

12.039 The major function of renal proximal tubules is:
   A. filtration
   B. manufacture of albumin
   C. charge-dependent permeability barrier
   D. sodium and water resorption
   E. renin production

D is correct.
Sodium and water resorption is the major function of the proximal renal tubules.

12.040 A patient with poststreptococcal glomerulonephritis typically presents with:
   A. elevated serum complement
   B. nephrotic syndrome
   C. nephritic syndrome
   D. decreased serum antistreptolysin O (ASO) titers
   E. WBC casts in the urine

C is correct.
The nephritic syndrome is the typical presentation of acute poststreptoccocal glomerulonephritis. This consists of microscopic hematuria, mild proteinuria, periorbital edema and mild hypertension.

12.041 Which of the following statements about adult polycystic kidney disease is TRUE?
   A. an abdominal mass is usually found at birth
   B. autosomal-dominant
   C. usually associated with Potter's syndrome
   D. patients usually present with the nephrotic syndrome
   E. 85–90% of these patients also have a dissecting aortic aneurysm

B is correct.
The pattern of inheritance of adult polycystic kidney disease is autosomal-dominant. The disease usually is not manifest until the fourth or fifth decade of life. Around 40% of patients have cysts in the liver, and 10–30% have 'berry' aneurysms in the circle of Willis.

12.042 Nephrolithiasis may be manifest with all of the following EXCEPT:
   A. hematuria
   B. RBC casts
   C. ureteral obstruction
   D. pain

B is correct.
Stones generally arise in the calyces of the renal pelvis. Although stones may cause bleeding, RBC casts are formed when red cells are present in the urine at the level of the renal tubules.

12.043 The risk of acute pyelonephritis is signifi-
cantly increased in all of the following EXCEPT:
  A. pregnant women
  B. men with prostatic hyperplasia
  C. patients with diabetes mellitus
  D. children with nephrotic syndrome

D is correct.
Diabetics have an increased susceptibility to infection. Pregnant women, due to pressure of the uterus
on the ureters, and men with prostatic hyperplasia
both have features of urinary tract obstruction which
predisposes to infection. There is no significant
increased predisposition to urinary tract infections
associated with the nephrotic syndrome.

12.044 Which one of the following renal diseases is
characterized by thickening of the glomerular capil-
lary wall with 'spike' formation?
  A. minimal-change disease
  B. membranous glomerulopathy
  C. Henoch–Schonlein purpura
  D. diabetic nephropathy
  E. IgA nephropathy (Berger's disease)

B is correct.
In membranous glomerulopathy, there is diffuse
thickening of the glomerular capillary wall. Electron
microscopy reveals irregular dense deposits between
the basement membrane and the visceral epithelial
cells. Basement membrane material is laid down
between the deposits, appearing as irregular spikes
protruding from the basement membrane.

12.045 All of the following conditions are asso-
ciated with the nephrotic syndrome EXCEPT:
  A. minimal-change disease
  B. membranous glomerulopathy
  C. poststreptococcal glomerulonephritis
  D. diabetic nephropathy
  E. IgA nephropathy (Berger's disease)

C is correct.
Poststreptococcal glomerulonephritis presents with
the nephritic syndrome and, although there is mild
proteinuria, the nephrotic syndrome is not a feature.
All of the other diseases listed may cause the
nephrotic syndrome.

12.046 The rapid onset of nephrotic syndrome in a
5-year-old child is MOST likely to be caused by:
  A. minimal-change disease
  B. membranous glomerulopathy
  C. Henoch–Schonlein purpura
  D. diabetic nephropathy
  E. IgA nephropathy (Berger's disease)

A is correct.
Minimal-change disease (lipoid nephrosis) is
responsible for approximately 65% of all cases of
nephrotic syndrome in children.

12.047 Which one of the following diseases usually
presents as asymptomatic hematuria in patients
15–35 years of age?
  A. minimal-change disease
  B. membranous glomerulopathy
  C. Henoch–Schonlein purpura
  D. diabetic nephropathy
  E. IgA nephropathy (Berger's disease)

E is correct.
IgA nephropathy is a very frequent cause of recurrent gross or microscopic hematuria. It is probably
the most common type of glomerulonephritis
worldwide. Mild proteinuria is usually present in the
condition. The nephrotic syndrome may occur.

12.048 Antibody-mediated injury is typically
involved in which one of the following renal dis-
eases?
  A. amyloidosis
  B. poststreptococcal glomerulonephritis
  C. minimal-change disease
  D. nephrolithiasis
  E. renal tubular acidosis

B is correct.
In poststreptococcal glomerulonephritis, circulating
antigen–antibody complexes are deposited on the
glomerular basement membrane, causing activation
of the complement system and ultimate injury to the
basement membrane.

12.049 Nephrotic syndrome in an otherwise healthy 6-year-old boy is MOST likely due to:
    A. amyloidosis
    B. poststreptococcal glomerulonephritis
    C. minimal-change disease
    D. membranous glomerulopathy
    E. lupus erythematosus

C is correct.
Minimal-change disease (lipoid nephrosis) is responsible for around 65% of cases of nephrotic syndrome in children.

12.050 Thickening of the glomerular basement membrane without the deposition of immune-complex material is characteristic of which one of the following diseases?
    A. diabetes mellitus
    B. poststreptococcal glomerulonephritis
    C. minimal-change disease
    D. membranous glomerulopathy
    E. lupus erythematosus

A is correct.
In diabetes mellitus, there is a diffuse glomerular basement membrane-thickening, but immune-complex material is not identified in the thickened basement membrane. There is no immune-complex material in minimal-change disease either, but the basement membrane is not thickened in this disease.

12.051 Hypercellular glomeruli with a neutrophilic infiltrate are typically seen in which one of the following renal diseases?
    A. amyloidosis
    B. poststreptococcal glomerulonephritis
    C. minimal-change disease
    D. membranous glomerulopathy
    E. IgA nephropathy

B is correct.
Typical histologic findings in poststreptococcal glomerulonephritis include hypercellularity of the glomerular tuft secondary to proliferation of endothelial, mesangial and, occasionally, epithelial cells along with an infiltrate of polymorphonuclear leukocytes.

12.052 The nephrotic syndrome in an otherwise healthy 35-year-old man is MOST likely to be secondary to which one of the following diseases?
    A. rapidly progressive glomerulonephritis
    B. diabetic nephropathy
    C. membranous nephropathy
    D. hereditary nephritis
    E. systemic lupus erythematosus

C is correct.
In adults with the nephrotic syndrome, around 40% are due to membranous nephropathy. This is by far the most common cause of nephrotic syndrome in adults.

12.053 A 45-year-old woman presents with dull abdominal pain and hematuria of 3 days' duration. She has had two similar episodes in the last 3 months. Other than these complaints, the patient has had no previous medical problems. Significant family history includes the death of her mother at age 42 years due to a ruptured berry aneurysm. Urinalysis reveals hematuria, but no RBC casts and mild proteinuria, BUN 47 (normal 10–20) mg/dl, and creatinine 2.3 (normal 0.6–1.1) mg/dl. Which one of the following diseases is MOST likely in this patient?
    A. ischemic acute tubular necrosis
    B. autosomal-dominant polycystic kidney
       disease
    C. nephrolithiasis
    D. Wilms' tumor
    E. renal cell carcinoma
    F. membranous glomerulopathy

B is correct.
Adult polycystic renal disease usually becomes manifest in the fourth or fifth decade of life. Presenting symptoms include hematuria, protein-uria, polyuria and hypertension. Around 10–30% of patients have associated berry aneurysms in the circle of Willis. As the disease has an autosomal-dominant transmission and the patient's mother died due to berry aneurysm, the history strongly suggests the diagnosis of polycystic renal disease. Nephro-lithiasis can cause hematuria, but is usually not asso-ciated with proteinuria, and elevated BUN and crea-tinine. Renal cell carcinoma does not present with proteinuria or elevated BUN and creatinine.

12.054   A 58-year-old man presents with gross hematuria of 2 days' duration. He states that he has noticed prominent weakness over the past 2 weeks. He also complains of low-grade fever intermittent during the last 4 months. On questioning, the patient notes a vague dull right-sided flank pain over the last 2 weeks. Urinalysis reveals hematuria, but no RBC casts and no proteinuria; BUN and creatinine normal; hemoglobin 18 (normal 14–16) g/dl; hematocrit 54% (normal 42–48%). Which one of the following diseases is MOST likely in this patient?

    A. ischemic acute tubular necrosis
    B. autosomal-dominant polycystic kidney disease
    C. nephrolithiasis
    D. Wilms' tumor
    E. renal cell carcinoma
    F. membranous glomerulopathy

E is correct.
Renal cell carcinoma occurs most frequently in the sixth and seventh decades of life. The usual presentation is hematuria. Flank pain and a palpable mass may also be present. Often, generalized constitutional symptoms occur with renal cell carcinoma and include fever, malaise, weakness, and weight loss. BUN and creatinine are usually normal. Several paraneoplastic syndromes may occur with renal cell carcinoma, including polycythemia. This would explain the elevated hemoglobin and hematocrit.

12.055   A 27-year-old woman presents with a 2-week history of fatigue, a facial rash and a 3-day history of joint pain and swelling in both hands. She is afebrile with a normal pulse and respiration, but her blood pressure is 160/95 mmHg. Previous blood pressure on a routine examination 1 year previously was 115/72 mmHg. Physical examination revealed the following positive findings: a flat erythematous rash over the facial malar eminences, and mild facial edema. Laboratory data included hemoglobin 9.5 (normal 12–16) g/dl with an elevated reticulocyte count; a WBC 3500 (normal 5000–10 000); serum creatinine 2 (normal 0.6–1.1) mg/dl; BUN 45 (normal 7–18) mg/dl. Urinalysis revealed 3+ protein, and 4+ blood with red cells and red cell casts. Serum complement and antinuclear–antibody levels were ordered and are pending. Renal biopsy showed cellular proliferation, but no crescent formation. Which one of the following conditions is the MOST likely in this patient?

    A. nephritic syndrome
    B. rapidly progressive glomerulonephritis
    C. nephrotic syndrome
    D. acute renal failure
    E. chronic renal failure
    F. renal tubular defect
    G. urinary tract infection
    H. nephrolithiasis

A is correct.
The patient probably has systemic lupus erythematosus (SLE). The findings of hypertension, azotemia, proteinuria, and hematuria with RBC casts define the nephritic syndrome. The absence of crescents on biopsy rules out rapidly progressive glomerulonephritis. The patient probably has diffuse proliferative glomerulonephritis secondary to SLE.

12.056 A 28-year-old man presents to the Emergency Room with severe cramping abdominal and flank pain, which awakened him from sleep around 30 min prior to admission. The patient has had no previous significant medical problems. Urinalysis reveals hematuria, but no RBC casts and no proteinuria. BUN and creatinine are normal. Which one of the following diseases is MOST likely in this patient?

    A. ischemic acute tubular necrosis
    B. autosomal-dominant polycystic kidney disease
    C. nephrolithiasis
    D. Wilms' tumor
    E. renal cell carcinoma
    F. membranous glomerulopathy

C is correct.
This is a typical history for renal stones, which usually present with sharp colicky pain and hematuria.

12.057 A 4-year-old boy presents with 'puffy face' and lower extremity edema of 3 days' duration. The mother states that the child has had no previous such episodes; his only previous illnesses were 2–3 episodes of otitis media when he was 2 years old. Blood pressure is normal. On physical examination, 1 + edema is seen on both the face and anterior lower extremities. The chest is clear. Cardiac and abdominal examinations are within normal limits. Pertinent laboratory data include normal glucose, BUN, creatinine, and electrolytes. Urinalysis shows 4 + protein with no casts, 24-hour urine protein 5 g / 24 h (normal < 0.35 g / 24 h), and serum albumin 2.1 (normal 3.5–5.5) g / dl. Which one of the following conditions is the MOST likely in this patient?

    A. nephritic syndrome
    B. rapidly progressive glomerulonephritis
    C. nephrotic syndrome
    D. acute renal failure
    E. chronic renal failure
    F. renal tubular defect
    G. urinary tract infection
    H. nephrolithiasis

C is correct.
This child has the typical clinical features of the nephrotic syndrome. These are edema, proteinuria > 3.5 g over a 24-hour period, and hypoproteinemia. Statistically, the most likely cause of the nephrotic syndrome in this child is minimal-change disease.

12.058 Renal failure is associated with each of the following EXCEPT:

    A. congestive heart failure
    B. renal ischemia
    C. renal cell carcinoma
    D. prostatic hyperplasia
    E. crescentic glomerulonephritis (rapidly progressive glomerulonephritis)

C is correct.
Renal cell carcinoma is typically unilateral and only affects a portion of the kidney. The remainder of the involved kidney and the other kidney will maintain function.

12.059 Each of the following statements about post-streptococcal glomerulonephritis is true EXCEPT:
   A. glomeruli contain group A beta-hemolytic streptococci
   B. glomeruli are hypercellular
   C. glomeruli contain a neutrophil infiltrate
   D. RBC casts are usually present in the urine
   E. >95% of children recover without sequelae

A is correct.
There is usually a recent history of a streptococcal infection. The infection subsides, and the circulating antigen–antibody complexes are deposited on the glomerular basement membrane. These complexes cause damage to the glomerulus. The bacteria themselves are not in the glomeruli.

12.060 The definition of the acute nephritic syndrome includes which one of the following?
   A. crescents
   B. hypoalbuminemia
   C. urinary frequency
   D. renal colic
   E. RBC casts

E is correct.
The nephritic syndrome is defined by mild proteinuria and edema, azotemia, hypertension, and hematuria with RBC casts in the urine.

12.061 White blood cell casts are MOST closely associated with which one of the following?
   A. ischemic acute renal failure
   B. pyelonephritis
   C. acute nephritic syndrome
   D. nephrotic syndrome
   E. chronic renal failure

B is correct.
Pyelonephritis is an acute suppurative infection of the renal parenchyma. The polymorphonuclear response is marked, and involves the interstitium and tubules predominantly. The leukocytes form a mold or 'cast' of the tubular lumen and are identified in the urine.

12.062 In patients with advanced hepatic failure, renal failure may also develop. This is called the 'hepatorenal syndrome'. Microscopic examination of a renal biopsy from such a patient is MOST likely to show:
   A. glomerular crescent formation
   B. basement membrane-thickening
   C. focal sclerosis
   D. endothelial and epithelial proliferation
   E. normal structure

E is correct.
The renal failure secondary to hepatic failure is believed to be due to altered blood flow to the renal cortex. There is no intrinsic morphologic or functional cause for the renal failure.

12.063 Each of the following renal diseases involves either antibody or antigen–antibody deposition on the glomerular basement membrane EXCEPT:
   A. poststreptococcal glomerulonephritis
   B. minimal-change disease
   C. membranous nephropathy
   D. Goodpasture's disease

B is correct.
In minimal-change disease, there is an absence of immune deposition.

12.064   Each of the following statements about membranous nephropathy is true EXCEPT:
A. a major cause of idiopathic nephrotic syndrome in adults
B. approximately 50% of the patients will progress to renal insufficiency
C. essentially no changes seen by light and immunofluorescent microscopy
D. around 15% of cases are secondary to another condition

C is correct.
Light-microscopy changes include a uniform diffuse thickening of the glomerular capillary wall. Immunofluorescent microscopy reveals a characteristic granular immunofluorescent deposition of IgG along the glomerular basement membrane. A typical 'spiking' pattern is seen.

12.065   Mesangial deposits of IgA are prominent in which one of the following diseases?
A. amyloidosis
B. Berger's disease
C. diabetic nephropathy
D. focal-segmental glomerulosclerosis
E. hereditary nephritis

B is correct.
Berger's disease (IgA nephropathy) demonstrates prominent IgA deposits in the mesangium.

12.066   Nodular glomerulosclerosis is a feature of which one of the following diseases?
A. amyloidosis
B. Berger's disease
C. diabetic nephropathy
D. focal-segmental glomerulosclerosis
E. hereditary nephritis

C is correct.
Nodular glomerulosclerosis or Kimmelstiel–Wilson disease is a feature of diabetic nephropathy. The glomerular lesions are in the form of spherical hyaline masses located in the periphery of the glomerulus.

12.067   Nerve deafness and asymptomatic hematuria are associated with which one of the following diseases?
A. amyloidosis
B. Berger's disease
C. diabetic nephropathy
D. focal-segmental glomerulosclerosis
E. hereditary nephritis

E is correct.
Hereditary nephritis refers to a group of hereditary familial renal diseases mainly associated with glomerular injury. Alport's syndrome is one of these diseases associated with nerve deafness and certain eye disorders. The most common presenting symptom is hematuria.

12.068   A 6-year-old child presents with edema of 1 week's duration. BUN and creatinine are normal. Urinalysis reveals 4 + protein, no blood and no casts. Glucose and electrolytes are normal; complete blood count is normal; serum albumin is low. Which one of the following diseases is the MOST likely in this patient?
A. acute nephritic syndrome
B. rapidly progressive glomerulonephritis
C. nephrotic syndrome
D. asymptomatic urinary abnormalities
E. urinary tract infection
F. nephrolithiasis

C is correct.
The nephrotic syndrome typically presents with edema, marked proteinuria, and hypoalbuminemia. Hyperlipidemia may also be present. Noticeably absent in uncomplicated nephrotic syndrome are hypertension, azotemia, and hematuria.

12.069 A 12-year-old boy presents with a main complaint of reddish-brown urine. BUN is 60 (normal 10–20) mg/dl; creatinine 2.1 (normal < 1.0) mg/dl; serum complement is low; complete blood count is normal; electrolytes are normal. Urinalysis shows numerous RBCs and RBC casts. Antistreptolysin O (ASO) titer is elevated. Which one of the following diseases is MOST likely in this patient?
   A. acute nephritic syndrome
   B. rapidly progressive glomerulonephritis
   C. nephrotic syndrome
   D. asymptomatic urinary abnormalities
   E. urinary tract infection
   F. nephrolithiasis

A is correct.
The nephritic syndrome is characterized by hematuria, mild proteinuria, azotemia, hypertension, and mild facial edema. The elevated ASO titer suggests that the patient has poststreptococcal glomerulonephritis.

12.070 Which one of the following diseases usually presents after a gastrointestinal or flu-like episode?
   A. Alport's syndrome
   B. acute pyelonephritis
   C. minimal-change disease
   D. hemolytic–uremic syndrome
   E. diffuse glomerulosclerosis

D is correct.
Childhood hemolytic–uremic syndrome consists of bleeding manifestations, oliguria, hematuria, a microangiopathic hemolytic anemia and, in some patients, neurologic changes. Typically, there is a sudden onset, usually following a gastrointestinal or flu-like episode.

12.071 A unilateral large abdominal mass in a 3-year-old girl is MOST likely to be which one of the following diseases?
   A. renal cell carcinoma
   B. transitional cell carcinoma
   C. autosomal-dominant polycystic renal disease
   D. Wilms' tumor
   E. angiolipoma

D is correct.
Children with Wilms' tumor usually present with a large abdominal mass. This is the most common primary renal tumor of childhood, usually occurring between the ages of 2 and 5 years.

12.072 The MOST common postrenal cause of acute renal failure is:
   A. exstrophy
   B. cystitis
   C. transitional cell carcinoma
   D. squamous cell carcinoma
   E. adenocarcinoma
   F. prostatic hyperplasia
   G. seminoma
   H. embryonal cell carcinoma
   I. testicular torsion
   J. syphilis

F is correct.
Acute renal failure secondary to postrenal causes is most commonly seen in acute urinary retention secondary to benign prostatic hyperplasia. The enlarged prostate encroaches on the prostatic urethra until complete obstruction occurs.

12.073 Goodpasture's syndrome is generally associated with which one of the following?
   A. nephritic syndrome
   B. rapidly progressive glomerulonephritis
   C. nephrotic syndrome
   D. acute renal failure
   E. renal tubular defect
   F. urinary tract infection
   G. nephrolithiasis

B is correct.
In Goodpasture's syndrome, antibodies are present which crossreact with the glomerular basement membrane and the alveolar basement membrane. Typical renal involvement presents as crescentic or rapidly progressive glomerulonephritis.

12.074   Group A beta-hemolytic streptococcus is associated with which one of the following?
  A. nephritic syndrome
  B. rapidly progressive glomerulonephritis
  C. nephrotic syndrome
  D. acute renal failure
  E. renal tubular defect
  F. urinary tract infection
  G. nephrolithiasis

A is correct.
Poststreptococcal glomerulonephritis typically presents with the nephritic syndrome, with hematuria, mild proteinuria and edema, azotemia, and hypertension.

12.075   Membranous nephropathy is associated with which one of the following?
  A. nephritic syndrome
  B. rapidly progressive glomerulonephritis
  C. nephrotic syndrome
  D. acute renal failure
  E. renal tubular defect
  F. urinary tract infection
  G. nephrolithiasis

C is correct.
Membranous nephropathy is the most common cause of the nephrotic syndrome in adults. The nephrotic syndrome consists of proteinuria $>3.5\,g$ over 24 hours, hypoalbuminemia, and edema. Hyperlipidemia may also be a feature.

12.076   Hypotension after severe burns is associated with which one of the following?
  A. nephritic syndrome
  B. rapidly progressive glomerulonephritis
  C. nephrotic syndrome
  D. acute renal failure
  E. renal tubular defect
  F. urinary tract infection
  G. nephrolithiasis

D is correct.
Severe burns may lead to shock due to massive loss of fluid and electrolytes or, later, secondary to infection. Secondary to the hypotension, renal blood flow may decrease significantly, leading to tubular necrosis and acute renal failure.

12.077   Minimal-change disease is associated with which one of the following?
  A. nephritic syndrome
  B. rapidly progressive glomerulonephritis
  C. nephrotic syndrome
  D. acute renal failure
  E. renal tubular defect
  F. urinary tract infection
  G. nephrolithiasis

C is correct.
Minimal-change disease is the most common cause of the nephrotic syndrome in children.

12.078   Positive antineutrophil cytoplasmic antibody (ANCA) is associated with which one of the following?
  A. nephritic syndrome
  B. rapidly progressive glomerulonephritis
  C. nephrotic syndrome
  D. acute renal failure
  E. renal tubular defect
  F. urinary tract infection
  G. nephrolithiasis

B is correct.
ANCAs are present in almost all cases of rapidly progressive glomerulonephritis with minimal or no immune deposition (pauci-immune crescentic glomerulonephritis).

12.079   Antibiotic-induced azotemia is associated with which one of the following?
A. nephritic syndrome
B. rapidly progressive glomerulonephritis
C. nephrotic syndrome
D. acute renal failure
E. renal tubular defect
F. urinary tract infection
G. nephrolithiasis

D is correct.
Toxic injury to the kidney, usually to the renal tubules, may occur in certain instances secondary to antibiotic therapy. An acute renal failure may occur.

12.080   Diabetes mellitus-associated proteinuria is associated with which one of the following?
A. nephritic syndrome
B. rapidly progressive glomerulonephritis
C. nephrotic syndrome
D. acute renal failure
E. renal tubular defect
F. urinary tract infection
G. nephrolithiasis

C is correct.
Diabetes mellitus, systemic lupus erythematosus and amyloidosis are the most frequent systemic causes of the nephrotic syndrome.

12.081   The alternate pathway of complement activation is associated with which one of the following renal diseases?
A. rapidly progressive glomerulonephritis
B. membranous glomerulopathy
C. type II membranoproliferative glomerulonephritis
D. diabetic glomerulosclerosis
E. acute proliferative glomerulonephritis

C is correct.
Type II membranoproliferative glomerulonephritis is associated with deposition of dense material of unclear composition in the glomerular basement membrane. It is often referred to as 'dense-deposit disease'. In type II membranoproliferative glomerulonephritis, there is a serum factor (C3 nephritic factor) which may activate the alternate complement pathway.

12.082   A 68-year-old man with flank pain, hematuria, an abdominal mass, and normal renal function is MOST likely to have which one of the following diseases?
A. testicular torsion
B. cryptorchidism
C. nodular hyperplasia
D. polycystic kidney disease
E. renal cell carcinoma
F. nephrolithiasis
G. Wilms' tumor
H. teratocarcinoma

E is correct.
Renal cell carcinomas occur most often in the sixth and seventh decades of life. Hematuria is present in almost all cases. Flank pain and a palpable mass may also be present.

12.083   Proteinuria of $>6\,g/24\,h$ is MOST likely to be found in which one of the following conditions?
A. cystitis
B. renal cell carcinoma
C. pyelonephritis
D. focal-segmental glomerulosclerosis
E. adult polycystic kidney disease
F. primary syphilis
G. crescentic glomerulonephritis
H. nephrolithiasis

D is correct.
Around 80% of patients with focal-segmental glomerulonephritis have the nephrotic syndrome. Nephrotic syndrome is, in part, defined by proteinuria $>3.5\,g/24\,h$.

12.084 Red blood cell casts are MOST likely to be found in which one of the following conditions?
  A. cystitis
  B. renal cell carcinoma
  C. pyelonephritis
  D. focal-segmental glomerulosclerosis
  E. adult polycystic kidney disease
  F. primary syphilis
  G. crescentic glomerulonephritis
  H. nephrolithiasis

G is correct.
Red cell casts are formed when there is bleeding into the renal tubules. This is a characteristic feature of the nephritic syndrome as well as of crescentic glomerulonephritis.

12.085 Prominent proliferation of visceral epithelial cells of Bowman's space is a prominent feature of which one of the following renal diseases?
  A. rapidly progressive glomerulonephritis
  B. membranous glomerulopathy
  C. type II membranoproliferative glomerulonephritis
  D. diabetic glomerulosclerosis
  E. acute proliferative glomerulonephritis

A is correct.
In rapidly progressive glomerulonephritis, there is a rapid progressive loss of renal function. The characteristic morphologic feature of this disease is the appearance of epithelial crescents in numerous glomeruli. These crescents are formed from proliferating parietal epithelial cells of Bowman's capsule.

12.086 Which one of the following renal diseases is characterized by a thickened glomerular basement membrane, but no immune deposits?
  A. rapidly progressive glomerulonephritis
  B. membranous glomerulopathy
  C. focal-segmental glomerulosclerosis
  D. diabetic glomerulosclerosis
  E. minimal-change disease

D is correct.
The glomerular lesions of diabetic nephropathy consist of capillary basement membrane thickening, diffuse glomerulosclerosis, and nodular glomerulosclerosis. Immune deposits are not associated with the glomerular changes. Minimal-change disease is not associated with immune deposits, but there is no thickening of the glomerular basement membrane in this disease. All of the other renal diseases listed are associated with immune deposits and thickening of the glomerular basement membrane.

12.087 The differential diagnosis of hematuria should include each of the following EXCEPT:
  A. poststreptococcal glomerulonephritis
  B. renal cell carcinoma
  C. cystitis
  D. minimal-change disease
  E. urolithiasis

D is correct.
Minimal-change disease characteristically presents with massive proteinuria and the nephrotic syndrome. Hematuria is not a feature.

12.088 Each of the following statements about the glomerulus is true EXCEPT:
  A. it is a size-selective filter
  B. a hallmark of glomerular disease is proteinuria $> 3.5\,g/24\,h$
  C. none are found in the normal renal medulla
  D. it is a charge-selective filter
  E. its major function is the resorption of sodium and water

E is correct.
Water and sodium resorption is a function of renal tubules.

12.089 All of the following predispose to urinary tract stone formation EXCEPT:
    A. hypercalcemia
    B. alkaline urine
    C. urinary tract obstruction
    D. nephrotic syndrome
    E. hyperuricemia

D is correct.
In the nephrotic syndrome, there is a massive proteinuria and possible lipiduria. However, there are no urine changes which predispose to the precipitation of salts resulting in stone formation.

12.090 Goodpasture's syndrome is BEST defined as:
    A. gastrointestinal hemorrhage and glomerulonephritis
    B. hepatosplenomegaly and acute renal failure
    C. pulmonary hemorrhage and crescentic glomerulonephritis
    D. cardiomegaly and nephrotic syndrome
    E. abdominal mass and hematuria

C is correct.
In Goodpastures's syndrome, there are antibodies that crossreact with glomerular and alveolar basement membranes. Clinically, these patients present with pulmonary hemorrhage and rapidly progressive (crescentic) glomerulonephritis.

12.091 Which one of the following is a feature of the acute nephritic syndrome?
    A. massive proteinuria
    B. urinary oval fat bodies
    C. elevated acid phosphatase
    D. elevated urine sodium
    E. hypertension

E is correct.
The nephritic syndrome consists of mild hypertension, proteinuria, edema, and azotemia.

12.092 Which of the following is characteristic of rapidly progressive glomerulonephritis?
    A. renal colic
    B. dysuria
    C. glomerular crescent formation
    D. hypoalbuminemia
    E. normal serum creatinine

C is correct.
The formation of widespread epithelial crescents in the glomerulus is a typical histologic finding in rapidly progressive glomerulonephritis. These crescents are formed by the proliferation of parietal epithelial cells together with monocytes and macrophages.

12.093 Creatinine is an endogenous substance released into the blood at a relatively constant rate and produced by metabolism of which one of the following?
    A. ingested protein
    B. nitrogenous waste products
    C. muscle creatine
    D. pancreatic amylase
    E. liver lactate dehydrogenase

C is correct.
Creatinine is an endogenous substance produced by the metabolism of creatine in muscle and released from muscle into the bloodstream at a relatively constant rate.

12.094 A 12-year-old boy presents with hematuria, occasional RBC casts and a rising creatinine over the last 5 days. Based on the available data, what is the MOST likely diagnosis?
    A. membranoproliferative glomerulonephritis type II
    B. Goodpasture's syndrome
    C. focal-segmental glomerulosclerosis
    D. Berger's disease
    E. poststreptococcal glomerulonephritis

E is correct.
The most common cause of red cell casts and azotemia in a child is poststreptococcal glomerulonephritis.

12.095   A 24-year-old woman presents with hematuria, numerous RBC casts and a positive antinuclear-antibody (ANA) titer. Her complement is low, and her creatinine has risen from 1 mg/dl to 4 mg/dl over the last 5 months. Her antineutrophil cytoplasmic antibody (ANCA) is negative. Based on the available data, what is the MOST likely diagnosis?

   A. minimal-change nephrotic syndrome

   B. hereditary nephritis (Alport's syndrome)

   C. immune complex-mediated rapidly progressive glomerulonephritis

   D. membranoproliferative glomerulonephritis type I

   E. non-immune (pauci-immune) crescentic glomerulonephritis

C is correct.

Diffuse proliferative glomerulonephritis is the most serious form of glomerulonephritis occurring in patients with systemic lupus erythematosus. This patient's positive ANA suggests a diagnosis of SLE. The low complement supports an immune-mediated glomerular injury. The rapidly rising creatinine indicates a rapidly progressive course.

12.096   An 18-year-old boy is brought to the Emergency Room following an auto accident. He has sustained multiple fractures of his left femur with a crush injury to the muscle. He also has first- and second-degree burns to his chest and upper extremities. Over the next 3 days, his BUN and creatinine rise rapidly, and he becomes oliguric. Urinalysis shows tubular epithelial cells and granular casts. The BEST diagnosis for his renal condition is which one of the following?

   A. acute tubular necrosis

   B. acute pyelonephritis

   C. rapidly progressive glomerulonephritis

   D. nephrocalcinosis

   E. unilateral renal infarcts

A is correct.

Acute tubular necrosis is a reversible condition seen in various settings, including severe trauma. Hypotension and shock result in inadequate blood flow to organs, including the kidneys. The renal tubular epithelial cells are sensitive to decreases in oxygen and undergo injury or necrosis. If the patient can be sustained, the tubular epithelial cells will regenerate.

12.097   Which one of the following statements is TRUE of nephrolithiasis (renal stones)?

   A. they may arise at any level, but most often form in the kidney

   B. the passage of small stones is usually painless

   C. bilateral 75% of the time

   D. women are affected around 4 times more often as men

   E. 80–85% of all renal stones are uric acid stones

A is correct.

Most stones are calcium-containing. They are most often unilateral, and affect men more frequently than women. They may arise anywhere in the urinary tract, but most arise in the renal calyces and pelves.

12.098   A 4-year-old girl with a unilateral abdominal mass, abdominal pain and hematuria is MOST likely to have which one of the following?

   A. transitional cell carcinoma

   B. adenomatous hyperplasia

   C. ovarian cystadenocarcinoma

   D. nephroblastoma

   E. adenocarcinoma

D is correct.

Nephroblastomas (Wilms' tumors) occur most frequently in young children. An abdominal mass is the usual presenting symptom. The other tumors listed occur in adults.

12.099   An 18-year-old boy is found to have asymptomatic hematuria with RBC casts on routine premilitary physical examination. Mesangial IgA deposits are seen on renal biopsy. This boy MOST likely has which one of the following conditions?
  A. membranous nephropathy
  B. minimal-change disease
  C. focal-segmental glomerulosclerosis
  D. diabetic nephropathy
  E. membranoproliferative glomerulonephritis
  F. Goodpasture's syndrome
  G. Wegener's granulomatosis
  H. poststreptococcal glomerulonephritis
  I. Berger's disease
  J. lupus nephritis

I is correct.
Berger's disease of IgA nephropathy is characterized by IgA deposits in the mesangial area of glomeruli. It is a frequent cause of recurrent gross or microscopic hematuria.

12.100   A 27-year-old woman presents with migratory arthritis, a facial rash and low-grade anemia. Renal biopsy reveals a proliferative glomerulonephritis with IgG, IgM, IgA, and C3 glomerular deposition. 'Wireloops' are also seen. This patient MOST likely has which one of the following?
  A. membranous nephropathy
  B. minimal-change disease
  C. focal-segmental glomerulosclerosis
  D. diabetic nephropathy
  E. membranoproliferative glomerulonephritis
  F. Goodpasture's syndrome
  G. Wegener's granulomatosis
  H. poststreptococcal glomerulonephritis
  I. Berger's disease
  J. lupus nephritis

J is correct.
The clinical history suggests a diagnosis of systemic lupus erythematosus. The finding of thickened glomerular capillaries ('wireloops') together with the wide spectrum of glomerular deposits strongly support a diagnosis of lupus nephritis.

12.101   Which one of the following morphologic alterations is characteristic of focal-segmental glomerulosclerosis?
  A. disruption of visceral epithelial cells
  B. ribbon-like electron-dense deposits in the glomerular basement membrane
  C. glomerular epithelial crescent formation
  D. 'spike-and-dome' pattern of glomerular basement membrane
  E. nodular glomerulosclerosis

A is correct.
In focal-segmental glomerulosclerosis, there is a characteristic disruption of visceral epithelial cells. Also present is hyalinosis and sclerosis due to entrapment of plasma proteins and lipids in foci of increased permeability. There is also a reactive mesangial cell proliferation.

12.102 A 29-year-old man presents with hemoptysis, alveolar infiltrates, hematuria, and RBC casts. His creatinine has risen over the last 4 months to 4.0 (normal < 1.0) mg/dl. Renal biopsy shows crescent formation. Which one of the following is MOST likely to be seen on special histologic examination of the glomeruli?
    A. linear IgG pattern
    B. mesangial IgA deposition
    C. granular IgG, IgM, and C3 deposits
    D. loss of epithelial cell foot processes with no immunoglobulins
    E. irregular spiking of glomerular basement membrane with deposits of immunoglobulins and complement

A is correct.
The hemoptysis together with hematuria and rapidly rising creatinine suggest Goodpasture's syndrome. In this disease, circulating antiglomerular basement-membrane antibodies are deposited in a linear pattern on the glomerular basement membrane.

12.103 Each of the following strongly supports the diagnosis of a acute urinary tract infection EXCEPT:
    A. WBC casts
    B. dysuria
    C. nephrotic-range proteinuria
    D. bacteriuria
    E. pyuria

C is correct.
White blood cell casts, dysuria, bacteriuria, and pyuria are all typical findings in acute urinary tract infection. Nephrotic-range proteinuria (urinary loss > 3.5 g/day) is a characteristic of the nephrotic syndrome, but is not seen in association with acute urinary tract infections.

12.104 The 'horseshoe' kidney is a consequence of:
    A. severe renovascular hypertension *in utero*
    B. fusion of the metanephric blastema during organogenesis
    C. obstruction of the renal collecting ducts during fetal life
    D. congenital neoplasia of the kidneys with soft tissue spread
    E. perinatal trauma with hemorrhage medial to the kidneys

B is correct.
Fusion of the upper or lower poles of the kidneys results in a horseshoe-shaped kidney. Ninety percent of these kidneys are fused at the lower pole and 10% at the upper pole.

12.105 The BEST radiographic method of staging renal cell carcinoma is:
    A. renal angiography
    B. computed tomography
    C. ultrasound scanning
    D. intravenous pyelogram with tomography
    E. nuclear medicine scanning

B is correct.
The use of computed tomography remains the best radiographic method of staging renal cell carcinoma.

12.106 A 19-year-old boy is found to have microscopic hematuria on a routine physical. The patient is asymptomatic, has normal complement levels and a negative ANA. Urinalysis is positive for RBCs, but negative for protein. He MOST likely has which one of the following diseases?
    A. poststreptococcal glomerulonephritis
    B. rapidly progressive glomerulonephritis
    C. minimal-change disease
    D. membranous glomerulopathy
    E. Berger's disease

E is correct.
Berger's disease, or IgA nephropathy, is a frequent cause of asymptomatic recurrent gross or microscopic hematuria.

SECTION 13: MALE GENITAL SYSTEM

13.001 Transitional cell carcinoma typically arises from each of the following locations EXCEPT:
    A. glans penis
    B. urinary bladder
    C. ureter
    D. renal pelvis
    E. renal calyx

A is correct.
The glans penis contains squamous epithelium, not transitional. All of the other sites listed are composed of transitional cell epithelium, hence carcinomas arising in these sites are typically of the transitional cell type.

13.002 Each of the following statements about testicular neoplasms is true EXCEPT:
    A. embryonal carcinomas are usually resistant to radiation therapy
    B. choriocarcinomas contain syncytiotrophoblastic and cytotrophoblastic areas
    C. teratocarcinomas are composed of cells derived from more than one germ-cell layer
    D. pure seminomas have the worst prognosis of all the testicular malignant neoplasms
    E. cryptorchidism increases the risk of developing a testicular neoplasm

D is correct.
Seminomas, which are histologically identical to dysgerminomas of the ovary, have the best prognosis of the primary testicular tumors.

13.003 Neoplasms of the penis are MOST often which one of the following types?
    A. embryonal carcinoma
    B. adenocarcinoma
    C. transitional cell carcinoma
    D. hemangiomas
    E. squamous cell carcinoma

E is correct.
Most carcinomas of the penis arise on the glans or inner surface of the prepuce near the coronal sulcus and are of squamous cell type.

13.004 The MOST common type of germinal tumor in the testis is:
    A. seminoma
    B. choriocarcinoma
    C. mature teratoma
    D. immature teratoma
    E. yolk sac tumor

A is correct.
Seminomas are the most common type of germinal tumor in the testis, representing about 30% of all cases.

13.005 Malignant neoplasms of the prostate are MOST likely to be of what morphologic type?
    A. squamous cell carcinoma
    B. transitional cell carcinoma
    C. adenocarcinoma
    D. leiomyosarcoma
    E. lymphoma

C is correct.
Most primary malignant prostatic neoplasms are adenocarcinomas.

13.006 Most neoplasms of the urinary bladder are of what morphologic type?
   A. squamous cell carcinoma
   B. transitional cell carcinoma
   C. adenocarcinoma
   D. leiomyosarcoma
   E. lymphoma

B is correct.
Over 90% of primary bladder tumors are of the transitional cell type.

13.007 Each of the following statements about the prostate is true EXCEPT:
   A. nodular hyperplasia is common in men ≥70 years of age
   B. nodular hyperplasia is not premalignant
   C. prostate carcinomas are 'rock-hard' on digital examination
   D. malignant neoplasms of the prostate are almost always adenocarcinomas
   E. prostate carcinoma rarely metastasizes to bone

E is correct.
Bone is a favored site of metastasis for prostatic adenocarcinoma. It especially spreads to the vertebrae.

13.008 Phimosis is a term which BEST describes:
   A. a fungal infection of the urinary bladder
   B. urethral opening on the dorsal surface of the penis
   C. a prepuce which cannot be retracted over the glans penis
   D. a viral infection of the glans penis

C is correct.
Phimosis refers to a condition where the orifice of the prepuce is too small to allow normal retraction over the glans penis. This condition is important in that, due to an inability to maintain proper hygiene, there is an increased susceptibility to secondary infections and possibly to the development of carcinoma of the penis.

13.009 The seminoma in the testis has an almost identical histologic counterpart in the ovary. This ovarian tumor is called:
   A. granulosa cell tumor
   B. yolk sac tumor
   C. Brenner tumor
   D. dysgerminoma

D is correct.
The dysgerminoma of the ovary is a germ cell tumor as is the seminoma of the testis. These two tumors are histologically nearly identical.

13.010 Each of the following statements about carcinoma of the urinary bladder is true EXCEPT:
   A. squamous cell carcinomas account for 85–90% of all bladder cancers
   B. the development of bladder cancer is associated with cigarette-smoking
   C. grade I neoplasms are fairly well differentiated
   D. bladder exstrophy is associated with an increased risk of development of bladder carcinoma

A is correct.
About 90% of all bladder cancers are transitional cell carcinomas. Remember that the bladder is lined by transitional cell epithelium.

13.011   Each of the following statements about carcinoma of the prostate is true EXCEPT:
A. adenocarcinomas account for >95% of all prostate carcinomas
B. skeletal metastases from prostatic carcinomas are usually osteoblastic
C. microscopic foci of carcinoma are found in 50% of prostates in men past the age of 80 years
D. symptoms of urinary obstruction occur early in the course of prostatic carcinoma

D is correct.
Most prostatic cancers begin in a subcapsular location distant from the prostatic urethra; therefore, symptoms of urethral obstruction occur late in the course of the disease.

13.012 Which one of the following terms describes a type of carcinoma in situ of the penis?
A. Bowen's disease
B. chancroid
C. condyloma acuminata
D. paraphimosis
E. phimosis

A is correct.
Bowen's disease is one form of carcinoma in situ of the penis. It presents as a plaque-like lesion on the penis. Other sites where Bowen's disease may occur are the vulva and oral mucosa.

13.013   Sudden onset of severe testicular pain is MOST likely to be seen in:
A. testicular torsion
B. seminoma
C. embryonal cell carcinoma
D. syphilis
E. hydrocele

A is correct.
Torsion of the spermatic cord leads to sudden ischemia, pain, and possible infarction.

13.014   The palpation of a 'rock-hard' prostatic nodule on rectal examination signifies the likelihood of which one of the following neoplasms?
A. clear cell carcinoma
B. squamous cell carcinoma
C. transitional cell carcinoma
D. adenocarcinoma
E. embryonal carcinoma

D is correct.
Carcinomas of the prostate often present as stony-hard masses which are palpated on rectal examination. Essentially all carcinomas of the prostate are adenocarcinomas. This stony-hard feature of the neoplasm is due to its prominent desmoplastic (fibrous) component.

13.015   A crusted ulcerated lesion on the penis is MOST likely to be which one of the following neoplasms?
A. clear cell carcinoma
B. squamous cell carcinoma
C. transitional cell carcinoma
D. adenocarcinoma
E. embryonal carcinoma

B is correct.
Primary neoplasms of the penis are essentially all squamous cell carcinomas. The lesion usually begins on the glans or on the inner surface of the prepuce.

13.016   Painless enlargement of the testicle is MOST likely due to which one of the following neoplasms?
   A. clear cell carcinoma
   B. squamous cell carcinoma
   C. transitional cell carcinoma
   D. adenocarcinoma
   E. embryonal carcinoma

E is correct.
Testicular tumors most commonly present as painless enlargement of the testis. Most testicular tumors are either seminomas, embryonal carcinomas, yolk sac tumors, choriocarcinomas, teratomas, or mixed types of these tumors.

13.017 The majority of testicular neoplasms are of which of the following types?
   A. choriocarcinoma
   B. embryonal carcinoma
   C. mixed germ cell tumors
   D. seminoma
   E. teratoma

C is correct.
Mixed germ cell tumors constitute approximately 60% of all testicular neoplasms.

13.018 The penile lesion 'erythroplasia of Queyrat' is BEST described as a:
   A. carcinoma in situ
   B. hemangioma
   C. variant of congenital syphilis
   D. verrucous carcinoma
   E. viral infection

A is correct.
Erythroplasia of Queyrat is a type of carcinoma in situ of the penis which presents as an erythematous area on the glans penis.

13.019 Which of the following is necessary for the development of nodular prostatic hyperplasia?
   A. chronic inflammation
   B. elevated serum acid phosphatase
   C. elevated serum prostate specific antigen
      (PSA)
   D. functioning testis
   E. chronic urinary obstruction

D is correct.
Androgens and estrogens both play a role in the development of nodular prostatic hyperplasia. Men who are castrated before puberty do not develop nodular hyperplasia of the prostate.

13.020 Condyloma acuminata are caused by:
   A. *Calymmatobacterium donovani*
   B. herpes simplex virus
   C. *Hemophilus ducreyi*
   D. human papillomavirus
   E. *Clamydia trachomatis*

D is correct.
Condyloma acuminata (venereal warts) are caused by human papillomavirus types 6 and 11. These lesions appear on the penis. They may also be found on the female genitalia.

13.021 The histologic finding of proliferating epithelial cells with hyperchromatic nuclei surrounded by a clear perinuclear halo in a biopsy of the penis is MOST characteristic of which one of the following?
   A. chancroid
   B. condyloma acuminata
   C. erythroplasia of Queyrat
   D. lymphogranuloma venereum
   E. transitional cell carcinoma

B is correct.
Condyloma acuminata appear as sessile or papillary proliferations near the coronal sulcus of the penis. The typical histologic appearance is that of proliferating epithelial cells with hyperchromatic nuclei surrounded by a clear perinuclear halo. These lesions are caused by human papillomavirus types 6 and 11.

13.022 A 15-year-old boy is observed to have one undescended testis, which is then surgically removed. Which of the following is MOST likely to be seen on histologic examination of the surgically removed testis?
  A. atrophy
  B. hemorrhage
  C. infarction
  D. malignant neoplasm
  E. normal architecture

A is correct.
Some degree of atrophy is obvious in an undescended testis by the time of puberty. There is a loss of tubules which is usually associated with a mild hyperplasia of the interstitial cells of Leydig. There is an increased risk of malignancy in an undescended testis, but the most frequent finding is atrophy.

13.023 The peak incidence of testicular neoplasms occurs in which one of the following age groups?
  A. 1–6 months
  B. 1–4 years
  C. 6–14 years
  D. 15–35 years
  E. 65–80 years

D is correct.
The peak age incidence for testicular neoplasms is 15–34 years.

13.024 Which one of the following is the MOST common primary testicular neoplasm in children <3 years of age?
  A. choriocarcinoma
  B. embryonal carcinoma
  C. seminoma
  D. teratoma
  E. yolk sac tumor

E is correct.
Yolk sac tumors are the most common primary testicular neoplasms in children <3 years of age. These neoplasms represent endodermal sinus differentiation of totipotential cells.

13.025 A 62-year-old man with urinary frequency, retention and difficulty starting urination MOST likely has which one of the following conditions?
  A. testicular torsion
  B. cryptorchidism
  C. nodular hyperplasia
  D. polycystic kidney disease
  E. renal cell carcinoma
  F. nephrolithiasis
  G. Wilms' tumor
  H. teratocarcinoma

C is correct.
The symptoms are classical for prostatic nodular hyperplasia with partial obstruction of the prostatic urethra by the enlarged nodular prostate.

13.026 Which one of the following testicular neoplasms contains significant infiltrates of lymphocytes?
  A. choriocarcinoma
  B. embryonal carcinoma
  C. seminoma
  D. teratoma
  E. yolk sac tumor

C is correct.
Seminomas consist of large cells with distinct borders and clear cytoplasm. The nuclei are round and contain prominent nucleoli. There is usually a prominent lymphocytic infiltrate present.

13.027 Each of the following is a classic feature of nodular hyperplasia of the prostate EXCEPT:
- A. difficulty initiating urine stream
- B. recurrent urinary tract infections
- C. nodular enlargement of lateral lobes of the prostate
- D. 'rock-hard' nodule on rectal examination
- E. increased glandular and fibromuscular tissue

D is correct.
The finding of a 'rock-hard' area in the prostate on digital rectal exam is more consistent with carcinoma that with benign hyperplasia.

13.028 Which one of the following is the BEST screening test for prostate cancer?
- A. skeletal X-rays
- B. cytology of prostate secretions
- C. serum acid phosphatase
- D. digital rectal examination
- E. radioisotope bone scan

D is correct.
Most prostatic carcinomas occur in the posterior lobe of the prostate gland, which is easily palpated on digital rectal examination. This screening test remains important in detecting prostate cancer.

SECTION 14: FEMALE GENITAL SYSTEM AND BREAST

14.001 All of the following are associated with an increased risk for endometrial carcinoma EXCEPT:
- A. obesity
- B. hypertension
- C. multiple sexual partners
- D. granulosa cell tumor
- E. thecoma of the ovary

C is correct.
Multiple sexual partners may place a woman at increased risk of cervical carcinoma due to the relationship of cervical carcinoma and human papillomavirus. No such association has been identified with endometrial carcinoma.

14.002 Factors that contribute to the development of toxemia of pregnancy include all of the following EXCEPT:
- A. increased placental thromboxane production
- B. decreased placental prostaglandin production
- C. increased placental renin production
- D. increased placental angiotensin production
- E. increased maternal catecholamine production

E is correct.
Toxemia of pregnancy is believed to be due to a decreased placental perfusion which induces the production of vasoconstrictor substances such as thromboxane and angiotensin, and the inhibition of vasodilator substances such as certain prostaglandins in the placenta. Maternal catecholamines are not implicated in toxemia.

14.003 A normally developing fetus is LEAST likely to be associated with which one of the following circumstances?
- A. an 18-year-old with multiple cervical condyloma
- B. a 32-year-old with a complete hydatidiform mole
- C. a 40-year-old primigravida with ductal carcinoma of the breast
- D. a 36-year-old nullipara with carcinoma in situ (CIN III) of the cervix
- E. a 25-year-old with multiple painful herpetic ulcers of the vagina and cervix

B is correct.
Hydatidiform mole is characterized by cystic swelling of the chorionic villi along with trophoblastic proliferation. Fetal parts may be seen in partial moles, but are never present in complete moles.

14.004 Invasive vulvar carcinoma is MOST strongly associated with a previous history of:
- A. breast carcinoma
- B. ovarian stromal tumors
- C. vulvar intraepithelial neoplasia
- D. pelvic inflammatory disease
- E. clear cell vaginal adenocarcinoma

C is correct.
There is a strong relationship between vulvar intraepithelial neoplasia or carcinoma in situ (Bowen's disease) and invasive vulvar carcinoma.

14.005 The MOST common cause of death in advanced cervical cancer is:
- A. brain metastasis
- B. lung metastasis
- C. vertebral fracture
- D. renal failure
- E. adrenal cortical failure

D is correct.
Most patients with invasive cervical carcinoma die due to the effects of local invasion. The tumor invades the bladder wall and surrounds the ureteral orifices into the bladder. This results in obstructive uropathy, pyelonephritis and, ultimately, uremia.

14.006 A 22-year-old woman complains of a greenish malodorous vaginal discharge. What is the MOST likely organism responsible for her discharge?

  A. *Trichomonas vaginalis*
  B. *Neisseria gonorrhea*
  C. *Treponema pallidum*
  D. herpes simplex virus
  E. *Candida albicans*

A is correct.

Trichomonas vaginalis is a flagellated unicellular protozoan which may cause infection of the lower genital tract. The mucosa is often markedly inflamed with a foamy, greenish, malodorous discharge.

14.007 Which one of the following tumors involving the female genital tract has the WORST prognosis?

  A. dysgerminoma in a 35-year-old
  B. fibroma in a 40-year-old
  C. uterine choriocarcinoma in a 25-year-old with a recent history of molar pregnancy
  D. granulosa cell tumor in a 40-year-old
  E. serous cystadenocarcinoma of the ovary in a 45-year-old

E is correct.

Around 75% of serous cystadenocarcinomas of the ovary are in an advanced stage at the time of diagnosis. These tumors have a worse prognosis than any of the other tumors listed.

14.008 Which of the following tumors is followed clinically by serum markers?

  A. dysgerminomas
  B. immature teratomas
  C. Brenner tumors
  D. yolk sac tumors
  E. lymphomas

D is correct.

Yolk sac, or endodermal sinus, tumors are thought to be derived from embryonal carcinomas by differentiation towards yolk sac structures. Similar to the yolk sac, these tumor cells produce α-fetoprotein and α_1-antitrypsin. These serum markers may aid in following these tumors clinically.

14.009 Morphologic changes typically include benign cysts, fibrous stroma, and epithelial hyperplasia in which one of the following conditions?

  A. atypical epithelial hyperplasia
  B. fibrocystic disease
  C. phyllodes tumor
  D. intraductal papilloma
  E. fibroadenoma

B is correct.

Fibrocystic disease of the breast is the most common alteration seen in the female breast. It consists of a fibrous stroma and dilated ducts with the formation of variable-sized cysts. Proliferation of ductal epithelium is usually present.

14.010 Which one of the following lesions is usually a low-grade neoplasm arising from intralobular stroma, but may occur as a high-grade malignant variant?

  A. atypical epithelial hyperplasia
  B. fibrocystic disease
  C. phyllodes tumor
  D. intraductal papilloma
  E. fibroadenoma

C is correct.

Phyllodes tumors arise from intralobular stroma and resemble the fibroadenoma. They are distinguishable from the fibroadenoma by their cellularity, mitotic rate, nuclear pleomorphism and infiltrative margins. These tumors are low-grade and usually behave in a benign manner. Rarely, however, high-grade aggressive tumors do occur.

14.011   Which one of the following lesions commonly presents as a serous or bloody discharge from the nipple of the breast?
    A. atypical epithelial hyperplasia
    B. fibrocystic disease
    C. phyllodes tumor
    D. intraductal papilloma
    E. fibroadenoma

D is correct.
Intraductal papillomas are usually solitary lesions found within the principal ducts or sinuses. They typically present clinically with an either serous or bloody discharge from the nipple.

14.012   Which one of the following lesions is a significant risk factor for the development of invasive carcinoma of the breast?
    A. atypical epithelial hyperplasia
    B. fibrocystic disease
    C. phyllodes tumor
    D. intraductal papilloma
    E. fibroadenoma

A is correct.
Epithelial hyperplasia increases the risk of developing carcinoma of the breast. The more severe and atypical the hyperplasia, the greater the risk of invasive cancer.

14.013   A 25-year-old white woman and her husband visit an infertility clinic. During the infertility work-up, an endometrial biopsy is performed. Histologic examination of the biopsy shows complex adenomatous hyperplasia. Which one of the following lesions is MOST likely to be present in this patient?
    A. immature teratoma
    B. corpus luteum
    C. Brenner tumor
    D. granulosa cell tumor
    E. serous adenocarcinoma

D is correct.
Granulosa cell tumors may secrete large amounts of estrogen. In adult women, this may result in endometrial hyperplasia and even endometrial carcinoma.

14.014   A 15-year-old girl presents with a large unilateral adnexal mass and ascites. Which one of the following lesions is MOST likely in this patient?
    A. immature teratoma
    B. corpus luteum
    C. Brenner tumor
    D. granulosa cell tumor
    E. serous adenocarcinoma

A is correct.
Immature teratomas consist of fetal or embryonic tissue. These ovarian tumors occur most commonly in prepubertal adolescents. They grow rapidly and frequently spread to the peritoneum, resulting in ascites. Many may metastasize to distant sites.

14.015   A 64-year-old woman presents to her gynecologist for a routine examination. Bilateral adnexal masses (approximately 10 cm) are palpated. Which one of the following lesions is MOST likely in this patient?
    A. immature teratoma
    B. corpus luteum
    C. Brenner tumor
    D. granulosa cell tumor
    E. serous adenocarcinoma

E is correct.
Serous cystadenocarcinomas are the most common malignant ovarian tumor. They tend to occur later in life. Bilaterality is somewhat common, occurring in around 65% of serous adenocarcinomas.

14.016 A 27-year-old gravida VIII para VII woman at 32 weeks of gestation is brought to the Emergency Room because of profound uterine bleeding and premature contractions. She indicates that she has not received any prenatal care. Which one of the following conditions is MOST likely in this patient?
    A. acute chorioamnionitis
    B. placenta previa
    C. spontaneous abortion
    D. ectopic pregnancy
    E. placental abruption

B is correct.
Insertion of the placenta in the lower uterine segment is known as placenta previa. It is associated with severe antepartum bleeding and premature labor.

14.017 A 32-year-old febrile woman, gravida I para 0, at 38 weeks of gestation, is admitted to the hospital in active labor. She indicates that her water had broken several hours prior to the admission. Which one of the following conditions is MOST likely in this patient?
    A. acute chorioamnionitis
    B. placenta previa
    C. spontaneous abortion
    D. ectopic pregnancy
    E. placental abruption

A is correct.
Premature rupture of membranes allows a portal of entry for bacteria. This may result in chorioamnionitis. The amniotic fluid may become cloudy and contain purulent exudates. The most common organisms involved are group B streptococci and *Escherichia coli.*

14.018 A 45-year-old woman, gravida V para V, seeks medical attention because of increased vaginal bleeding. On physical examination, her uterus appears to be normal in size. Which one of the following lesions is MOST likely in this patient?
    A. leiomyoma
    B. invasive endometrioid adenocarcinoma
    C. leiomyosarcoma
    D. adenomyosis
    E. simple hyperplasia

E is correct.
Simple hyperplasia of the endometrium may cause abnormal vaginal bleeding. It is typically not associated with uterine enlargement. The other conditions listed would cause a clinically enlarged uterus.

14.019 A 54-year-old obese woman is seen in the clinic because of recent-onset vaginal bleeding. She is found to have hypertension and diabetes mellitus. Her uterus is enlarged, but no distinct masses are palpated. Which one of the following lesions is MOST likely in this patient?
    A. leiomyoma
    B. invasive endometrioid adenocarcinoma
    C. leiomyosarcoma
    D. adenomyosis
    E. simple hyperplasia

B is correct.
Vaginal bleeding is an important clinical sign for endometrial carcinomas. Obesity, hypertension, and diabetes are all associated with an increased incidence of endometrial carcinoma. In more advanced stages, the uterus is often diffusely enlarged.

14.020 A 32-year-old woman complains of dysmenorrhea. Her uterus is uniformly enlarged. No masses are palpated. Which one of the following lesions is MOST likely in this patient?

    A. adenomyosis
    B. endometriosis
    C. leiomyoma
    D. leiomyosarcoma

A is correct.

Adenomyosis is a condition in which endometrial glands extend deep into the myometrium. The condition causes enlargement of the uterine wall, forming isolated nests of glandular epithelium. Hemorrhage within these nests often results in dysmenorrhea or painful menstruation. Endometriosis may produce similar symptoms as adenomyosis, but involves tissues other than the uterus; hence, there would be no uterine enlargement.

14.021 A 35-year-old woman is admitted to the Emergency Room because of gastrointestinal obstruction. Her past medical history is remarkable for severe dysmenorrhea. Which one of the following lesions is MOST likely in this patient?

    A. adenomyosis
    B. endometriosis
    C. leiomyoma
    D. leiomyosarcoma

B is correct.

Endometriosis consists of the presence of endometrial glands or stroma in locations outside the uterus, frequently involving the ovaries, uterine ligaments, rectovaginal septum, and pelvic peritoneum. It causes infertility, dysmenorrhea, and pelvic pain. The endometrial foci undergo cyclic hemorrhage with menstruation. When extensive, the hemorrhage undergoes organization, forming numerous adhesions, which may serve as points where intestine may twist, thereby causing obstruction.

14.022 The MOST common anatomic site of origin of papillary serous cystadenocarcinoma is:

    A. ovary
    B. endometrium
    C. myometrium
    D. uterine cervix
    E. vagina
    F. labia majora

A is correct.

Cystadenocarcinomas typically arise from ovarian surface epithelium.

14.023 The MOST common anatomic site of origin of leiomyosarcoma is:

    A. ovary
    B. endometrium
    C. myometrium
    D. uterine cervix
    E. vagina
    F. labia majora

C is correct.

Leiomyosarcomas of the female genital tract usually arise in the myometrium of the uterus.

14.024 The MOST common anatomic site of origin of squamous cell carcinoma is:

    A. ovary
    B. endometrium
    C. myometrium
    D. uterine cervix
    E. vagina
    F. labia majora

D is correct.

The most common site of origin of squamous cell carcinomas in the female genital tract is the uterine cervix.

14.025   An 18-year-old sexually active woman presents with several painless elevated papillary wart-like lesions on the vulva and the vagina. A biopsy showed clearing of the epithelial cell cytoplasm, but no intranuclear or cytoplasmic inclusions. The MOST likely cause of her condition is:

   A. *Neisseria gonorrhea*
   B. *Treponema pallidum*
   C. *Calymmatobacterium granulomatis*
   D. *Haemophilus ducreyi*
   E. *Gardnerella vaginalis*
   F. *Mycoplasma* spp
   G. *Candida albicans*
   H. herpes simplex virus
   I. molluscum contagiosum
   J. *Trichomonas vaginalis*
   K. human papillomavirus (HPV)
   L. human T-cell leukemia/lymphoma virus (HTLV) III [human immunodeficiency virus (HIV)-1]
   M. *Actinomyces israelii*

K is correct.

Human papillomavirus is associated with the development of raised or wart-like conditions of the vulva, such as condyloma acuminatum. HPV is a sexually transmitted disease. On histology, the lesions consist of a branching proliferation of squamous cells supported by a fibrous stroma. Prominent perinuclear vacuolization of the epithelial cells is present.

14.026   A 30-year-old pregnant woman presents with a creamy vaginal exudate. Visual examination reveals whitish patches on the vaginal mucosa. A wet smear discloses yeasts with pseudohyphae. The MOST likely cause of her condition is:

   A. *Neisseria gonorrhea*
   B. *Treponema pallidum*
   C. *Calymmatobacterium granulomatis*
   D. *Haemophilus ducreyi*
   E. *Gardnerella vaginalis*
   F. *Mycoplasma* spp
   G. *Candida albicans*
   H. herpes simplex virus
   I. molluscum contagiosum
   J. *Trichomonas vaginalis*
   K. human papillomavirus (HPV)
   L. human T-cell leukemia/lymphoma virus (HTLV) III [human immunodeficiency virus (HIV)-1]
   M. *Actinomyces israelii*

G is correct.

Candidal infections of the lower genital tract are common. Infections are manifested by white patches on the surface, accompanied by leukorrhea and pruritus. The finding of typical yeast forms on smear confirms the diagnosis.

14.027 A 32-year-old woman presents with a chief complaint of vaginal itching and a cloudy vaginal discharge. Wet smear shows motile single-celled organisms with whip-like flagellae. The MOST likely cause of her condition is:
  A. *Neisseria gonorrhea*
  B. *Treponema pallidum*
  C. *Calymmatobacterium granulomatis*
  D. *Haemophilus ducreyi*
  E. *Gardnerella vaginalis*
  F. *Mycoplasma* spp
  G. *Candida albicans*
  H. herpes simplex virus
  I. molluscum contagiosum
  J. *Trichomonas vaginalis*
  K. human papillomavirus (HPV)
  L. human T-cell leukemia/lymphoma virus (HTLV) III [human immunodeficiency virus (HIV)-1]
  M. *Actinomyces israelii*

J is correct.
Trichomonas vaginalis is a large flagellated protozoan. It is a common cause of lower genital tract infections and is typically associated with discomfort and a vaginal discharge.

14.028 The MOST common type of carcinoma of the female breast at the time of diagnosis is:
  A. invasive lobular carcinoma
  B. lobular carcinoma in situ (intralobular carcinoma)
  C. invasive ductal carcinoma
  D. ductal carcinoma in situ (intralobular carcinoma)
  E. tubular carcinoma

C is correct.
Invasive ductal carcinoma represents around 75% of all invasive carcinomas of the female breast.

14.029 Which one of the following is associated with involvement of the epidermis by malignant cells?
  A. phyllodes tumor
  B. Paget's disease of the breast
  C. lobular carcinoma
  D. tubular carcinoma
  E. comedo-type intraductal carcinoma

B is correct.
Paget's disease of the breast is a type of ductal carcinoma arising in the main ducts and extending intraepithelially, involving the skin of the nipple and areola.

14.030 Which of the following organisms is associated with the toxic shock syndrome?
  A. *Actinomyces israelii*
  B. *Haemophilus ducreyi*
  C. *Neisseria gonorrhea*
  D. *Staphylococcus aureus*
  E. *Trichomonas vaginalis*

D is correct.
The toxin of toxic shock syndrome is secreted by *Staphylococcus aureus* which have colonized the vagina of women using tampons.

14.031 Which of the following is NOT associated with pelvic inflammatory disease?
   A. intestinal obstruction
   B. peritonitis
   C. arthritis
   D. ovarian carcinoma
   E. infertility

D is correct.
There is no known association of ovarian carcinoma with pelvic inflammatory disease.

14.032 Which of the following ovarian tumors has the WORST prognosis?
   A. dysgerminoma
   B. immature teratoma
   C. granulosa cell tumor
   D. Brenner tumor
   E. choriocarcinoma

E is correct.
Unlike choriocarcinomas arising in the placenta, ovarian choriocarcinomas are highly aggressive tumors that are typically unresponsive to chemotherapy and associated with a very high fatality rate.

14.033 Which of the following lesions is MOST typically associated with dysmenorrhea?
   A. fibroma
   B. endometrioma
   C. thecoma
   D. leiomyoma
   E. condyloma

B is correct.
Endometrioma is a term sometimes used to describe a large nodule of endometriosis. Endometriosis typically presents clinically with prominent dysmenorrhea, or painful menstruation.

14.034 Which one of the following serum markers is MOST routinely used to follow patients with papillary serous carcinomas?
   A. CEA
   B. CA-19
   C. CA-125
   D. HCG
   E. α-fetoprotein

C is correct.
The majority of patients with serous carcinoma of the ovary have elevated serum tumor marker CA-125. CA-125 levels are used to monitor the disease course of the patient.

14.035 Which one of the following tumors is the MOST common germ cell tumor?
   A. mature teratoma
   B. fibroma
   C. serous cystadenoma
   D. dysgerminoma
   E. yolk sac tumor

A is correct.
Benign cystic (mature) teratomas are by far the most common germ cell tumor. These tumors are benign.

14.036 Which one of the following tumors elaborates human chorionic gonadotropin?
   A. granulosa cell tumor
   B. embryonal carcinoma
   C. immature teratoma
   D. choriocarcinoma
   E. Sertoli–Leydig cell tumor

D is correct.
Choriocarcinomas represent extraembryonic differentiation of malignant germ cells. Whether of placental or ovarian origin, these tumors produce high levels of chorionic gonadotropin.

14.037 A 10-year-old girl presents with abnormal uterine bleeding and precocious puberty. These findings are MOST likely to be associated with:
    A. immature teratoma
    B. choriocarcinoma
    C. fibroma
    D. granulosa cell tumor
    E. endometrioid adenofibroma

D is correct.
Granulosa cell tumors of the ovary may occur at any age. These tumors may secrete high levels of estrogen, which may cause precocious puberty in preadolescent girls. The high estrogen levels will also cause endometrial hyperplasia, which often presents with abnormal bleeding.

14.038 Which one of the following tumors is MOST common in a 60-year-old obese woman with a history of diabetes mellitus?
    A. leiomyosarcoma
    B. endocervical adenocarcinoma
    C. endometrial adenocarcinoma
    D. papillary serous carcinoma
    E. clear cell carcinoma of endocervix

C is correct.
An increased frequency of endometrial carcinoma is seen with obesity, diabetes mellitus, and hypertension. Infertility is also associated with an increased incidence of this neoplasm.

14.039 Which one of the following conditions is NOT associated with an enlarged uterus?
    A. adenomyosis
    B. invasive endometrial adenocarcinoma
    C. leiomyoma
    D. hydatidiform mole
    E. endometriosis

E is correct.
Endometriosis consists of endometrial glands or stroma in an extrauterine location. The uterus itself is not involved in endometriosis.

14.040 A 37-year-old woman in her third trimester is brought to the Emergency Room because of a seizure. She is found to have severe edema and hypertension. What is the MOST likely diagnosis?
    A. placental abruption
    B. eclampsia
    C. cerebral mass
    D. toxic shock
    E. placenta previa

B is correct.
Eclampsia consists of severe hypertension, proteinuria and edema, usually arising in the third trimester of pregnancy. Convulsions may occur.

14.041 A 22-year-old woman is brought to the Emergency Room with severe tenderness in the left lower abdomen. She is also found to be hypotensive. She states that she missed her last menstrual period. There has been no abnormal vaginal bleeding. What is the MOST likely underlying cause of her condition?
    A. endometrioma
    B. placenta previa
    C. spontaneous abortion
    D. hydatidiform mole
    E. tubal pregnancy

E is correct.
Most ectopic pregnancies are tubal in location. The typical clinical picture is of a woman in her reproductive years presenting with severe abdominal pain around 6 weeks after a normal menstrual period. Often, the tubal pregnancy ruptures, causing peritoneal bleeding. If sufficiently severe, hypotension and shock may ensue.

14.042 A 16-year-old girl in her second trimester is brought to the Emergency Room with vaginal bleeding. On physical examination, her uterus appears to be large for the gestational age. Ultrasound studies do not reveal any fetal parts. Endometrial curettage reveals a large amount of blood and grape-like masses of tissue. This condition is the MOST common precursor of:
  A. placenta previa
  B. placental abruption
  C. choriocarcinoma
  D. endometrial carcinoma
  E. cervical carcinoma

C is correct.
Approximately half of all choriocarcinomas arise in hydatidiform moles. Around one-fourth arise in previous abortions and around 22% arise in normal pregnancies.

14.043 A 7-lb newborn is found to have pneumonia with group B streptococci. What is the MOST likely predisposing factor?
  A. premature rupture of membranes
  B. placental abruption
  C. toxemia
  D. maternal pneumonia
  E. unsanitary condition during delivery

A is correct.
Premature rupture of the membranes opens a portal for bacteria. Group B streptococci are commonly involved as a cause of chorioamnionitis in premature rupture. Effects on the fetus include pneumonia.

14.044 Which of the following patients is MOST likely to develop invasive endometrial adenocarcinoma? A patient with:
  A. cystic hyperplasia
  B. endometrial polyp
  C. endocervical polyp
  D. atypical hyperplasia
  E. microglandular hyperplasia

D is correct.
Around 25% of patients with atypical hyperplasias eventually develop adenocarcinoma of the endometrium. This histologic type is more likely to progress to carcinoma than are the other lesions listed.

14.045 A 4-year-old girl presents with a large vaginal mass. What is the MOST likely diagnosis?
  A. sarcoma botryoides
  B. leiomyosarcoma
  C. squamous cell carcinoma
  D. clear cell carcinoma
  E. malignant melanoma

A is correct.
Sarcoma botryoides or embryonal rhabdomyosarcoma is an uncommon vaginal tumor which occurs most often in infants and in children <5 years of age. It presents as a bulky vaginal mass in the form of grape-like clusters.

14.046 A 65-year-old woman presents with a reddish pruritic vulvar lesion. Biopsy shows large cells with abundant cytoplasm infiltrating the epidermis. The cytoplasm of these cells contains neutral and acidic mucopolysaccharides. What is your diagnosis?
  A. squamous cell carcinoma
  B. malignant melanoma
  C. metastatic carcinoma
  D. verrucous carcinoma
  E. Paget's disease

E is correct.
This neoplasm presents with a pruritic red crusted zone, usually on the labia majora. On microscopy, large anaplastic tumor cells can be seen lying within the epidermis. The tumor cells contain mucopolysaccharides as detected by special stains. This is sometimes called extramammary Paget's disease to contrast it with Paget's disease of breast, which is associated with intraductal carcinoma.

14.047   The WORST prognosis in patients with endometrial carcinoma is found in patients with tumor involvement of the:
A. uterine cervix
B. upper vagina
C. bladder mucosa
D. parametrium

C is correct.
Involvement of the bladder mucosa constitutes a stage IV tumor. The other examples given are either stage II or III. The more advanced the stage of a tumor, the worse the prognosis.

14.048   Which of the following ovarian masses is MOST likely to be associated with ascites?
A. mucinous cystadenoma
B. mature teratoma
C. papillary serous carcinoma
D. dysgerminoma

C is correct.
Serous carcinomas may seed the peritoneal cavity, resulting in ascites.

14.049   A risk factor for the development of ductal carcinoma of the breast is:
A. lobular carcinoma
B. cystosarcoma phyllodes
C. intraductal papilloma
D. medullary carcinoma of the breast
E. atypical ductal hyperplasia

E is correct.
Atypical ductal epithelial hyperplasia is considered a risk factor for the development of ductal carcinoma. The more severe the atypical hyperplasia, the greater the risk.

14.050   Inspissated secretions in the ducts of the female breast with subsequent ductal dilation and rupture BEST describes which one of the following conditions?
A. fibrocystic change
B. acute mastitis
C. chronic mastitis
D. mammary duct ectasia
E. sclerosing adenosis

D is correct.
Mammary duct ectasia consists of a non-bacterial inflammatory process of the breast. The main excretory ducts contain inspissated breast secretions with ductal dilation and rupture. The surrounding breast tissue is the site of an inflammatory reaction with prominent lymphocytic and plasma cell infiltrates. Granulomas may occur in the periductal stroma.

14.051   Which one of the following lesions is a variant of invasive ductal carcinoma with a better prognosis than conventional invasive ductal carcinoma?
A. lobular carcinoma
B. cystosarcoma phyllodes
C. intraductal papilloma
D. medullary carcinoma of the breast
E. atypical ductal hyperplasia

D is correct.
Medullary carcinoma of the breast is a fleshy tumor that is a variant of invasive ductal carcinoma. These tumors do not have the extensive fibrous stroma as seen with typical ductal carcinoma. The tumor has a lymphocytic infiltrate which is believed to be associated with the better prognosis with these tumors compared with the typical ductal carcinomas.

14.052   Which one of the following lesions is MOST associated with an increased risk for bilateral breast carcinoma?
A. lobular carcinoma
B. cystosarcoma phyllodes
C. intraductal papilloma
D. medullary carcinoma of the breast
E. atypical ductal hyperplasia

A is correct.
Lobular carcinoma is manifested by the proliferation of abnormal cells in one or more terminal ducts and/or acini of the breast. There is a high incidence of bilateral involvement with this condition.

14.053 Which one of the following lesions appears histologically as a biphasic tumor with a stromal component which may be malignant?
   A. lobular carcinoma
   B. cystosarcoma phyllodes
   C. intraductal papilloma
   D. medullary carcinoma of the breast
   E. atypical ductal hyperplasia

B is correct.
Phyllodes tumor of the breast arises from intra-lobular stroma, and consists of both stroma and glandular epithelium. Unlike the fibroadenoma, some of these tumors may behave aggressively, with metastases from malignant stromal cells.

14.054 All of the following tumors are most commonly unilateral EXCEPT:
   A. dysgerminoma
   B. yolk sac tumor
   C. Krukenberg's tumor
   D. Brenner tumor
   E. thecoma

C is correct.
Metastatic gastrointestinal tumors to the ovaries are termed 'Krukenberg's tumor'. These tumors are bilateral metastases containing signet-ring cells and are most often of gastric origin.

14.055 All of the following microorganisms can cause intrauterine fetal demise or perinatal death EXCEPT:
   A. rubella togavirus
   B. cytomegalovirus
   C. *Treponema pallidum*
   D. *Listeria*
   E. human papillomavirus

E is correct.
Human papillomavirus is sexually transmitted and causes condyloma acuminatum, a verrucous lesion of the vulva. It is not associated with fetal death.

14.056 All of the following are associated with increased risk for endometrial carcinoma EXCEPT:
   A. obesity
   B. hypertension
   C. multiple pregnancies
   D. adenomatous hyperplasia of the endometrium
   E. granulosa-theca cell tumors of the ovary

C is correct.
Women who develop endometrial carcinoma are generally single and nulliparous.

14.057 All of the following conditions can present with abnormal bleeding EXCEPT:
   A. endometrial hyperplasia
   B. invasive squamous cell carcinoma of the cervix
   C. endometrial adenocarcinoma
   D. benign endometrial polyp
   E. vaginal adenosis

E is correct.
Vaginal adenosis is a condition in which glandular epithelium appears beneath the squamous epithelium of the vagina. It is not associated with bleeding.

14.058 Which of the following is the MOST likely diagnosis in a 32-year-old woman who presents with a unilateral adnexal mass and pleural effusion?
   A. ovarian fibroma
   B. pelvic inflammatory disease
   C. ectopic pregnancy
   D. ovarian mature teratoma
   E. Krukenberg's tumor

A is correct.
In approximately 40% of cases of fibroma–thecomas of the ovary, there is an associated ascites. Some of these patients also have a hydrothorax, usually on the right side. This combination of findings is termed 'Meigs' syndrome'. The pathogenesis of the syndrome is unknown.

14.059 A 30-year-old postpartum woman presents to the obstetrician because of new onset of hemorrhage. Her temperature is reported to be 103°F. This is MOST likely due to:
A. ruptured uterus
B. invasive cervical carcinoma
C. granulomatous endometritis
D. retained placental parts
E. tubal gestation

D is correct.
Postpartum bleeding and fever should arouse suspicion of retained placental fragments. These fragments of placenta are a source of bleeding and may become infected.

14.060 Which one of the following features is MOST commonly seen in malignant smooth muscle tumors of the myometrium?
A. numerous well-defined masses
B. abnormal uterine bleeding
C. a single 10-cm mass protruding from the cervical os
D. marked enlargement during pregnancy
E. a single large, ill-defined, soft fleshy mass

E is correct.
Leiomyosarcomas arise *de novo* in the uterine wall. They appear as bulky, fleshy masses which invade the uterine wall, creating an ill-defined border.

14.061 Which of the following tumors has the WORST prognosis?
A. grade I endometrial adenocarcinoma involving the inner third of the myometrium
B. low-grade stromal sarcoma with no evidence of metastasis
C. clear cell carcinoma involving the endometrium and cervix
D. malignant mixed mesodermal tumor involving the outer half of the myometrium
E. choriocarcinoma of the ovary

E is correct.
Choriocarcinomas of the ovary are usually found in association with other germ cell tumors. They are very aggressive tumors which metastasize widely to the lungs, liver, bone and elsewhere, at an early stage. Unlike placental choriocarcinomas, ovarian tumors are generally unresponsive to chemotherapy.

14.062 Which of the following is associated with a POORER prognosis in female patients who have invasive ductal carcinoma of the breast?
A. presence of estrogen/progesterone receptors on the tumor cells
B. presence of lymph node metastasis
C. presence of tubular carcinoma subtype
D. presence of medullary carcinoma subtype

B is correct.
Patients with no involvement of lymph nodes have a 5-year survival rate of around 80%. If one node is involved, the survival rate drops to 50%.

14.063 The MOST common benign tumor of the female breast is:
A. Paget's disease
B. fibroadenoma
C. phyllodes tumor
D. intraductal papilloma
E. sclerosing adenosis

B is correct.
The fibroadenoma is the most common benign tumor of the female breast. It is believed to develop secondary to increased estrogen activity. These benign neoplasms usually occur in young women, with a peak incidence in the third decade of life. Clinically, fibroadenomas present as a solitary, discrete, freely movable mass. They may enlarge in response to increased estrogen, such as during pregnancy.

14.064 A 25-year-old white woman and her husband visit an infertility clinic. Their infertility
work-up is negative except for bilateral obliteration
of both Fallopian tubes. Which of the following
organisms is known to be MOST associated with
this complication?

    A. papillomavirus

    B. *Trichomonas vaginalis*

    C. *Treponema pallidum*

    D. *Neisseria gonorrhoeae*

    E. *Candida*

D is correct.

Gonococcal infections usually begin in the vestibular or periurethral glands, and spread to involve the
tubes and tuboovarian regions. The tubal infection
may lead to fibrous scarring, with tubal obliteration
and sterility.

14.065 A 17-year-old woman presents to the clinic
because of generalized painless papules. Papules are
also noted on her palms and raised papules are
noted in the perineal region. Which of the following
organisms is the MOST likely etiology for her
condition?

    A. papillomavirus

    B. *Trichomonas vaginalis*

    C. *Treponema pallidum*

    D. *Neisseria gonorrhoeae*

    E. *Candida*

C is correct.

In the secondary stage of syphilis, there is typically
a diffuse rash, which usually affects the palms and
soles.

14.066 A 22-year-old comatose woman is admitted
to the ER. Her blood pressure is 60/40 mmHg and
her hematocrit is 18 (normal value is 35). This
patient MOST likely has:

    A. acute chorioamnionitis

    B. placenta previa

    C. spontaneous abortion

    D. ectopic pregnancy

    E. toxemia of pregnancy

D is correct.

Ectopic pregnancies usually occur in the tubes.
They may rupture, causing peritoneal hemorrhage
and shock.

14.067 A 23-year-old gravida 1, para 0 woman
is admitted to the hospital for observation. At the
time of admission, her blood pressure is 150/
95 mmHg and she has 3+ proteinuria. This patient
MOST likely has:

    A. acute chorioamnionitis

    B. placenta previa

    C. spontaneous abortion

    D. ectopic pregnancy

    E. toxemia of pregnancy

E is correct.

Toxemia of pregnancy is a syndrome of hypertension, proteinuria and edema. It most commonly
appears in the third trimester of pregnancy and is
more usually seen in primiparous than in multi-
parous women.

14.068   A 45-year-old woman who is gravida 5, para 5, seeks medical attention for severe postcoital bleeding. On physical examination, a 4-cm indurated cervical mass is identified. This patient MOST likely has:
  A. condyloma acuminatum
  B. invasive squamous cell carcinoma of the cervix
  C. cervical intraepithelial neoplasia
  D. microglandular hyperplasia
  E. sarcoma botryoides

B is correct.
Invasive carcinoma of the cervix may cause postcoital bleeding. The finding of a cervical mass is most consistent with this diagnosis.

14.069 Ovarian neoplasms MOST commonly arise from:
  A. coelomic epithelium
  B. non-specific mesenchyme
  C. specialized gonadal stroma
  D. primitive germ cells
  E. follicular epithelium

A is correct.
The majority of ovarian neoplasms arise from surface epithelium (coelomic epithelium). Malignant ovarian neoplasms arising from coelomic epithelium represent around 90% of all ovarian malignancies. Ovarian neoplasms arising from coelomic epithelium include serous, mucinous, endometrioid, clear cell, Brenner tumors and cystadenofibromas.

14.070 A 17-year-old girl presents with a 30-cm unilateral adnexal mass. The CT scan shows marked retroperitoneal lymphadenopathy. The MOST likely diagnosis is:
  A. papillary serous cystadenocarcinoma
  B. immature teratoma
  C. polycystic ovaries
  D. follicular cyst
  E. granulosa cell tumor

B is correct.
Immature teratomas are uncommon tumors which form tissues that resemble those in the embryo. These tumors are usually found in young girls (mean age 18 years). The lymphadenopathy suggests metastatic neoplasm. These tumors grow rapidly and metastasize early. Cystadenocarcinomas tend to occur in older age groups.

14.071   A 24-year-old woman presents with a 4-cm unilateral adnexal mass. The MOST likely diagnosis is:
  A. papillary serous cystadenocarcinoma
  B. immature teratoma
  C. polycystic ovaries
  D. follicular cyst
  E. granulosa cell tumor

D is correct.
A unilateral 4-cm adnexal mass in a 24-year-old woman is most likely to be a follicular cyst. Cystic follicles originate from unruptured Graafian follicles. They are usually multiple and range up to 2 cm in size. On occasions, these cystic follicles grow to be > 2 cm and are termed 'follicular cysts'.

14.072 A 59-year-old woman presents with ascites and large bilateral adnexal masses. The MOST likely diagnosis is:
  A. papillary serous cystadenocarcinoma
  B. immature teratoma
  C. polycystic ovaries
  D. follicular cyst
  E. granulosa cell tumor

A is correct.
Tumors of coelomic epithelium of the ovaries are the most common tumors of the ovary. Cystadenocarcinomas occur later in life. Around 65% of these neoplasms are bilateral. They tend to seed the peritoneum, causing ascites.

14.073 A 10-year-old girl is seen by the pediatrician for precocious sexual development. The MOST likely diagnosis is:
   A. papillary serous cystadenocarcinoma
   B. immature teratoma
   C. polycystic ovaries
   D. follicular cyst
   E. granulosa cell tumor

E is correct.
Granulosa cell tumors usually occur in postmenopausal women, but may occur at any age. They are associated with a large production of estrogens which may cause precocious puberty in prepubertal girls.

14.074 All of the following are correct statements as regards cervical carcinoma EXCEPT:
   A. preinvasive lesions can usually be detected by a routine test
   B. more commonly seen in women with multiple partners
   C. the vast majority of cases are squamous in nature
   D. cervical carcinomas progress more rapidly in HIV-positive patients
   E. commonly metastasize to distant organs

E is correct.
Invasive cervical carcinoma tends to invade contingent structures and spread to regional lymph nodes rather than metastasize outside the pelvis.

14.075 All of the following are associated with increased risk for endometrial carcinoma EXCEPT:
   A. adenomatous endometrial hyperplasia
   B. hypertension
   C. history of invasive cervical carcinoma
   D. granulosa cell tumor
   E. thecoma of the ovary

C is correct.
There is no association between endometrial carcinoma and cervical carcinoma.

14.076 Clear cell carcinoma of the vagina is thought to be caused by:
   A. human papillomavirus (HPV)
   B. high level of estrogen
   C. exposure *in utero* to diethylstilbestrol
   D. unopposed progesterone stimulation
   E. herpesvirus

C is correct.
Clear cell adenocarcinomas of the vagina are most frequently seen in teenage girls whose mothers took diethylstilbestrol during pregnancy.

14.077 A 22-year-old woman attends the Family Planning Clinic. During routine physical examination, a non-tender indurated ulcer is noted on her labia minora. What is the MOST likely causative microorganism?
   A. *Treponema pallidum*
   B. herpesvirus
   C. human papillomavirus
   D. *Chlamydia trachomatis*
   E. molluscum contagiosum

A is correct.
Primary syphilis presents as a single firm, non-tender, raised lesion at the site of invasion by *Treponema pallidum*, usually on the labia.

14.078   Which of the following is a variant of breast carcinoma which occurs MORE often in younger women and is MORE likely to be bilateral than conventional invasive ductal carcinoma?
    A. lobular carcinoma
    B. ductal carcinoma in situ
    C. phyllodes tumor (cystosarcoma phyllodes)
    D. intraductal papilloma
    E. gynecomastia

A is correct.
Lobular carcinoma arises from the terminal ductules of the breast. These tumors are often bilateral and tend to be multicentric.

14.079   Malignant tumor cells remain confined to the duct in which of the following breast cancers?
    A. lobular carcinoma
    B. ductal carcinoma in situ
    C. phyllodes tumor (cystosarcoma phyllodes)
    D. intraductal papilloma
    E. gynecomastia

B is correct.
Ductal carcinoma in situ refers to non-invasive carcinoma confined to the ductal epithelium.

14.080   A hysterectomy specimen from a 40-year-old woman shows multiple discrete, sharply circumscribed, firm gray-white masses ranging from 5 mm to 8 cm in size. What is the MOST likely diagnosis?
    A. leiomyosarcoma
    B. leiomyoma
    C. endometriosis
    D. endometrial stromal sarcoma
    E. fibroma

B is correct.
The description is classic for leiomyoma. These are the most common benign tumors found in women. They are present in up to 50% of women during reproductive life. Estrogens stimulate the growth of leiomyomas. The most frequent clinical symptom of leiomyoma is menorrhagia. It is unlikely that leiomyomas become malignant.

14.081   A 35-year-old woman presented to the Infertility Clinic. Her diagnostic work-up was negative except for a sessile intrauterine mass which was seen at the time of hysteroscopy. The MOST likely diagnosis is:
    A. leiomyoma
    B. invasive endometrioid adenocarcinoma
    C. leiomyosarcoma
    D. adenomyosis
    E. simple endometrial hyperplasia

A is correct.
Leiomyomas, or benign neoplasms of smooth muscle, are common in the myometrium. On occasions, they may protrude into the uterine cavity on a sessile stalk. In this situation, they may contribute to infertility.

SECTION 15: ENDOCRINE SYSTEM

15.001   Of the following hypertensive patients, which one is MOST likely to have a decreased peripheral venous renin concentration?
- A. a patient with chronic glomerulonephritis
- B. a patient with atherosclerotic plaques in both renal arteries
- C. a patient with primary hyperaldosteronism due to adrenal adenoma
- D. a patient with secondary hyperaldosteronism due to liver disease
- E. a patient with essential hypertension taking diuretics for reduction in plasma volume

C is correct.
A patient with primary aldosteronism has suppressed plasma renin that is resistant to stimulation by sodium deprivation because aldosterone is being produced autonomously.

15.002   Adrenal neuroblastomas may undergo differentiation to become:
- A. schwannomas
- B. ganglioneuromas
- C. pheochromocytomas
- D. glioblastomas
- E. adenomas

B is correct.
Neuroblastomas can and do differentiate either partially or totally into ganglioneuromas, especially in infants.

15.003 A 45-year-old man has moderate sustained hypertension, with low plasma renin resistant to stimulation by acute volume depletion and persistently low serum potassium levels. Urine 24-h metanephrine and vanillylmandelic acid levels are normal as are plasma 0600-h and 1800-h cortisol levels. The MOST likely pathologic lesion resulting in this syndrome is:
- A. bilateral adrenocortical hyperplasia
- B. bilateral adrenomedullary hyperplasia
- C. unilateral adrenopheochromocytoma
- D. unilateral adrenocortical adenoma
- E. unilateral adrenocortical carcinoma

D is correct.
At least 75% of all cases of primary hyperaldosteronism are due to a small unilateral adrenocortical adenoma.

15.004 Following a camping trip, an 18-year-old girl develops a high fever and a disseminated purpuric rash. Treatment with antibiotics is instituted but, on the next day, profound circulatory collapse develops, followed by death. The adrenal glands are MOST likely to reveal:
- A. multiple adenomatous nodules
- B. granulomatous disease
- C. hemorrhagic necrosis
- D. atrophy with lymphoid infiltrates
- E. bilateral diffuse cortical hyperplasia

C is correct.
Both rickettsial and meningococcal sepsis may result in disseminated intravascular coagulation leading to fatal bilateral hemorrhagic adrenal necrosis.

15.005 A 50-year-old woman presents mainly with complaints of weight loss, fatigue and cutaneous hyperpigmentation. She has tachycardia. Her serum Na^+ is low, but serum K^+ is elevated; serum cortisol is low with absence of diurnal variation; and serum thyroxine (T_4), triiodothyronine (T_3) and PTH levels are normal. A nuclear-medicine study shows greatly diminished total intravascular volume. Urine studies show greatly increased sodium excretion. An abdominal MRI shows no mass lesions and the adrenal glands are very small bilaterally. Which of the following will give the MOST definitive diagnosis of this patient's condition?

    A. a dexamethasone suppression test for Cushing's disease

    B. an ACTH stimulation test for Addison's disease

    C. an ADH stimulation test for diabetes insipidus

    D. an insulin stimulation test for pituitary insufficiency

    E. an adrenal biopsy for malignancy

B is correct.

An ACTH stimulation test to assess the extent of adrenal reserve is needed. Failure to respond by significant increases in plasma cortisol and urine 24-h free cortisol establishes the diagnosis.

15.006 A 50-year-old man presents mainly with complaints of headache, dizziness and palpitations. Physical examination reveals a blood pressure of 190/105 mmHg. Postural hypotension is present. The retina shows 3+ hypertensive changes. Serum glucose is mildly elevated, but electrolytes, calcium, BUN, creatinine, cortisol and thyroxine are all normal. His 24-h urine shows elevated levels of vanillylmandelic acid. The pathologic process resulting in this syndrome is MOST likely to be:

    A. bilateral hyperplasia

    B. bilateral benign neoplasia

    C. unilateral benign neoplasia

    D. unilateral malignant neoplasia

    E. unilateral hyperplasia

C is correct.

Unilateral benign neoplasia (pheochromocytoma) accounts for 80–90% of cases with presentations similar to this one.

15.007 A 45-year-old woman presents with a main complaint of a 50-lb weight gain over 6 months. Abdominal cutaneous striae are present. Laboratory results show elevated plasma cortisol and elevated 24-h urinary free cortisol. An MRI of the abdomen shows mild bilateral adrenal enlargement without mass lesions. Which of the following laboratory tests is MOST likely to reveal the definitive cause of this patient's problem?

    A. glucose tolerance test

    B. dexamethasone suppression test

    C. water-deprivation test

    D. ACTH stimulation test

    E. TRH stimulation test

B is correct.

Elevated plasma cortisol which is suppressed with high- (8 mg/day), but not low- (2 mg/day), dose dexamethasone is diagnostic of pituitary-based hypercortisolism (Cushing's disease).

15.008 A normotensive 15-year-old girl presents with hirsutism, male distribution of pubic hair and primary amenorrhea. Physical examination reveals an enlarged clitoris, with a small but palpable uterus and adnexa. Serum electrolytes show mildly depressed serum Na^+ and mildly elevated serum K^+. An abdominal MRI shows bilateral adrenal enlargement, but the ovaries are small. Plasma ACTH is mildly elevated. Overproduction of which of the following hormones directly by the adrenal cortex is MOST likely the cause of this syndrome?

    A. cortisol

    B. aldosterone

    C. corticosterone

    D. dehydroepiandrosterone

    E. 1,25-dihydrocholecalciferol

D is correct.

Dehydroepiandrosterone, an androgen, is being overproduced because plasma ACTH is increased to compensate for the underproduction of cortisol (usually due to 21-hydroxylase deficiency).

15.009 A 50-year-old man presents with a history of moderately severe sustained hypertension. His serum K^+ is depressed, plasma renin levels are suppressed and resistant to stimulation by volume depletion using a loop diuretic, and plasma free catecholamine and urine vanillylmandelic acid levels are within normal limits. A 24-h urine shows elevated levels of aldosterone. Renal vein catheterization discloses a 7 : 1 ratio between aldosterone concentrations on the left compared with the right. The pathologic lesion resulting in this syndrome is MOST likely to be:

    A. a small unilateral adrenocortical adenoma

    B. a large unilateral adrenocortical carcinoma

    C. bilateral adrenal hyperplasia

    D. a pituitary adenoma

    E. an oat-cell carcinoma of the lung

A is correct.

Primary hyperaldosteronism is usually due to a unilateral adenoma. The ratio for plasma aldosterone between the left and right renal veins confirms the laterality of the neoplasm.

15.010 A 4-year-old child presents with weight loss, bone pain and a palpable left lower abdominal mass. Although the child is normotensive, plasma free catecholamines and urinary 24-h vanillylmandelic acid are both increased. Multiple lytic bone lesions are present in the skull, spine and pelvis. Which of the following is the MOST likely diagnosis?

    A. neuroblastoma

    B. ganglioneuroma

    C. pheochromocytoma

    D. adrenocortical adenoma

    E. adrenocortical cell carcinoma

A is correct.

In a child of this age, an abdominal mass coupled with increased plasma catecholamines and lytic bone lesions is virtually diagnostic of neuroblastoma.

15.011   A 54-year old man presents with severe episodic hypertension punctuated by attacks of dizziness accompanied by orthostatic hypotension. Serum glucose is mildly elevated, but all other serum chemistries, including cortisol, are normal. An MRI discloses a 3-cm ovoid mass in the right adrenal gland. Which of the following diagnostic tests is MOST likely to result in a definitive diagnosis of this patient's condition?

   A. plasma renin determination

   B. glucose tolerance test

   C. dexamethasone suppression test

   D. 24-h urinary vanillylmandelic acid determination

   E. water-deprivation test with ADH

D is correct.

An elevated 24-h urinary vanillylmandelic acid determination would establish that a pheochromocytoma is the cause of the hypertension.

15.012   A 50-year-old man presents with a history of recent weight loss and fatigue. He is plethoric and short of breath, and mildly hypertensive. Serum chemistries show increased glucose and potassium. Serum cortisol is somewhat elevated with loss of diurnal variation. Radiographic studies show bilateral enlargement of the adrenal glands without nodules and a CT scan of the pituitary is normal. A chest X-ray shows a right upper lobe mass invading the mediastinum, and sputum cytology shows undifferentiated small malignant cells. Which of the following combinations of endocrine abnormalities is this patient MOST likely to have?

   A. very high ACTH with suppression by dexamethasone

   B. very high ACTH without suppression by dexamethasone

   C. low-to-absent ACTH with suppression by dexamethasone

   D. low-to-absent ACTH without suppression by dexamethasone

   E. low-to-absent ACTH with increase after dexamethasone

B is correct.

The plasma ACTH will be very elevated and will not be suppressed by high-dose dexamethasone treatment.

15.013   A moderately obese 45-year-old man presents with recent onset of blurred vision, excessive urine output and fatigue. The remainder of the physical examination is within normal limits. Fasting serum glucose is elevated. Other serum chemistries are normal, including plasma insulin, cortisol and serum creatinine levels. No insulin antibodies are present in the serum. Urinalysis is normal except for a positive glucose reaction. This patient MOST likely has:

   A. secondary diabetes mellitus due to a glucagon-secreting adenoma
   B. secondary diabetes mellitus due to a pituitary adenoma secreting ACTH
   C. early type II diabetes due to a relative lack of insulin and peripheral insulin resistance
   D. late type II diabetes with terminal renal failure and neuropathy
   E. early type I diabetes due to a viral infection and autoimmunity

C is correct.
Early type II (primary) diabetes is associated with relative insulin deficiency and peripheral insulin resistance. The plasma insulin may be normal, as in this case, but the release of insulin after a glucose load is delayed. This, together with deficiencies in insulin receptor activity, is responsible for the elevated serum glucose.

15.014   A 42-year-old woman presents with a history of paroxysmal attacks of sweating, heart palpitations, anxiety, weakness and hunger. She states that she has lost consciousness during these attacks. Physical examination is within normal limits, including pulse and blood pressure. Serum glucose is normal as are plasma insulin and C peptide levels. All other routine laboratory chemistry determinations are normal. The MOST appropriate next diagnostic maneuver is to:

   A. provoke hypoglycemia by overnight fasting
   B. perform a dexamethasone suppression test
   C. perform an ACTH stimulation test
   D. order an MRI of the pituitary
   E. measure the right and left renal vein renin levels

A is correct.
As insulin release from a pancreatic islet cell adenoma is usually paroxysmal, patients are frequently asymptomatic when examined. A 12–24-h fast with mild exercise will provoke an attack in 75% of such patients.

15.015   A 54-year-old male attorney has been followed in your clinic for 15 years for type II diabetes. He has required therapy with insulin-releasing agents. Although he has been only mildly hyperglycemic on his visits, his hemoglobin A_{1C} levels have been consistently somewhat elevated. Although he has a negative physical examination and chest X-ray, he is febrile. He now has a mildly elevated BUN and creatinine with mild proteinuria. Numerous white blood cell casts are noted on micro-scopic examination of the urine. He is at greatest immediate risk for which of the following devastat-ing complications of diabetes mellitus:
   A. ketoacidosis
   B. hyperosmolar non-ketotic coma
   C. renal papillary tip necrosis
   D. disseminated (miliary) tuberculosis
   E. nodular glomerulosclerosis

C is correct.
Due to the microvascular thickening seen in diabetes mellitus, acute pyelonephritis results in renal papillary tip infarction with sloughing into the ureter. This is a devastating complication of renal infection in diabetes.

15.016 Type I diabetes mellitus shows an epidem-iological association with previous infection by:
   A. cytomegalovirus
   B. measles paramyxovirus
   C. *Streptococcus viridans*
   D. rubella togavirus
   E. Epstein–Barr virus

D is correct.
Rubella-induced cellular cytotoxicity is implicated in the destruction of beta cells preceding type I diabetes mellitus. Some cases have occurred due to vaccine strains.

15.017 A 46-year-old woman is diagnosed with Zollinger–Ellison syndrome after a long history of intractable peptic ulcer disease. As an astute clini-cian, you take a detailed family history and find that her mother had a pituitary adenoma and an uncle had bilateral adrenal hyperplasia. What OTHER organ or tissue do you suspect of harboring neoplasms in this patient or other family members?
   A. adrenal medulla
   B. parathyroid glands
   C. peripheral nerves
   D. thymus
   E. carotid body

B is correct.
Parathyroid adenomas are associated with both multiple endocrine neoplasia syndromes – type I (MEN I) and type IIa (MEN IIa).

15.018   A 45-year-old woman presents mainly with a complaint of recurrent midepigastric pain. Endoscopy reveals an ulcer in the first portion of the duodenum with a possible second ulcer in the second portion of the duodenum. Serum calcium is elevated and serum phosphorus is depressed. BUN, creatinine, glucose and electrolytes in the serum are all normal. It would be BEST to order which of the following pairs of serum hormone determinations?

   A. parathyroid hormone and insulin
   B. parathyroid hormone and gastrin
   C. parathyroid hormone and glucagon
   D. calcitonin and gastrin
   E. 1,25-dihydroxycholecalciferol and serotonin

B is correct.

The combination of elevated serum calcium and depressed serum phosphorus strongly suggests primary hyperparathyroidism for which a PTH level is diagnostic. Furthermore, the duodenal ulcers suggest the possibility of Zollinger–Ellison syndrome due to a gastrin-secreting pancreatic neoplasm (MEN I).

15.019   A 16-year-old patient develops severe hyperglycemia associated with undetectable plasma insulin levels. The patient has an identical twin whose parents are well-read and ask you for an explanation for why only 33% of identical twins of index patients subsequently develop this syndrome. The BEST answer is:

   A. inheritance of type I diabetes is polygenic
   B. type I diabetes is an autoimmune disorder occurring after a viral infection in susceptible individuals
   C. type I diabetes occurs after somatic mutation in the pancreatic islets; one twin has developed the mutation
   D. type I diabetes shows no genetic predisposition and the 33% is merely a coincidence
   E. type I diabetes is induced by dietary fads that were probably different between the two twins

B is correct.

Type I diabetes is an autoimmune disorder, but it requires an environmental interaction, such as a viral infection, to trigger the selective beta cell destruction in susceptible individuals. Hence, only some subjects carrying the gene develop the disease.

15.020   A 56-year-old woman is under your care for type II diabetes mellitus for several years; treatment is with dietary restriction and drugs promoting insulin release from the pancreas. Her serum glucose is frequently borderline elevated and her hemoglobin A_{1C} is consistently so. She complains of decreasing visual acuity. An ocular examination discloses bilateral cataracts. Accumulation and subsequent binding of which of the following in the lens is MOST responsible for the cataracts?

   A. insulin
   B. glucagon
   C. sorbitol
   D. mannitol
   E. glycogen

C is correct.

The hyperglycemia results in an increased passive diffusion of glucose into several tissues, including the lens. Sorbitol levels are also increased by metabolism of glucose. Sorbitol binds to collagen in the lens to produce opacification. Sorbitol is also implicated in diabetic neuropathy.

15.021 A 55-year-old woman presents with attacks of dizziness, confusion and seizures relieved by glucose administration. Plasma insulin levels are elevated, but other pancreatic islet hormones are normal. An overnight fast with exercise provokes profound hypoglycemia associated with marked elevation of plasma insulin concentration. Based on the relative frequencies of the lesions causing this syndrome, the pathology MOST likely to be found in the pancreas is:

    A. a single islet cell adenoma

    B. multiple islet cell adenomas

    C. a single islet cell carcinoma

    D. multiple islet cell carcinomas

    E. diffuse hyperplasia of the islets

A is correct.

The most common lesion associated with paroxysmal bouts of hypoglycemia associated with elevated plasma insulin levels is a single pancreatic islet cell adenoma.

15.022 Which of the following endocrine neoplasms is the MOST likely to pursue a malignant course?

    A. a parathyroid neoplasm secreting parathyroid hormone

    B. an intra-adrenal pheochromocytoma secreting norepinephrine

    C. a basophilic pituitary neoplasm secreting ACTH

    D. an islet cell tumor secreting gastrin

    E. an islet cell tumor secreting insulin

D is correct.

Up to 67% of all cases of Zollinger–Ellison syndrome (primary hypergastrinism) are due to islet cell carcinomas.

15.023 A 20-year-old woman first develops elevated fasting and 2-h postprandial plasma glucose concentrations during the third trimester of pregnancy. One month after delivery, both her fasting and 2-h postprandial blood glucose concentrations are normal. Which of the following is the MOST likely diagnosis?

    A. type I diabetes mellitus (IDDM)

    B. type II diabetes mellitus (NIDDM)

    C. mature-onset diabetes mellitus of the young (MODY)

    D. gestational diabetes mellitus

    E. secondary diabetes mellitus

    F. diabetes insipidus

D is correct.

Gestational diabetes mellitus is diagnosed when an elevated blood glucose ($<165\,mg/dl$ 2-h postprandial) level is first observed during pregnancy. Up to 50% of these women will subsequently develop permanent diabetes.

15.024   A 16-year-old girl presents with short stature, patchy calcifications of the skin, and mucocutaneous whitish patches in the mouth and vagina. Her serum calcium is low; the serum phosphorus is high; and levels of serum parathyroid hormone (PTH) are also elevated. A PTH infusion fails to result in an increase in cyclic AMP in the urine. This patient is MOST likely to have:

A. primary hypoparathyroidism
B. secondary hypoparathyroidism
C. pseudohypoparathyroidism
D. pseudopseudohypoparathyroidism
E. primary hyperparathyroidism

C is correct.
Pseudohypoparathyroidism presents with low serum calcium and high serum phosphorus, short stature and failure of PTH to increase cyclic AMP in the urine.

15.025   A 48-year-old woman presents to your clinic with her third episode of renal 'colic' due to passage of kidney stones. Deposition of a ring of calcium is noted around the corneal limbus in both eyes. Her serum calcium and parathyroid hormone are both elevated. The pathologic lesion(s) MOST likely to result in this syndrome is/are:

A. a single parathyroid adenoma
B. a single parathyroid carcinoma
C. primary hyperplasia of all four parathyroid glands
D. secondary hyperplasia of all four parathyroid glands
E. multiple parathyroid adenomas

A is correct.
Primary hyperparathyroidism is most often due to a single hyperfunctioning adenoma.

15.026   In which of the following disease states is the serum parathyroid hormone concentration MOST likely to be low in relation to the serum calcium?

A. primary hyperparathyroidism
B. secondary hyperparathyroidism
C. tertiary hyperparathyroidism
D. pseudohypoparathyroidism
E. malignancy-associated hypercalcemia (pseudohyperparathyroidism)

E is correct.
In malignancy-associated hypercalcemia, parathyroid hormone levels are low despite the elevated serum calcium. This situation is due to non-parathyroid mediators of bone resorption, such as so-called parathyroid hormone-like protein.

15.027   A 55-year-old man who has chronic renal failure due to glomerulonephritis is maintained by chronic hemodialysis. Serum calcium is depressed and serum phosphorus increased. An immuno-reactive serum parathyroid hormone level is also increased as is the 24-h urinary hydroxyproline excretion. Skeletal X-rays show multiple cystic lesions, especially in the pelvic bones. The cause of this pathophysiology is loss of an enzyme in the:

A. kidney
B. parathyroid
C. thyroid
D. small intestine
E. bone

A is correct.
The loss or suppression of 1-hydroxylase activity (conversion of 25-hydroxy-vitamin D_3 to the active form 1,25-dihydroxy-vitamin D_3) in the kidney is a principal factor in the calcium wasting syndrome in this patient.

15.028   A 50-year-old man with chronic mild hypertension complains of weakness, constipation and frequent bouts with renal stones. His serum calcium is increased and serum phosphorus is decreased. Serum creatinine, BUN and potassium are all normal. Bone films show demineralization with multiple small cystic areas. The primary cause of this patient's disease MOST likely lies in the:

    A. kidney

    B. bone

    C. adrenal glands

    D. parathyroid gland

    E. pituitary gland

D is correct.
The parathyroid glands are autonomously producing excessive parathyroid hormone, most probably due to a single hyperfunctioning adenoma.

15.029   A 45-year-old woman presents with a history of increasing glove and shoe sizes, and generalized joint pain. She has coarse features. Serum chemistries disclose an elevated fasting blood glucose. Physical examination reveals no abdominal cutaneous striae, 'buffalo hump' or galactorrhea. She has a reduced range of motion in all major joints. A CT scan discloses enlargement of the sella turcica. Hypersecretion of which of the following has MOST likely resulted in this syndrome?

    A. adrenocorticotropic hormone

    B. antidiuretic hormone

    C. thyroid-stimulating hormone

    D. somatotropin

    E. follicle-stimulating hormone

D is correct.
Somatotropin hypersecretion results in overgrowth of the hands and feet, generalized arthritis and insulin resistance with hyperglycemia.

15.030 A 52-year-old man presents with complaints of headache and decreased libido. He denies any weight gain or loss, change in shoe size, polyuria or heat intolerance. Visual field analysis shows bitemporal hemianopia. An MRI of the pituitary shows sellar enlargement. Routine clinical chemistry determinations are within normal limits. Plasma determination of which of the following hormones is MOST likely to be elevated?

    A. insulin

    B. somatostatin

    C. prolactin

    D. adrenocorticotropic hormone

    E. testosterone

C is correct.
Prolactin is the most common hormone secreted by pituitary adenomas and results in the syndrome seen in this patient.

15.031 The syndrome of inappropriate antidiuretic hormone secretion (SIADH) is MOST commonly seen with neoplasms of the:

    A. kidney

    B. adrenal

    C. liver

    D. lung

    E. brain

D is correct.
SIADH is most commonly seen in patients with small-cell undifferentiated pulmonary carcinoma.

15.032   Which one of the following hormones is deficient in primary adrenal insufficiency due to intrinsic adrenal disease, but NOT in secondary adrenal insufficiency due to pituitary disease?

   A. cortisol
   B. corticosterone
   C. aldosterone
   D. estrogen
   E. testosterone

C is correct.
Aldosterone is deficient in primary, but not in secondary, adrenal insufficiency.

15.033   The first clinical manifestation of Sheehan's syndrome is MOST commonly:

   A. hypothyroidism
   B. hypokalemia
   C. failure of lactation
   D. hypocalcemia
   E. hyperglycemia

C is correct.
Failure of lactation in the postpartum state is the usual first clinical manifestation of Sheehan's syndrome.

15.034   A 40-year-old woman presents with a history of a 40-lb weight gain, hirsutism and poor wound-healing. Physical examination reveals abdominal striae and centripetal obesity with a 'buffalo hump'. A CT scan shows bilateral adrenal enlargement without nodules; a chest X-ray is normal. The MOST likely combination of laboratory studies from the plasma is:

   A. increased cortisol, decreased ACTH, aldosterone normal
   B. increased cortisol, increased ACTH, aldosterone normal
   C. decreased cortisol, increased ACTH, decreased aldosterone
   D. cortisol normal, increased ACTH, increased aldosterone
   E. decreased cortisol, ACTH normal, increased aldosterone

B is correct.
Both plasma cortisol and ACTH will be increased, but plasma aldosterone will be normal.

15.035   A 28-year-old woman develops lethargy, amenorrhea, failure of lactation, and loss of libido following vaginal delivery of a 4.5-kg infant preceded by prolonged labor. Two months later, all of the following plasma hormone levels are markedly depressed EXCEPT:

   A. cortisol
   B. aldosterone
   C. thyroxine (T_4)
   D. prolactin
   E. follicle-stimulating hormone

B is correct.
Aldosterone is not depressed following pituitary infarction (Sheehan's syndrome), because its production is primarily under the control of the renin–angiotensin system rather than of ACTH.

15.036   A pregnant woman suffers hypovolemic shock at delivery secondary to placenta previa. Six months later, she has amenorrhea, low serum thyroxine (T$_4$) and TSH, and low ACTH. An insulin test for pituitary reserve confirms that the pituitary is not functioning. The pathologic process that has led to this syndrome is MOST likely to be:

   A. a large chromophobe adenoma developing during pregnancy

   B. autoimmune-mediated atrophy of the anterior pituitary

   C. hemorrhagic infarction of the anterior pituitary

   D. destruction of the posterior pituitary stalk

   E. infarction of the supraoptic nucleus in the hypothalamus

C is correct.

Hemorrhagic infarction of the pituitary due to shock during or around delivery is the most likely pathologic lesion. The infarction is hemorrhagic because the pituitary has a dual blood supply (an arterial and a portal venous system).

15.037   A 68-year-old woman presents to your clinic with a history of a mass in the right anterior midneck in the region occupied by the thyroid gland. The mass has attained a diameter of 5 cm over approximately 3 months. She is hospitalized and the mass is biopsied. The histology shows undifferentiated spindle and giant cells with a high mitotic rate. Although no colloid- or follicle-forming cells are seen, the neoplasm is histologically present in the strap muscle. The patient's son asks you for his mother's prognosis. Which of the following is the MOST accurate statement you can make to the son?

   A. this process may appear aggressive, but it is highly likely to undergo spontaneous remission

   B. this neoplasm has a tendency to spread to regional lymph nodes, which can be removed with a good possibility of cure

   C. this neoplasm is malignant and usually spreads to the liver and lungs, where chemotherapy is effective

   D. this highly malignant neoplasm grows so rapidly that it will compromise the airways before it metastasizes, resulting in death within a few weeks

   E. radiation, radical surgery and chemotherapy will produce a good response, but the patient will die within several years

D is correct.

This rapidly growing carcinoma (undifferentiated carcinoma) compromises the airways and kills in a matter of weeks.

15.038 A hypertensive 25-year-old woman presents with firm, 2-cm masses in both the right and left upper poles of the thyroid gland. A radioiodine thyroid scan discloses 'cold' nodules corresponding to the physical finding. Serum T_4, T_3, cortisol, BUN, creatinine and electrolytes are all normal. Serum calcitonin is elevated on two different occasions. What other organ is MOST likely to harbor a primary neoplasm in this patient?

    A. pancreas
    B. adrenal
    C. pituitary
    D. thymus
    E. ovary

B is correct.
This patient is at great risk for MEN II, in which 50% of the patients have adrenal pheochromocytomas.

15.039 A 32-year-old woman presents with a history of weight loss, palpitations, sleeplessness and heat intolerance. Her thyroid gland is diffusely enlarged without nodules and is non-tender. A bruit is heard over the gland. Serum T_4 and T_3 resin uptake are both markedly elevated. Radioiodine uptake by the gland is diffusely increased on a thyroid scan. If the thyroid gland were to be surgically removed, which of the following histologic descriptions is the MOST likely to be seen?

    A. acute inflammation and nodules of giant cells ingesting colloid
    B. increased height of thyroid acinar cells with no colloid present and marked hypervascularity
    C. an area of papillary growths with psammoma bodies
    D. lymphoid follicles, scarring and conversion of thyroid cells to oncocytes
    E. areas of hemorrhage and lakes of colloid with attenuated thyroid epithelial cells surrounding large follicles

B is correct.
Increased thyroid acinar cell height and hypervascularity are characteristic of Graves' disease (diffuse toxic goiter).

15.040 A 4-year-old girl is brought to your clinic by her parents, who have recently immigrated to the USA from a country in the Andes mountains. The child shows profound mental and growth retardation. The parents say she was 'normal' at birth. Her attempts at speech reveal a coarse voice, and deep tendon reflexes are depressed. She has a peculiar periorbital edema and a blank facial expression. A palpable mass is present in the anterior midneck surrounding the infraglottic trachea. A serum or plasma level of which hormone is MOST likely to be depressed?

    A. thyroxine (T_4)

    B. somatotropin (STH)

    C. thyroid-releasing hormone (TRH)

    D. thyroid-stimulating hormone (TSH)

    E. adrenocorticotropic hormone (ACTH)

A is correct.

Serum thyroxine (T_4) will be low in this child, who has congenital hypothyroidism or 'cretinism'.

15.041 A 40-year-old woman presents with features suggestive of early hypothyroidism. The MOST sensitive laboratory test to confirm the diagnosis is:

    A. T_3 resin uptake

    B. T_4 resin uptake

    C. plasma total T_4 level

    D. plasma thyroid-binding globulin level

    E. plasma TSH level

E is correct.

The plasma TSH will rise even before the plasma T_4 is significantly lowered as an attempt at compensation for the developing hypothyroidism.

15.042 A 25-year-old woman presents with a single firm nodule of the thyroid gland. A needle biopsy reveals papillary glandular fragments with a clear appearance to the nuclei and multilaminated extracellular calcified spherules. The MOST likely organ or tissue to also contain similar cells is:

    A. liver

    B. bone

    C. lymph node

    D. lung

    E. adrenal

C is correct.

Papillary thyroid carcinomas typically metastasize to the ipsilateral lymph nodes.

15.043 A 40-year-old woman who is HLA-DR5[+] has autoimmune thyroiditis (Hashimoto's disease). Her chances of developing which one of the following is markedly INCREASED?

    A. follicular carcinoma

    B. anaplastic (undifferentiated) carcinoma

    C. medullary carcinoma

    D. fibrosarcoma

    E. malignant lymphoma

E is correct.

The development of malignant lymphoma (B-cell type) is increased approximately 67-fold in patients with Hashimoto's disease.

15.044   A 45-year-old woman with a diffusely enlarged thyroid presents with clinical features of hypothyroidism. The MOST likely diagnosis is:
   A. de Quervain's disease (subacute granulomatous thyroiditis)
   B. Hashimoto's disease (chronic autoimmune thyroiditis)
   C. Graves' disease (diffuse toxic hyperplasia)
   D. Plummer's disease (toxic nodular goiter)
   E. Riedel's struma (ligneous thyroiditis)

B is correct.
Hashimoto's disease is the most common cause of hypothyroidism associated with an enlarged thyroid gland.

15.045   A 35-year-old woman presents with recent weight loss, heat intolerance and sleep disturbances. Physical examination reveals tachycardia and hyperactive deep tendon reflexes. Bilateral ocular proptosis and brawny patches of thickening of the pretibial skin are clearly present. Serum T_4 and T_3 resin uptake are both markedly elevated. The MOST likely condition leading to this pathophysiology is a:
   A. 'toxic' thyroid adenoma
   B. toxic thyroid nodular goiter
   C. diffuse toxic thyroid hyperplasia
   D. pituitary adenoma
   E. hypothalamic hyperplasia

C is correct.
The clinical picture and laboratory data suggest thyroid hyperfunction. The finding of bilateral ocular proptosis is not seen in cases of thyrotoxicosis except for Graves' disease (diffuse toxic thyroid hyperplasia).

15.046   A 32-year-old woman presents with a history of cold intolerance, weight gain and difficulty in performing her job as an accountant. Her face is edematous, and her hair is coarse and stiff. She has bradycardia with depressed deep tendon reflexes. Which of the following serum hormone determinations is MOST likely to be elevated?
   A. antidiuretic hormone (ADH)
   B. thyroid-stimulating hormone (TSH)
   C. adrenocorticotropic hormone (ACTH)
   D. somatotropin (STH)
   E. prolactin (PRL)

B is correct.
The clinical symptoms described are most likely associated with hypothyroidism. Laboratory evaluation of thyroid-stimulating hormone will probably provide confirmative information for a diagnosis.

15.047   Which of the following sets of screening laboratory data is MOST suggestive of hypoparathyroidism?
   A. low serum potassium in a hypertensive patient
   B. low serum glucose provoked by exercise
   C. low serum calcium and high serum phosphorus
   D. high serum glucose 2 h after a meal
   E. low serum chloride in a peptic ulcer patient

C is correct.
Parathyroid hormone mobilizes calcium from bone, increases renal tubular resorption of calcium and lowers serum phosphate by enhancing phosphate loss in the urine. Decreased concentrations of parathyroid hormone result in lowered serum calcium and increased serum phosphorus levels.

15.048 A 45-year-old woman is undergoing hemodialysis for chronic renal failure. Her serum calcium is chronically low in spite of dietary supplements. Serum parathyroid hormone is markedly elevated. Several lytic areas in the pelvic bones and long bones are noted. The microscopic appearance of these bone lesions is MOST likely to resemble:
    A. giant cell tumor of bone
    B. breast carcinoma
    C. small-cell undifferentiated carcinoma
    D. colon carcinoma
    E. Hodgkin's disease

A is correct.
The clinical condition in this case is that of secondary hyperparathyroidism. Elevated levels of parathyroid hormone initiate mediators that stimulate osteoclast activity. The resulting osteoclastic bone resorption appears on histology as increased numbers of osteoclasts, reactive fibrous tissue, cystic degeneration and hemosiderin pigmentation secondary to microhemorrhages. This histologic picture is similar to that of giant cell tumors of bone.

15.049 In the USA, which of the following clinical situations is the MOST common cause of secondary hyperparathyroidism?
    A. dietary calcium deficiency
    B. dietary vitamin D deficiency
    C. pseudohypoparathyroidism
    D. chronic renal failure
    E. malnutrition

D is correct.
Secondary hyperparathyroidism is most often due to chronic renal failure.

15.050 A 25-year-old primigravida woman experiences excessive blood loss, shock and disseminated intravascular coagulation during delivery. She recovers but, 6 months later, she has not begun menstruating and appears to be depressed with cold skin. The causative lesion in this patient is MOST likely to be located in the:
    A. adrenal glands
    B. anterior pituitary gland
    C. ovaries
    D. thyroid gland
    E. hypothalamus

B is correct.
This patient has Sheehan's syndrome or postpartum pituitary necrosis. This condition is caused by infarction of the anterior lobe of the pituitary. In pregnancy, the anterior pituitary enlarges, causing some compression of its vascular supply. Systemic hypotension secondary to blood loss causes vasospasm of vessels resulting in ischemic infarction.

15.051 A 30-year-old woman presents to your clinic with a history of a 20-lb weight loss, nervousness and excessive sweating. The thyroid gland is diffusely enlarged, but painless. Her deep tendon reflexes are increased and non-pitting edema is noted in the pretibial soft tissues bilaterally. Both eyes show mild proptosis. The substance stimulating the thyroid gland is being produced by:
    A. hypothalamic neurons
    B. anterior pituitary cells
    C. B lymphocytes / plasma cells
    D. splenic macrophages
    E. thymic neuroendocrine cells

C is correct.
The diagnosis in this case is Graves' disease or diffuse toxic thyroid hyperplasia. Evidence suggests that the changes in the thyroid gland are initiated by IgG antibodies against some portion of the TSH receptors. These antibodies are, of course, products of B lymphocytes and / or plasma cells.

15.052   An abnormally short 16-year-old girl presents with hypotension and attacks of tetany. She has patchy calcific plaques in the skin, calcification in the basal ganglia on a skull X-ray, and curiously short fourth metacarpal and metatarsal bones. Clinical laboratory studies reveal a low serum calcium, high serum phosphorus and an elevated serum parathyroid hormone (PTH) on several occasions. Serum creatinine, BUN and potassium are all normal. This patient's metabolic condition is MOST likely due to:

   A. parathyroid neoplasm
   B. renal tubular unresponsiveness to parathyroid hormone
   C. chronic renal failure
   D. dietary deficiency of calcium
   E. congenital absence of parathyroid glands

B is correct.
The diagnosis in this case is pseudohypoparathyroidism, a condition with hypocalcemia and hyperphosphatemia as the result of variable degrees of end-organ unresponsiveness to PTH. Serum levels of PTH are either normal or elevated.

15.053   A 55-year-old woman is referred to your office with a 10-year history of hypothyroidism. The thyroid gland has recently begun to diffusely and markedly enlarge, and antithyroid antibodies are present in high titers in her serum. On physical examination, you note bilateral enlargement of the cervical and supraclavicular lymph nodes. You perform needle aspiration of a cervical lymph node. Which of the following is the MOST likely finding?

   A. papillary fragments with psammoma bodies
   B. neuroendocrine cells and amyloid
   C. neoplastic thyroid acini
   D. dysplastic monoclonal B lymphocytes
   E. myeloblasts and immature granulocytes

D is correct.
This case typifies a patient with autoimmune thyroiditis, or Hashimoto's disease. In this condition, there is an increased prevalence of lymphoma usually of the non-Hodgkin's type. Most are of a large-cell immunoblastic pattern with B-cell lineage.

15.054 A 42-year-old hypertensive woman presents with a history of a 50-lb weight gain over the past year. Serum glucose and plasma cortisol are both elevated. Plasma and urine cortisol fail to suppress with either high- or low-dose dexamethasone infusions, and the plasma ACTH is undetectable. The lesion causing this patient's condition is MOST likely in the:

   A. hypothalamus
   B. anterior pituitary
   C. lung
   D. adrenal cortex
   E. adrenal medulla

D is correct.
Low-dose dexamethasone fails to suppress plasma and urine cortisol levels in patients with hypersteroidism secondary to pituitary hyperfunction or to adrenal neoplasm. High-dose dexamethasone suppresses cortisol levels in cases of pituitary hyperfunction, but not adrenal neoplasms. Therefore, failure to suppress with both low and high doses of dexamethasone indicate that the lesion is primary in the adrenal cortex.

15.055 A 50-year-old malpractice attorney presents with a history of headache and weakness. Physical examination discloses an elevated blood pressure of 160/108 mmHg on three separate days. Serum sodium is elevated and serum potassium is depressed. Plasma renin is suppressed and does not increase with acute volume depletion by diuretics. Plasma ADH and catecholamines are normal. The lesion causing this patient's syndrome is MOST likely to be in the:

    A. hypothalamus
    B. anterior pituitary
    C. posterior pituitary
    D. adrenal cortex
    E. adrenal medulla

D is correct.

Acute volume depletion with diuretics is used as a screening test in patients with hypertension, and low serum potassium and low peripheral venous renin concentrations. Normal subjects will stimulate renin whereas a patient with primary hyperaldosteronism will not. Most cases of primary hyperaldosteronism are due to a single unilateral adenoma in the adrenal cortex.

15.056 A 28-year-old pregnant woman is observed to have a fasting blood glucose of 220 mg/dl. She fails to keep her clinic appointments and is delivered by Cesarean section of an 11.8-lb (5.4-kg) infant after 35 weeks of gestation. The baby's large size is the result of overproduction of:

    A. maternal insulin
    B. maternal growth hormone
    C. maternal gonadotropins
    D. fetal insulin
    E. fetal gonadotropins

D is correct.

The maternal hyperglycemia stimulates hyperplasia of fetal islet cells. The increased fetal insulin production is responsible for the increased birth weight.

15.057 Which of the following risk factors is MORE important in the pathogenesis of type I (insulin-dependent) than in type II (non-insulin-dependent) diabetes mellitus?

    A. HLA-DR3/DQ3.2 heterozygosity
    B. obesity
    C. decrease in number of insulin receptors
    D. impaired activity of glucose transport units
    E. defects in insulin receptor tyrosine kinase activity

A is correct.

In type I diabetes, there is an altered immune regulation linked to HLA-DR3/DQ3.2 leading to autoimmunity to islet B cells. There is no HLA linkage with type II diabetes mellitus.

15.058 A 38-year-old woman presents with a 40-lb weight gain over the last 6 months, mild hirsutism and abdominal cutaneous striae. On physical examination, you think you palpate an abdominal mass in the left upper quadrant, but it may be the spleen. Plasma and 24-h urine cortisol determinations are both elevated, and both are suppressed by high, but not low, doses of dexamethasone infusions. The MOST likely site for the lesion causing this patient's symptoms is:

    A. lung
    B. anterior pituitary
    C. adrenal cortex
    D. adrenal medulla
    E. pancreas

B is correct.

Elevated plasma cortisol, which suppresses with high- (8 mg/day), but not low- (2 mg/day), dose dexamethasone is diagnostic of pituitary-based hypercortisolism (Cushing's disease).

15.059 A 21-year-old woman presents with a firm palpable nodule in the right upper lobe of the thyroid gland. A radioiodine (^{131}I) scan of her neck shows a single hypofunctioning nodule in the thyroid, but also several small foci of uptake in the right cervical lymph nodes. The process in the thyroid gland is MOST likely to be:

    A. follicular carcinoma

    B. follicular adenoma

    C. papillary carcinoma

    D. medullary carcinoma

    E. malignant lymphoma

C is correct.

The uptake in the cervical nodes suggests metastatic thyroid carcinoma. Papillary carcinomas are the most frequent form of thyroid carcinoma and have often metastasized to the cervical lymph nodes at the time of diagnosis.

15.060 A 15-year-old girl is brought to your office by her mother because of primary amenorrhea. On physical examination, the adolescent shows poor development of breast tissue, male pubic hair distribution and male pattern skin creases at the elbows. Plasma testosterone is normal, but plasma androstanedione and other C_{19} androgens are elevated. Plasma ACTH is markedly increased. An abdominal CT scan shows bilateral suprarenal masses. Administration of cortisol produces a marked decrease in C_{19} androgens. The primary defect in this patient is an enzyme defect in the:

    A. hypothalamus

    B. anterior pituitary

    C. ovaries

    D. adrenal cortex

    E. adrenal medulla

D is correct.

This patient has congenital adrenal hyperplasia (adrenogenital syndrome). A deficiency of an enzyme involved in the biosynthesis of corticosteroids is found in this disease. Because of the block in steroid synthesis, there is a low cortisol level, increased secretion of ACTH and resulting adrenocortical hyperplasia. The metabolic compounds in steroid metabolism are redirected toward other pathways, resulting in an increased production of androgens.

15.061 A 45-year-old man presents with a history of fatigue and weight loss. On physical examination, he is thin with hyperpigmentation of the skin and oral mucous membranes. He is hypotensive with a definite tachycardia. Serum chemistry studies show normal serum calcium, phosphorus and creatinine, but serum glucose and sodium are low, and potassium is elevated. The plasma morning cortisol level is low on several occasions and does not rise after ACTH administration. An abdominal CT scan discloses small adrenal glands bilaterally. This patient is MOST likely to have a(n):

    A. autoimmune disorder

    B. metastatic carcinoma

    C. pituitary neoplasm

    D. granulomatous infection

    E. congenital enzyme deficiency

A is correct.

This patient has primary chronic adrenocortical insufficiency (Addison's disease). Autoimmune adrenalitis is responsible for most of these cases.

15.062 A 52-year-old woman presents with breast cancer widely metastatic to bone with resulting hypercalcemia due to release of prostaglandin E_2 by tumor cells directly into the bone interstitium, where osteoclasts are then activated. This is an example of which of the following types of cellular secretory activity?

   A. endocrine

   B. paracrine

   C. neurocrine

   D. autocrine

   E. exocrine

B is correct.

Paracrine secretion is the release of a hormone into the interstitium to act locally. Endocrine secretion is the release of hormone into the blood to act systemically. Neurocrine secretion is the release through nerve synapses, and autocrine secretion is the release of hormones by a cell for its own receptors.

15.063 Which of the following 'stimulation' tests is used to confirm the presence of diabetes insipidus?

   A. insulin-induced hypoglycemia test

   B. parathyroid hormone provocation test

   C. water-deprivation test with and without antidiuretic hormone

   D. ACTH stimulation test

   E. glucose tolerance test

C is correct.

Dysfunction of the posterior pituitary gland manifests as antidiuretic hormone (ADH) deficiency, leading to diabetes insipidus, which consists of abnormal regulation of water excretion.

15.064 A 48-year-old woman presents to your clinic for a preemployment examination. She has recently moved to Arkansas from Montana, where she has lived her entire life. You note bilateral painless enlargement of her thyroid gland bearing several palpable nodules. Plasma thyroxine (T_4) and triiodothyronine (T_3) are normal, but plasma TSH is mildly elevated. No serum antithyroid antibodies are detected. Which of the following is the BEST presumptive diagnosis for this patient?

   A. non-toxic multinodular goiter

   B. toxic nodular goiter

   C. chronic autoimmune thyroiditis

   D. subacute granulomatous thyroiditis

   E. diffuse toxic goiter

A is correct.

Painless nodular enlargement of the thyroid with a euthyroid state is most likely due to multinodular goiter. This condition develops from a diffuse goiter due to differences among thyroid cells in terms of response to TSH and ability to replicate. Goiter is caused by a basic deficiency of iodine intake. The incidence is increased in certain geographic locations.

15.065   A 38-year-old woman presents to your clinic with a history of 30-lb (13.6-kg) weight gain over the last year. Her skin and hair are coarse, and her deep tendon reflexes are depressed. The thyroid gland is diffusely enlarged with no nodules or tenderness. Her plasma TSH is markedly elevated and total serum thyroxine (T_4) is depressed. Which of the following laboratory tests is MOST likely to give specific information as to the etiology of this patient's disorder?
   A. serum free T_4 determination
   B. serum antithyroid antibody determination
   C. TRH stimulation test
   D. serum T_3 determination
   E. serum T_3 uptake test

B is correct.
This is a case of Hashimoto's thyroiditis (chronic autoimmune thyroiditis). In this condition, there is production of thyroid autoantibodies by B cells resulting in high levels of circulating autoantibodies with affinity for the TSH receptor.

15.066   A 30-year-old woman presents to your clinic with a history of a 20-lb weight loss, nervousness and excessive sweating. The thyroid gland is diffusely enlarged and a soft bruit can be heard over the gland. Her deep tendon reflexes are increased. Other than her thyroid gland, which of the following tissues is MOST likely to contain lymphoid infiltrates related to her basic disease state?
   A. orbital extraocular tissues
   B. brain
   C. liver
   D. parathyroid glands
   E. pituitary gland

A is correct.
In Graves' disease, there may be orbital edema, mucopolysaccharide deposits, fibrosis and lymphocytic infiltrates resulting in exophthalmos.

15.067   In a patient with true hypoparathyroidism, the etiology is MOST frequently:
   A. renal failure
   B. previous thyroidectomy / parathyroidectomy
   C. congenital absence
   D. idiopathic atrophy
   E. vitamin D deficiency

B is correct.
Most cases of true hypoparathyroidism are secondary to surgical removal of all parathyroid glands during thyroidectomy, or the removal of too much parathyroid tissue during surgical treatment for primary parathyroid hyperplasia.

15.068   A 55-year-old man is being treated with hemodialysis for chronic glomerulonephritis with renal insufficiency. His serum calcium is in the low-normal range whereas his serum phosphorus remains high. He is at GREATEST risk for which of the following conditions?
   A. parathyroid adenoma
   B. parathyroid carcinoma
   C. parathyroid hyperplasia
   D. parathyroid atrophy
   E. pseudohypoparathyroidism

C is correct.
Phosphate retention and hypocalcemia associated with chronic renal disease result in compensatory hyperplasia of the parathyroid glands.

15.069 A 54-year-old man presents with severe episodic hypertension punctuated by attacks of dizziness and cardiac arrhythmias accompanied by orthostatic hypotension. His serum glucose is mildly elevated, but all other serum chemistries, including cortisol and aldosterone, are normal. An MRI discloses a 3-cm ovoid mass in the right adrenal gland. Which of the following conditions is MOST likely to explain all of the pathophysiology seen in this patient?

    A. adrenocortical adenoma
    B. adrenocortical hyperplasia
    C. pituitary adenoma
    D. islet cell adenoma
    E. pheochromocytoma

E is correct.
The findings of episodic hypertension, attacks of dizziness and cardiac arrhythmias, and orthostatic hypotension along with a mass in the adrenal gland strongly suggest a diagnosis of pheochromocytoma.

15.070 A 54-year-old male attorney has been followed in your clinic for 15 years for type II diabetes. Thus far, he has required therapy with diet and oral insulin-releasing agents. Although he is only mildly hyperglycemic on his clinic visits at 3-month intervals, he is developing proteinuria and a mild increase in serum creatinine, so you are concerned about the extent of his hyperglycemia between visits. The BEST laboratory test to answer this question is:

    A. serum level of insulin-releasing drug
    B. simultaneous serum insulin and peptide C levels
    C. urine albumin quantitation
    D. hemoglobin A_{1C} level
    E. plasma cortisol level

D is correct.
The amount of enzymatic glycosylation is directly related to the level of blood glucose. Determination of glycosylated hemoglobin (hemoglobin A_{1C}) concentration in the plasma is helpful in determining the degree of hyperglycemia over a period of time.

15.071 A 50-year-old man presents to your clinic with a complaint of 'blind spots' in his work as a truck driver. Visual field analysis shows bitemporal hemianopsia. An MRI shows a large expansile mass in the sella turcica. Clinical laboratory studies show depressed levels of all anterior pituitary hormones. The function of which of the following endocrine tissues is LEAST likely to be impaired by this patient's disease and its subsequent surgical treatment?

    A. testes
    B. thyroid gland
    C. parathyroid gland
    D. adrenal cortex
    E. posterior pituitary 'gland'

C is correct.
Parathyroid hormone is secreted by chief cells of the parathyroid glands. The case described here is a pituitary neoplasm. Parathyroid hormone production is not affected by destruction of the pituitary by neoplasm or by surgical removal of the pituitary gland.

15.072   A 10-year-old child develops meningo-coccal septicemia with disseminated intravascular coagulopathy. The child is at GREATEST risk for which of the following endocrine catastrophes?
A. parathyroid infarction
B. hemorrhagic infarction of the pituitary
C. hemorrhagic infarction of the adrenal glands
D. acute postinfectious diabetes mellitus
E. acute Graves' disease

C is correct.
Overwhelming septicemic infection, such as meningococcal, may result in massive, bilateral adrenal hemorrhage and acute adrenocortical insufficiency. This is called the Waterhouse–Friderichsen syndrome.

15.073   A 12-year-old boy is diagnosed with a large craniopharyngioma compressing the third ventricle and invading the inferior hypothalamus. All of the following are expected complications of this process EXCEPT:
A. growth arrest
B. hypogonadism
C. diabetes insipidus
D. diabetes mellitus

D is correct.
Craniopharyngiomas may result in hypo- or hyperfunction of the anterior pituitary as well as cause diabetes insipidus. Diabetes mellitus involves the pancreas.

15.074   The release of thyroxine (T_4) from thyroid acinar cells directly into the blood is considered to be which type of hormonal secretion?
A. endocrine
B. paracrine
C. neurocrine
D. autocrine

A is correct.
Endocrine secretion is the release of hormone into the blood to act systemically whereas paracrine secretion is the release of hormone through the interstitium to act locally. Neurocrine secretion is the release through nerve synapses whereas autocrine secretion is the release of hormone by a cell for its own receptors.

SECTION 16: SKIN

16.001 A 50-year-old man has been treated for chronic osteomyelitis of the tibia for several years without success. Multiple draining sinus tracts have been noted on the skin surface over the tibia. Over the past 6 months, a necrotic mass $3 \times 3\,cm$ in size has formed at the site of the sinus tracts. A biopsy shows dysplastic cells with eosinophilic cytoplasm. Which of the following is the MOST likely diagnosis of the skin neoplasm in this patient?
- A. squamous cell carcinoma
- B. basal cell carcinoma
- C. Bowen's disease
- D. Paget's disease
- E. malignant melanoma, superficial spreading type
- F. malignant melanoma, nodular type
- G. dermatofibrosarcoma protuberans
- H. Kaposi's sarcoma
- I. mycosis fungoides

A is correct.

Chronic ulcers, draining osteomyelitis and old burn scars are all implicated as predisposing factors in the development of squamous cell carcinoma at the site of the disease process.

16.002 A 50-year-old white farmer presents with a pearly nodule on his forehead containing a central necrotic ulcerated area. A biopsy shows palisading basophilic cells in sheets, cords and nests in the dermis. Which of the following is the MOST likely diagnosis of the skin neoplasm in this patient?
- A. squamous cell carcinoma
- B. basal cell carcinoma
- C. Bowen's disease
- D. Paget's disease
- E. malignant melanoma, superficial spreading type
- F. malignant melanoma, nodular type
- G. dermatofibrosarcoma protuberans
- H. Kaposi's sarcoma
- I. mycosis fungoides

B is correct.

Basal cell carcinomas tend to occur in areas with chronic exposure to sunlight. The typical clinical appearance of these tumors is a pearly white nodule with dilated subepidermal blood vessels. Older lesions may ulcerate. Histologically, these tumors appear as cords and islands of basophilic cells with hyperchromatic nuclei. Cells making up the peripheral layer tend to line up radially (palisading).

16.003   A 30-year-old white man presents with a history of weight loss and difficulty in breathing. A chest X-ray reveals a diffuse five-lobe infiltrate. A bronchoalveolar lavage specimen contains *Pneumocystis carinii*. Physical examination reveals multiple reddish-purple slightly raised macules over the chest, back and arms. A biopsy of one of these lesions shows dysplastic spindle cells in the dermis with interspersed red blood cells. Which of the following is the MOST likely diagnosis of the skin neoplasm in this patient?

   A. squamous cell carcinoma
   B. basal cell carcinoma
   C. Bowen's disease
   D. Paget's disease
   E. malignant melanoma, superficial
      spreading type
   F. malignant melanoma, nodular type
   G. dermatofibrosarcoma protuberans
   H. Kaposi's sarcoma
   I. mycosis fungoides

H is correct.

Kaposi's sarcoma may occur in association with AIDS. The typical clinical presentation is the appearance of reddish-purple macules, papules and plaques on the skin surface. The nodules have no predilection for any particular site. On histology, plump spindle-shaped stromal cells associated with irregular slit-like spaces lined with endothelium and containing red cells are seen.

16.004   A 32-year-old red-haired woman presents with a slightly raised pigmented lesion on her back. Close examination reveals that the lesion has an irregular border and areas of depigmentation near the center. A biopsy shows clumps of ovoid cells with prominent nuclei and cytoplasmic pigment predominantly located in the dermoepidermal junction. These cells are seen invading the superficial papillary dermis and as single cells in the epidermis at the edges of the lesion. Which of the following is the MOST likely diagnosis of the skin neoplasm in this patient?

   A. squamous cell carcinoma
   B. basal cell carcinoma
   C. Bowen's disease
   D. Paget's disease
   E. malignant melanoma, superficial
      spreading type
   F. malignant melanoma, nodular type
   G. dermatofibrosarcoma protuberans
   H. Kaposi's sarcoma
   I. mycosis fungoides

E is correct.

Melanomas show marked variations in pigmentation and zones of hypopigmentation may be present. Borders are usually irregular. Growth of the tumor within the epidermal and superficial dermal layers indicates a horizontal growth phase. Such tumors are called 'superficial spreading melanomas'. During this stage of growth, the tumor cells do not metastasize.

16.005   A 58-year-old man presents with multiple reddish plaques over the trunk, arms and legs. The regional lymph nodes are enlarged. A skin biopsy shows ovoid dysplastic round cells with indented nuclei infiltrating the epidermis and forming loose clusters in the dermis. Examination of the peripheral blood reveals similar cells in significant numbers. The dysplastic cells are marked as T lymphocytes by immunocytochemistry. Which of the following is the MOST likely diagnosis of the skin neoplasm in this patient?

    A. squamous cell carcinoma

    B. basal cell carcinoma

    C. Bowen's disease

    D. Paget's disease

    E. malignant melanoma, superficial
       spreading type

    F. malignant melanoma, nodular type

    G. dermatofibrosarcoma protuberans

    H. Kaposi's sarcoma

    I. mycosis fungoides

I is correct.

Mycosis fungoides is a type of cutaneous T-cell lymphoma. T-helper cells (Sézary–Lutzner cells) form aggregates in the superficial dermis. In late stages, these cells may seed into the lymphatic and peripheral blood systems.

16.006   A 50-year-old man develops a generalized skin eruption characterized by bullous separation of the epidermis. A skin biopsy shows that the bullae are intraepithelial and a characteristic zone of epithelial cells has separated from the epidermis, but remains attached to the dermal basement membrane. Direct immunofluorescence studies show that IgG antibody directed against the epithelial desmosomes is present. Which one of the following diagnoses is the MOST likely in this patient?

    A. allergic contact dermatitis

    B. atopic eczematous dermatitis

    C. pemphigus vulgaris

    D. erythema multiforme

    E. dermatitis herpetiformis

    F. impetigo

    G. herpes zoster

    H. chloracne

    I. psoriasis

    J. sarcoidosis

    K. discoid lupus erythematosus

    L. systemic lupus erythematosus

    M. scleroderma

C is correct.

Pemphigus is an autoimmune disorder resulting from the loss of integrity of intercellular attachments within the epidermis as well as mucosa. Acantholysis, or lysis of intercellular adhesion sites in the squamous epithelial surface, is characteristic of this disease. The process selectively involves the cells immediately above the basal cell layer.

16.007 A 30-year-old woman presents to her physician with a severe dermatitis of the hands. The skin is red and fissured, and the process is most severe along the lateral edges of the fingers and in the skin fold between the fingers. A biopsy shows acute and chronic inflammatory cells in the dermis with marked spongiosis of the epidermis. Which one of the following diagnoses is the MOST likely in this patient?

    A. allergic contact dermatitis
    B. atopic eczematous dermatitis
    C. pemphigus vulgaris
    D. erythema multiforme
    E. dermatitis herpetiformis
    F. impetigo
    G. herpes zoster
    H. chloracne
    I. psoriasis
    J. sarcoidosis
    K. discoid lupus erythematosus
    L. systemic lupus erythematosus
    M. scleroderma

A is correct.

Allergic contact dermatitis is a type of acute eczematous dermatitis resulting from contact with certain substances. There is marked itching and burning with erythema, and often with blistering and oozing of the skin surface as well. On histology, there is a lymphocytic (and sometimes eosinophilic) infiltrate together with marked edema primarily in the stratum spinosum. This gives a 'spongy' appearance to the epidermis, hence the term 'spongiosis'.

16.008 A 60-year-old woman is undergoing chemotherapy for chronic lymphoid leukemia. After several days of a burning, itching sensation along the distribution of the eighth intercostal nerve on the right, several raised crusting pustules appear in a line in this area. A biopsy of one of these lesions shows ballooning degeneration, giant cell formation and intranuclear inclusions. Which one of the following diagnoses is the MOST likely in this patient?

    A. allergic contact dermatitis
    B. atopic eczematous dermatitis
    C. pemphigus vulgaris
    D. erythema multiforme
    E. dermatitis herpetiformis
    F. impetigo
    G. herpes zoster
    H. chloracne
    I. psoriasis
    J. sarcoidosis
    K. discoid lupus erythematosus
    L. systemic lupus erythematosus
    M. scleroderma

G is correct.

When replication of the varicella-zoster virus is reactivated in ganglion cells, the virus travels down the sensory nerve serving a dermatome. The virus then infects the epidermis of the dermatome, resulting in a painful localized vesicular eruption. Risk of reactivation of the virus increases with advanced age and any factor which may impair cell-mediated immunity.

16.009 A 24-year-old woman presents to her physician with a generalized rash, which had appeared immediately after she had eaten seafood. She has a history of 'asthma' as a child. A skin biopsy shows acute inflammation of the dermis, spongiosis of the epidermis and degranulation of mast cells. Which one of the following diagnoses is the MOST likely in this patient?

    A. allergic contact dermatitis
    B. atopic eczematous dermatitis
    C. pemphigus vulgaris
    D. erythema multiforme
    E. dermatitis herpetiformis
    F. impetigo
    G. herpes zoster
    H. chloracne
    I. psoriasis
    J. sarcoidosis
    K. discoid lupus erythematosus
    L. systemic lupus erythematosus
    M. scleroderma

B is correct.
Atopic dermatitis is a form of acute eczematous dermatitis occurring in susceptible subjects. Sensitization is by contact with the skin, gastrointestinal tract or respiratory tract. There is an immediate-type hypersensitivity mechanism involved with fixation of IgE to mast cells and degranulation of mast cells upon exposure to the antigen.

16.010 A 24-year-old woman presents to her physician with multiple small yellowish bumps on the skin of her arms and legs. A skin biopsy shows non-caseating granulomas in the dermis. A chest X-ray shows multiple reticulogranular densities and hilar adenopathy. Which one of the following diagnoses is the MOST likely in this patient?

    A. allergic contact dermatitis
    B. atopic eczematous dermatitis
    C. pemphigus vulgaris
    D. erythema multiforme
    E. dermatitis herpetiformis
    F. impetigo
    G. herpes zoster
    H. chloracne
    I. psoriasis
    J. sarcoidosis
    K. discoid lupus erythematosus
    L. systemic lupus erythematosus
    M. scleroderma

J is correct.
Skin lesions may occur in patients with sarcoidosis. The clinical presentation is usually the appearance of discrete subcutaneous nodules, elevated erythematous plaques or flat lesions. On histology, typical non-caseating granulomas are seen.

16.011 An 18-year-old female freshman college student has a brown raised pigmented spot on her face. The lesion is removed. Microscopic examination shows nests of round-to-oval pigment-containing cells in the dermoepidermal junction and extending into the upper portion of the dermis. No mitotic activity is present. This patient MOST likely has which one of the following diagnoses?

    A. squamous cell carcinoma

    B. basal cell carcinoma

    C. verruca vulgaris

    D. junctional nevocellular nevus

    E. compound nevocellular nevus

    F. radial growth phase (superficial spreading) malignant melanoma

    G. vertical growth phase (nodular) malignant melanoma

    H. acral lentiginous malignant melanoma

    I. dermatofibrosarcoma (protuberans)

    J. Kaposi's sarcoma

    K. hemangioma

    L. mycosis fungoides

E is correct.

Nevocellular nevi are formed from melanocytes. The melanocytes (or nevus cells) become round-to-oval in shape and occur in nests along the dermo-epidermal junction. Their nuclei are uniform and there is little or no mitotic activity. Such nevi are called 'junctional nevi'. Eventually, most of these junctional nevi extend down into the dermis and are then referred to as 'compound nevi'.

16.012 A 46-year-old man suffered from severe burns on his lower legs while fighting a brushfire 16 years earlier. Scars had developed but, recently, one of them has undergone ulceration. A biopsy shows dysplastic keratinized cells with mitotic activity invading the subcutaneous tissue. The popliteal and femoral lymph nodes are enlarged. This patient MOST likely has which one of the following diagnoses?

    A. squamous cell carcinoma

    B. basal cell carcinoma

    C. verruca vulgaris

    D. junctional nevocellular nevus

    E. compound nevocellular nevus

    F. radial growth phase (superficial spreading) malignant melanoma

    G. vertical growth phase (nodular) malignant melanoma

    H. acral lentiginous malignant melanoma

    I. dermatofibrosarcoma (protuberans)

    J. Kaposi's sarcoma

    K. hemangioma

    L. mycosis fungoides

A is correct.

Chronic ulcers, draining osteomyelitis and old burn scars are all implicated as predisposing factors in the development of squamous cell carcinoma at the site of the disease process. The finding of dysplastic keratinized cells with enlarged regional nodes suggests metastases and supports the diagnosis of squamous cell carcinoma.

16.013 A 14-year-old adolescent boy is brought to your clinic because of rapidly enlarging cutaneous nodules on his right distal third and fourth fingers. Biopsies of both lesions show hyperkeratosis with extreme elongation of the rete ridges and marked vacuolization of the nuclei of the cells in the granular layer of the epidermis. This patient MOST likely has which one of the following diagnoses?

    A. squamous cell carcinoma
    B. basal cell carcinoma
    C. verruca vulgaris
    D. junctional nevocellular nevus
    E. compound nevocellular nevus
    F. radial growth phase (superficial spreading) malignant melanoma
    G. vertical growth phase (nodular) malignant melanoma
    H. acral lentiginous malignant melanoma
    I. dermatofibrosarcoma (protuberans)
    J. Kaposi's sarcoma
    K. hemangioma
    L. mycosis fungoides

C is correct.

Verruca vulgaris is a common type of wart caused by papillomaviruses. The most frequent site of occurrence is on the hands. Typical microscopic features include epidermal hyperplasia and cytoplasmic vacuolization.

16.014 A highly successful attorney presents to your office with the main complaint of a recurrent, intensely pruritic, erythematous scaling rash that is worse over the elbows, knees, buttocks and scrotum. Upon questioning, the patient notes that the rash is definitely worse in the winter and is sometimes accompanied by joint pains. The rash is scaling and, when gently abraded, discharges thin silvery patches of skin. A biopsy shows hyperkeratosis, parakeratosis and a 'sawtooth' pattern of the rete ridges, together with dyskeratotic cells and increased mitotic activity in the upper epidermis. This patient MOST likely has which one of the following diagnoses?

    A. allergic contact dermatitis
    B. atopic eczematous dermatitis
    C. pemphigus vulgaris
    D. erythema multiforme
    E. dermatitis herpetiformis
    F. impetigo
    G. herpes zoster
    H. chloracne
    I. psoriasis
    J. sarcoidosis
    K. discoid lupus erythematosus
    L. systemic lupus erythematosus
    M. scleroderma

I is correct.

Psoriasis is a chronic inflammatory condition of the skin which typically affects the elbows, knees, scalp and lumbosacral areas. Psoriatic arthritis may occur. The skin lesions typically present as well-demarcated pink plaques covered by whitish/silvery scales. On histology, acanthosis and downward elongation of the rete ridges is seen. There is thinning of the stratum granulosum and a marked overlying parakeratotic scale.

16.015 An 8-year-old girl presents to your clinic with several erythematous raised, pustular, crusting lesions on the chin and neck. You are able to express pus-like material. Gram stain of the material shows numerous gram-positive cocci in chains. Several weeks earlier, an older sister had had a similar rash, followed by the development of acute renal failure requiring dialysis. This patient MOST likely has which one of the following diagnoses?

    A. allergic contact dermatitis

    B. atopic eczematous dermatitis

    C. pemphigus vulgaris

    D. erythema multiforme

    E. dermatitis herpetiformis

    F. impetigo

    G. herpes zoster

    H. chloracne

    I. psoriasis

    J. sarcoidosis

    K. discoid lupus erythematosus

    L. systemic lupus erythematosus

    M. scleroderma

F is correct.

Impetigo is a superficial infection of the skin most often caused by staphylococci or streptococci. Nephritogenic strains of streptococcus may cause impetigo. Clinically, the skin lesions present as multiple small pustules following the appearance of erythematous macules.

16.016 A 25-year-old man is being treated with a high dose of a synthetic penicillin analogue for pneumonia. After 10 days of therapy, he develops widespread skin and mucous membrane lesions consisting of macules, papules, vesicles and bullae with a characteristic red border and a pale eroded center resembling a target. Biopsy shows necrosis of a central zone surrounded by cytotoxic CD8-positive lymphocytes. This patient MOST likely has which one of the following diagnoses?

    A. allergic contact dermatitis

    B. atopic eczematous dermatitis

    C. pemphigus vulgaris

    D. erythema multiforme

    E. dermatitis herpetiformis

    F. impetigo

    G. herpes zoster

    H. chloracne

    I. psoriasis

    J. sarcoidosis

    K. discoid lupus erythematosus

    L. systemic lupus erythematosus

    M. scleroderma

D is correct.

Erythema multiforme is most probably a hypersensitivity response to certain infections and drugs. Penicillin is known to be associated with the condition. The typical clinical presentation is the appearance of macules, papules, vesicles and bullae. A characteristic lesion consists of a red macule or papule with a pale center (target lesion). On histology, there is necrosis of keratinocytes and a surrounding accumulation of cytotoxic CD8-positive lymphocytes.

SECTION 17: MUSCULOSKELETAL SYSTEM AND SOFT TISSUES

17.001 Ankylosing spondylitis is characterized by all of the following EXCEPT:

    A. enthesopathy
    B. chronic iritis
    C. presence of HLA-B27
    D. presence of rheumatoid factor
    E. ossification of periarticular tendons

D is correct.
Rheumatoid factor is not found in patients with ankylosing spondylitis.

17.002 Histopathologic characteristics of osteoarthritis involve all of the following EXCEPT:

    A. fibrillation
    B. connective tissue vasculitis
    C. chondrocytic proliferation
    D. subchondral pseudocysts
    E. osteophyte formation

B is correct.
Connective tissue vasculitis is not seen in primary osteoarthritis of any type.

17.003 All of the following are characteristic of Sjögren's syndrome EXCEPT:

    A. xerostomia
    B. relatively mild rheumatoid arthritis
    C. keratoconjunctivitis sicca
    D. increased incidence of lymphoma
    E. leg ulcers

E is correct.
Leg ulcers are characteristic of Felty's, and not Sjögren's, syndrome.

17.004 A 28-year-old female forest ranger, who is 6 months postpartum, presents with painful, mildly swollen joints in the hands and feet. All of the following are reasonable diagnostic considerations EXCEPT:

    A. rheumatoid arthritis
    B. gonorrheal arthritis
    C. gouty arthritis
    D. Lyme arthritis
    E. lupus erythematosus arthritis

C is correct.
Gouty arthritis almost never occurs in healthy women prior to the menopause.

17.005 In patients with rheumatoid arthritis, all of the following are increased in incidence compared with the general population EXCEPT:

    A. Sjögren's syndrome
    B. amyloidosis
    C. Felty's syndrome
    D. synoviosarcoma
    E. malignant non-Hodgkin's lymphoma

D is correct.
Synoviosarcomas are highly malignant soft tissue neoplasms that are not associated with joint disease in general or with rheumatoid arthritis in particular.

17.006   A 38-year-old woman presents with a history of morning stiffness and fatigue. Several firm subcutaneous nodules are palpable on her arms. A serum determination for rheumatoid factor is positive. She is likely to have involvement of all of the following joints EXCEPT:

A. proximal interphalangeal joints
B. distal interphalangeal joints
C. metacarpophalangeal joints
D. hips
E. knees

B is correct.
Distal interphalangeal involvement is very rare in rheumatoid arthritis, but is common in generalized osteoarthritis and psoriatic arthritis.

17.007   The severe secondary osteoarthritis that follows aseptic necrosis of the femoral head is primarily due to:

A. pannus-mediated cartilage lysis
B. immune synovitis
C. ischemic necrosis of articular cartilage
D. collapse of underlying subchondral bone
E. sensory neuropathy

D is correct.
The collapse of the underlying subchondral bone in aseptic necrosis allows the cartilage to buckle and, subsequently, be abraded from the surface.

17.008   The full expression of the complete triad of hypertrophic osteoarthropathy is MOST characteristic of:

A. ulcerative colitis
B. congenital heart disease
C. pulmonary neoplasia
D. hyperparathyroidism
E. hypoparathyroidism

C is correct.
The full triad (clubbing, generalized arthritis and periostitis) is seen only with pulmonary neoplasias, including primary and metastatic carcinomas, sarcomas and mesotheliomas.

17.009   The amyloid protein associated with long-standing rheumatoid arthritis is composed of:

A. amyloid-associated protein (AA)
B. immunoglobulin light chain fragments (AL)
C. prealbumin variants (AF)
D. precalcitonin (AE)
E. β_2-microglobulin (AH)

A is correct.
The amyloid associated with rheumatoid arthritis is composed largely of amyloid-associated protein, which has a serum antecedent (SAA) produced in the liver in response to interleukin-1 (IL-1).

17.010   A 25-year-old man presents with low back pain and stiffness, and mild but painful arthritis of the hip and shoulder joints. Radiographs of the pelvis show bilateral sacroiliitis. Serum rheumatoid factor is negative. This patient is MOST likely to develop:

A. rheumatoid nodules
B. rheumatoid pneumonitis
C. lupus erythematosus nephritis
D. chronic iritis
E. hypersplenism syndrome

D is correct.
Chronic iritis is characteristic of ankylosing spondylitis patients such as the one described here.

17.011   A 44-year-old woman develops enlarged hands and feet, peripheral arthritis, an enlarging head with coarse facial features and diabetes mellitus, over a 5-year period. The MOST likely site of origin for this disease process is the:
  A. thyroid gland
  B. parathyroid gland
  C. adrenal gland
  D. pituitary gland
  E. endocrine pancreas

D is correct.
Acromegaly due to a somatotropinoma of the pituitary gland leads to secondary osteoarthritis due to joint deformity as a result of overgrowth of the bone ends.

17.012   Which one of the following diseases has the LEAST likelihood of resulting in chronic destructive arthropathy?
  A. rheumatoid arthritis
  B. juvenile rheumatoid arthritis
  C. rheumatic fever
  D. psoriasis
  E. gout

C is correct.
Rheumatic fever 'licks the joints and bites the heart', but almost never causes permanent destructive arthropathy.

17.013   Which one of the following histopathologic changes is MOST characteristic of osteoarthritis?
  A. subcutaneous nodules with necrosis
  B. fibrillation of cartilage
  C. granulomas in synovium
  D. fibrinoid necrosis of synovium
  E. synovial lymphoid nodules

B is correct.
Fibrillation (or cracking) is characteristic of early osteoarthritis.

17.014   A 56-year-old stockbroker presents with a psoriasiform rash and destructive peripheral arthropathy in the hands with distal interphalangeal involvement. Which one of the following laboratory tests is the MOST informative as to his likelihood of developing spinal involvement by this disorder?
  A. HLA-B27 determination
  B. serum rheumatoid factor titer
  C. erythrocyte sedimentation rate (ESR)
  D. serum complement level
  E. plasma antidouble-stranded DNA titer

A is correct.
A positive HLA-B27 indicates that the patient is more likely to develop spondylitis as a component of his psoriatic arthritis.

17.015   Which one of the following bits of diagnostic information is MOST helpful in establishing a diagnosis of gouty arthritis?
  A. polyarticular joint swelling
  B. oligoarticular joint swelling
  C. subcutaneous nodules
  D. serum hyperuricemia
  E. urate crystals in joint aspirate

E is correct.
Urate crystals in a joint aspirate are diagnostic of gouty arthritis. Their presence inside granulocytes indicates acute gout.

17.016   Pseudogout is an arthritic disorder associated with granulocyte phagocytosis of:
   A. calcium pyrophosphate crystals
   B. calcium urate crystals
   C. calcium oxalate crystals
   D. ferric oxide crystals
   E. copper sulfate crystals

A is correct.
Pseudogout is caused by granulocytic release of inflammatory substances after phagocytosis of calcium pyrophosphate crystals.

17.017   A 30-year-old woman presents to your clinic with a chief complaint of morning stiffness of approximately 1 year's duration along with a subjective feeling of fatigue. On further questioning, she relates problems with dry eyes and mouth. Her parotid glands are enlarged bilaterally. Her hands show fusiform swellings around the metacarpophalangeal joints, and bilateral knee effusions are present. No skin or genitourinary abnormalities are noted. A serum rheumatoid factor is positive and an ESR is elevated. A serum test for antibody against SS-B antigen is also positive. All other routine hematology and chemistry determinations are normal. This patient undoubtedly has the early signs of:
   A. Charcot's arthropathy
   B. Reiter's syndrome
   C. Felty's syndrome
   D. Sjögren's syndrome
   E. Marie–Strümpell disease (rheumatoid spondylitis)

D is correct.
Sjögren's syndrome typically manifests in patients as a relatively mild rheumatoid arthritis, with dry eyes, dry mouth, and enlarged parotid glands.

17.018   A 50-year-old woman presents to your clinic with a chief complaint of pain in the hands, shoulders, back, and legs. Physical examination reveals bony enlargements of the distal interphalangeal joints bilaterally. The remainder of the physical examination is non-contributory. Radiography shows joint space narrowing with osteophytes in numerous joints, including the thoracic spine, knees, elbows, and hips. Her mother and an older sister had similar complaints. An ESR is normal and serum rheumatoid factor is negative. The BEST diagnosis for this woman's condition is:
   A. rheumatoid arthritis
   B. post-traumatic arthritis
   C. generalized osteoarthritis
   D. psoriatic arthritis
   E. neuropathic arthritis

C is correct.
Generalized osteoarthritis is associated with widespread joint pain and osteophytes, particularly in the distal interphalangeal joints (Heberden's nodes).

17.019 A 34-year-old man presents with a history of several years of back pain with a feeling of stiffness. Physical examination reveals limitation of motion in the lower and middle spine as well as restriction of chest expansion. Joint effusions are present in both hips, but there is no evidence of peripheral arthritis in the small joints nor any skin lesions. A radiograph of the pelvis discloses bilateral sacroiliitis with erosion of the bone, and periarticular bone bridging the joints bilaterally. Serum rheumatoid factor is negative, but his lymphocytes are positive for HLA-B27. The BEST diagnosis for this patient's condition is:

    A. rheumatoid arthritis

    B. generalized osteoarthritis

    C. ankylosing spondylitis

    D. gout

    E. psoriatic arthritis

C is correct.

Ankylosing spondylitis usually presents in young men with back pain and stiffness, and limitation of chest expansion. These patients are rheumatoid factor-negative and HLA-B27-positive.

17.020 A 22-year-old man has pronounced bilateral conjunctivitis and iritis, and a pustular skin rash with accentuation over the palms and soles. He complains of multiple joint pains. Physical examination reveals swelling of multiple joints, especially in the wrists and hands. Although rheumatoid factor is negative, a high titer of antibodies against *Chlamydia trachomatis* is detected in the serum. The patient is HLA-B27-positive. Bacterial cultures of the genital tract, urine, and blood are negative. What is the MOST appropriate diagnosis?

    A. primary generalized osteoarthritis (GOA)

    B. secondary osteoarthritis

    C. rheumatoid arthritis

    D. juvenile rheumatoid arthritis (Still's disease)

    E. ankylosing spondylitis

    F. Reiter's syndrome

    G. psoriatic arthritis

    H. rheumatic fever arthritis

    I. Lyme arthritis

    J. enteropathic spondyloarthritis

    K. pseudogout

    L. gout

    M. gonococcal arthritis

    N. tuberculous arthritis

    O. Sjögren's syndrome

F is correct.

This combination of physical findings and laboratory results is extremely suggestive of Reiter's syndrome.

17.021   A 35-year-old woman presents with a history of bilateral stiffness and pain in her hands. Physical examination reveals inflamed and mildly swollen proximal interphalangeal and metacarpophalangeal joints bilaterally. Effusions are present in both knees. Several painless, firm, subcutaneous nodules are noted around the elbows. The ESR is elevated as is the serum titer for rheumatoid factor. What is the MOST appropriate diagnosis?

   A. primary generalized osteoarthritis (GOA)
   B. secondary osteoarthritis
   C. rheumatoid arthritis
   D. juvenile rheumatoid arthritis (Still's disease)
   E. ankylosing spondylitis
   F. Reiter's syndrome
   G. psoriatic arthritis
   H. rheumatic fever arthritis
   I. Lyme arthritis
   J. enteropathic spondyloarthritis
   K. pseudogout
   L. gout
   M. gonococcal arthritis
   N. tuberculous arthritis
   O. Sjögren's syndrome

C is correct.

This combination of physical findings and laboratory results is characteristic of early rheumatoid arthritis.

17.022   A 60-year-old man's chief complaint is a painful swollen knee. Physical examination reveals a mildly inflamed knee joint with moderate effusion. X-rays reveal some loss of cartilage with soft calcification in the menisci and periarticular tissues. Examination of the joint fluid reveals many PMNs containing intracytoplasmic rhomboid-shaped crystals that show weak positive birefringence. What is the MOST appropriate diagnosis?

   A. primary generalized osteoarthritis (GOA)
   B. secondary osteoarthritis
   C. rheumatoid arthritis
   D. juvenile rheumatoid arthritis (Still's disease)
   E. ankylosing spondylitis
   F. Reiter's syndrome
   G. psoriatic arthritis
   H. rheumatic fever arthritis
   I. Lyme arthritis
   J. enteropathic spondyloarthritis
   K. pseudogout
   L. gout
   M. gonococcal arthritis
   N. tuberculous arthritis
   O. Sjögren's syndrome

K is correct.

This combination of physical and radiographic findings, and laboratory results is characteristic of pseudogout.

17.023 A 50-year-old woman has developed severe arthritis in the right hip. X-rays show marked joint space narrowing with abnormal angulation of the femoral neck. In an automobile accident 15 years earlier, she had fractured her right femoral neck, which required open reduction with a plate and screws. Radiography reveals no arthritic changes in other joints. What is the MOST appropriate diagnosis?

    A. primary generalized osteoarthritis (GOA)
    B. secondary osteoarthritis
    C. rheumatoid arthritis
    D. juvenile rheumatoid arthritis (Still's disease)
    E. ankylosing spondylitis
    F. Reiter's syndrome
    G. psoriatic arthritis
    H. rheumatic fever arthritis
    I. Lyme arthritis
    J. enteropathic spondyloarthritis
    K. pseudogout
    L. gout
    M. gonococcal arthritis
    N. tuberculous arthritis
    O. Sjögren's syndrome

B is correct.

This combination of patient history, radiographic appearances, and physical findings is extremely characteristic of severe localized post-traumatic secondary osteoarthritis.

17.024 A 62-year-old hypertensive man taking thiazide diuretics has a painful swollen red great toe on the left foot. Several firm subcutaneous nodules are noted around the ankles. Aspiration of the first metatarsal–phalangeal joint space reveals a marked infiltrate of PMNs. Gram stain is negative, but polarized microscopy reveals needle-shaped negatively birefringent crystals within WBCs. What is the MOST appropriate diagnosis?

    A. primary generalized osteoarthritis (GOA)
    B. secondary osteoarthritis
    C. rheumatoid arthritis
    D. juvenile rheumatoid arthritis (Still's disease)
    E. ankylosing spondylitis
    F. Reiter's syndrome
    G. psoriatic arthritis
    H. rheumatic fever arthritis
    I. Lyme arthritis
    J. enteropathic spondyloarthritis
    K. pseudogout
    L. gout
    M. gonococcal arthritis
    N. tuberculous arthritis
    O. Sjögren's syndrome

L is correct.

This combination of patient history, physical examination findings, and laboratory results is diagnostic of gouty arthritis of the secondary type. Thiazides reduce excretion of urates in the distal convoluted tubules of the kidney and provoke gout in susceptible individuals.

17.025 A 9-year-old boy's elbow, wrist, and knee joints are swollen, warm, and tender. He has a maculopapular skin rash and hepatosplenomegaly. The mother has noted the rash and occasional fever over the last 3 months. No bone erosion is seen on X-rays. Serum studies for Lyme, antistreptococcal, and anti-DNA antibodies, and rheumatoid factors, are all negative. A joint aspirate shows no crystals or bacteria. What is the MOST appropriate diagnosis?

    A. primary osteoarthritis
    B. secondary osteoarthritis
    C. calcium pyrophosphate arthropathy
    D. gouty arthropathy
    E. hypertrophic pulmonary osteoarthropathy
    F. rheumatoid arthritis
    G. Still's disease
    H. Reiter's syndrome
    I. ankylosing spondylitis
    J. enteropathic spondyloarthritis
    K. Lyme arthritis
    L. tuberculous arthritis
    M. gonorrheal arthritis
    N. rheumatic fever arthritis
    O. systemic lupus arthritis
    P. psoriatic arthritis
    Q. staphylococcal arthritis

G is correct.
This combination of patient history, physical findings, and laboratory results is extremely characteristic of Still's disease (juvenile rheumatoid arthritis) of the systemic type.

17.026 A 53-year-old man has a history of intermittent joint pain in the feet and toes. The right great and second toes are red, warm, swollen, and tender. Several firm non-tender nodules are seen on the ankles. X-rays show soft periarticular calcification and destruction of the metatarsotarsal joints. A joint aspirate shows negatively birefringent needle-like crystals. What is the MOST appropriate diagnosis?

    A. primary osteoarthritis
    B. secondary osteoarthritis
    C. calcium pyrophosphate arthropathy
    D. gouty arthropathy
    E. hypertrophic pulmonary osteoarthropathy
    F. rheumatoid arthritis
    G. Still's disease
    H. Reiter's syndrome
    I. ankylosing spondylitis
    J. enteropathic spondyloarthritis
    K. Lyme arthritis
    L. tuberculous arthritis
    M. gonorrheal arthritis
    N. rheumatic fever arthritis
    O. systemic lupus arthritis
    P. psoriatic arthritis
    Q. staphylococcal arthritis

D is correct.
This combination of historical, physical, radiographic, and laboratory findings is diagnostic of acute gouty arthropathy.

17.027 A 50-year-old man has a history of chronic cough and a 20-lb weight loss. He has smoked cigarettes for many years, but quit about 6 months ago because of his cough. He also complains of bilateral swollen, painful knees and elbows. Physical examination shows dullness over the right midlung and 'clubbing' of the fingers. X-rays show a right pulmonary hilar mass, and consolidation in the right upper and lower lobes. Periosteal new-bone formation is noted on his knee X-rays. What is the MOST likely type of arthritis in this patient?

    A. primary osteoarthritis
    B. secondary osteoarthritis
    C. calcium pyrophosphate arthropathy
    D. gouty arthropathy
    E. hypertrophic pulmonary osteoarthropathy
    F. rheumatoid arthritis
    G. Still's disease
    H. Reiter's syndrome
    I. ankylosing spondylitis
    J. enteropathic spondyloarthritis
    K. Lyme arthritis
    L. tuberculous arthritis
    M. gonorrheal arthritis
    N. rheumatic fever arthritis
    O. systemic lupus arthritis
    P. psoriatic arthritis
    Q. staphylococcal arthritis

E is correct.

This combination of patient history, physical examination, and radiographic findings is diagnostic of hypertrophic pulmonary osteoarthropathy. A diagnosis of primary lung carcinoma is confirmed by bronchoscopic biopsy.

17.028 A 25-year-old married mother of two young children presents to your office with a chief complaint of fatigue and joint pain. Her past medical history indicates a febrile illness about 3 months ago after a camping trip with her husband and children. She recalls a painful red area on her leg with a surrounding blanched, pale zone. Physical examination shows mild swelling and warmth of multiple small joints. Antistreptolysin O, rheumatoid and antinuclear factors, and anti-Epstein–Barr virus nuclear antigen are all negative. Borrelial antibodies are positive. What is the MOST likely type of arthritis in this patient?

- A. primary osteoarthritis
- B. secondary osteoarthritis
- C. calcium pyrophosphate arthropathy
- D. gouty arthropathy
- E. hypertrophic pulmonary osteoarthropathy
- F. rheumatoid arthritis
- G. Still's disease
- H. Reiter's syndrome
- I. ankylosing spondylitis
- J. enteropathic spondyloarthritis
- K. Lyme arthritis
- L. tuberculous arthritis
- M. gonorrheal arthritis
- N. rheumatic fever arthritis
- O. systemic lupus arthritis
- P. psoriatic arthritis
- Q. staphylococcal arthritis

K is correct.

This combination of patient history, physical examination, and laboratory findings is diagnostic of Lyme arthritis. These patients are easily misdiagnosed as rheumatoid arthritis by the unwary.

17.029   A 60-year-old male attorney presents to your clinic with a chief complaint of an extremely painful left hip. Past medical history reveals moderately heavy consumption of alcohol. There is no history of trauma. He is currently taking corticosteroid therapy for severe recurrent allergies. Clinical laboratory studies are negative for rheumatoid factor or hyperuricemia. Radiography shows loss of the joint space in the left hip with a wedge-like zone of collapse in the femoral head; no osteophytes are present. The right hip appears normal as do the knees and hands. What is the MOST likely type of arthritis in this patient?

    A. primary osteoarthritis

    B. secondary osteoarthritis

    C. calcium pyrophosphate arthropathy

    D. gouty arthropathy

    E. hypertrophic pulmonary osteoarthropathy

    F. rheumatoid arthritis

    G. Still's disease

    H. Reiter's syndrome

    I. ankylosing spondylitis

    J. enteropathic spondyloarthritis

    K. Lyme arthritis

    L. tuberculous arthritis

    M. gonorrheal arthritis

    N. rheumatic fever arthritis

    O. systemic lupus arthritis

    P. psoriatic arthritis

    Q. staphylococcal arthritis

B is correct.

This combination of patient history, radiographic findings, and laboratory results is diagnostic of severe secondary osteoarthritis due to avascular necrosis associated with chronic ethanolism.

17.030   A 32-year-old woman presents to her physician with a chief complaint of morning bilateral stiffness and pain in her hands. Her past medical history is non-contributory, but she has recently been pregnant and delivered a normal full-term infant 6 months previously. Physical examination reveals fusiform swellings and warmth in the metacarpophalangeal and proximal interphalangeal joints bilaterally. Effusions are present in both knee joints and several painless subcutaneous nodules are noted around the elbows. Periarticular bone erosion is seen on radiographs of the hands, but the distal interphalangeal joints are spared. The ESR is markedly elevated and a Lyme titer is negative. A joint aspirate reveals a high granulocyte count, but is negative for crystals or bacteria. What is the MOST likely type of arthritis in this patient?

    A. primary osteoarthritis
    B. secondary osteoarthritis
    C. calcium pyrophosphate arthropathy
    D. gouty arthropathy
    E. hypertrophic pulmonary osteoarthropathy
    F. rheumatoid arthritis
    G. Still's disease
    H. Reiter's syndrome
    I. ankylosing spondylitis
    J. enteropathic spondyloarthritis
    K. Lyme arthritis
    L. tuberculous arthritis
    M. gonorrheal arthritis
    N. rheumatic fever arthritis
    O. systemic lupus arthritis
    P. psoriatic arthritis
    Q. staphylococcal arthritis

F is correct.

Such a patient history, when complemented by physical findings of symmetric polyarthritis, periarticular bone erosions, elevated ESR, and negative results for other arthropathies, is highly characteristic of early rheumatoid arthritis.

17.031   A 45-year-old woman's chief complaint is fatigue. Bilateral knee effusions are present. Serum chemistries show elevated calcium, decreased phosphorus, and normal creatinine values. A serum PTH determination is elevated. X-rays of the knees show soft periarticular and meniscal calcification. A joint-fluid aspirate reveals positively birefringent rhomboid-shaped crystals in granulocytes What is the MOST likely type of arthritis in this patient?

A. primary osteoarthritis
B. secondary osteoarthritis
C. calcium pyrophosphate arthropathy
D. gouty arthropathy
E. hypertrophic pulmonary osteoarthropathy
F. rheumatoid arthritis
G. Still's disease
H. Reiter's syndrome
I. ankylosing spondylitis
J. enteropathic spondyloarthritis
K. Lyme arthritis
L. tuberculous arthritis
M. gonorrheal arthritis
N. rheumatic fever arthritis
O. systemic lupus arthritis
P. psoriatic arthritis
Q. staphylococcal arthritis

C is correct.

This combination of physical examination, radiographic, and laboratory findings is diagnostic of pseudogout of the secondary type, associated with primary hyperparathyroidism.

17.032 A febrile 22-year-old woman has a warm swollen wrist joint. An aspirate shows a marked increase in WBCs, 95% of which are granulocytes. Gram-negative diplococci are seen in the cytoplasm of several WBCs. Other than a left-shifted, raised blood WBC count, routine blood studies are negative. What is the MOST likely type of arthritis?

    A. primary osteoarthritis
    B. secondary osteoarthritis
    C. calcium pyrophosphate arthropathy
    D. gouty arthropathy
    E. hypertrophic pulmonary osteoarthropathy
    F. rheumatoid arthritis
    G. Still's disease
    H. Reiter's syndrome
    I. ankylosing spondylitis
    J. enteropathic spondyloarthritis
    K. Lyme arthritis
    L. tuberculous arthritis
    M. gonorrheal arthritis
    N. rheumatic fever arthritis
    O. systemic lupus arthritis
    P. psoriatic arthritis
    Q. staphylococcal arthritis

M is correct.

The physical examination and laboratory findings are diagnostic of *Neisseria gonorrhea* arthritis. Joint aspiration is the key to the diagnosis.

17.033   A 50-year-old man presents with pain and limited motion in the right knee. No other joints appear to be involved. Radiographs show marked joint destruction and narrowing with involvement of the bone on both sides of the joint. No osteophytes are seen. Routine chest X-ray shows bilateral fibrotic cavities in both apices and a calcified hilar lymph node. Needle biopsy of the right knee joint shows caseating granulomas in the synovium. What is the MOST likely type of arthritis in this patient?

    A. primary osteoarthritis
    B. secondary osteoarthritis
    C. calcium pyrophosphate arthropathy
    D. gouty arthropathy
    E. hypertrophic pulmonary osteoarthropathy
    F. rheumatoid arthritis
    G. Still's disease
    H. Reiter's syndrome
    I. ankylosing spondylitis
    J. enteropathic spondyloarthritis
    K. Lyme arthritis
    L. tuberculous arthritis
    M. gonorrheal arthritis
    N. rheumatic fever arthritis
    O. systemic lupus arthritis
    P. psoriatic arthritis
    Q. staphylococcal arthritis

L is correct.

The physical examination, radiographic, and laboratory results of this patient are virtually diagnostic of tuberculous arthritis. Confirmation is by acid fast stain, culture or, best of all, by polymerase chain reaction (PCR).

17.034   Which one of the following pathogenetic mechanisms is the MOST likely in Charcot's arthropathy?

    A. autoimmune synovitis
    B. improper alignment after fracture healing
    C. disintegration of joint due to sensory nerve damage
    D. avascular necrosis of supporting bone
    E. abnormal remodeling of underlying bone
    F. developmental anomaly of joint
    G. abnormal or repetitive stress pattern of joint use
    H. aging changes in cartilage-matrix molecules
    I. chemical alteration of proteoglycans by accumulation of homogentisic acid
    J. heritable abnormalities of cartilage (type II) collagen
    K. crystal-induced synovitis with joint destruction due to enzyme release.

C is correct.

The mechanism of Charcot's arthropathy is disintegration of the joint due to minor repetitive trauma after sensory denervation.

17.035 Which one of the following pathogenetic mechanisms is the MOST likely in rheumatoid arthritis?

A. autoimmune synovitis
B. improper alignment after fracture healing
C. disintegration of joint due to sensory nerve damage
D. avascular necrosis of supporting bone
E. abnormal remodeling of underlying bone
F. developmental anomaly of joint
G. abnormal or repetitive stress pattern of joint use
H. aging changes in cartilage-matrix molecules
I. chemical alteration of proteoglycans by accumulation of homogentisic acid
J. heritable abnormalities of cartilage (type II) collagen
K. crystal-induced synovitis with joint destruction due to enzyme release.

A is correct.

Rheumatoid arthritis is fundamentally an auto-immune synovitis arising in genetically susceptible individuals carrying HLA-DR4 (including DW4, DW14, and DW15), all of which have a common sequence.

17.036 Which one of the following pathogenetic mechanisms is the MOST likely in gout arthropathy?

A. autoimmune synovitis
B. improper alignment after fracture healing
C. disintegration of joint due to sensory nerve damage
D. avascular necrosis of supporting bone
E. abnormal remodeling of underlying bone
F. developmental anomaly of joint
G. abnormal or repetitive stress pattern of joint use
H. aging changes in cartilage-matrix molecules
I. chemical alteration of proteoglycans by accumulation of homogentisic acid
J. heritable abnormalities of cartilage (type II) collagen
K. crystal-induced synovitis with joint destruction due to enzyme release

K is correct.

Gouty arthropathy is due to crystal-induced synovitis, which causes granulocytes and macrophages to release inflammatory mediators.

17.037   Which one of the following pathogenetic mechanisms is the MOST likely in osteoarthritis secondary to congenital hip dysplasia?
  A. autoimmune synovitis
  B. improper alignment after fracture healing
  C. disintegration of joint due to sensory nerve damage
  D. avascular necrosis of supporting bone
  E. abnormal remodeling of underlying bone
  F. developmental anomaly of joint
  G. abnormal or repetitive stress pattern of joint use
  H. aging changes in cartilage-matrix molecules
  I. chemical alteration of proteoglycans by accumulation of homogentisic acid
  J. heritable abnormalities of cartilage (type II) collagen
  K. crystal-induced synovitis with joint destruction due to enzyme release.

F is correct.

The developmental anomaly results in excess force on a small joint surface, leading to precocious secondary osteoarthritis with loss of cartilage.

17.038   Which one of the following pathogenetic mechanisms is the MOST likely in autosomal-dominant osteoarthritis with spondylodysplasia?
  A. autoimmune synovitis
  B. improper alignment after fracture healing
  C. disintegration of joint due to sensory nerve damage
  D. avascular necrosis of supporting bone
  E. abnormal remodeling of underlying bone
  F. developmental anomaly of joint
  G. abnormal or repetitive stress pattern of joint use
  H. aging changes in cartilage-matrix molecules
  I. chemical alteration of proteoglycans by accumulation of homogentisic acid
  J. heritable abnormalities of cartilage (type II) collagen
  K. crystal-induced synovitis with joint destruction due to enzyme release.

J is correct.

Various heritable abnormalities of the type II collagen chain structure prevent normal triple-helix formation, resulting in precocious osteoarthritis in families with this disorder.

17.039   Which one of the following pathogenetic mechanisms is the MOST likely in ochronotic spondyloarthropathy?
   A. autoimmune synovitis
   B. improper alignment after fracture healing
   C. disintegration of joint due to sensory nerve damage
   D. avascular necrosis of supporting bone
   E. abnormal remodeling of underlying bone
   F. developmental anomaly of joint
   G. abnormal or repetitive stress pattern of joint use
   H. aging changes in cartilage-matrix molecules
   I. chemical alteration of proteoglycans by accumulation of homogentisic acid
   J. heritable abnormalities of cartilage (type II) collagen
   K. crystal-induced synovitis with joint destruction due to enzyme release.

I is correct.
Chemical alteration of proteoglycans by homogentisic acid polymers interferes with water binding of the cartilage and eventually results in ochronotic arthropathy.

17.040   Which one of the following pathogenetic mechanisms is the MOST likely in pseudogout arthropathy?
   A. autoimmune synovitis
   B. improper alignment after fracture healing
   C. disintegration of joint due to sensory nerve damage
   D. avascular necrosis of supporting bone
   E. abnormal remodeling of underlying bone
   F. developmental anomaly of joint
   G. abnormal or repetitive stress pattern of joint use
   H. aging changes in cartilage-matrix molecules
   I. chemical alteration of proteoglycans by accumulation of homogentisic acid
   J. heritable abnormalities of cartilage (type II) collagen
   K. crystal-induced synovitis with joint destruction due to enzyme release.

K is correct.
Crystal-induced synovitis with joint destruction due to inflammatory mediator and enzyme release is the cause of pseudogout.

17.041 All of the following are true of malignant fibrous histiocytoma EXCEPT:

A. the most common malignant soft tissue tumor of adults

B. may occur in the retroperitoneum and deep soft tissues of an extremity

C. storiform–pleomorphic subtype is the most common

D. commonly associated with characteristic translocation involving chromosomes 11 and 12

D is correct.

Ewing's sarcoma of bone may be associated with a translocation between chromosomes 11 and 22. There is no association between malignant fibrous histiocytoma and a translocation of chromosomes 11 and 12.

17.042 Which of the following sites is the MOST characteristic of metastatic carcinoma?

A. distal femoral metaphysis

B. proximal tibial metaphysis

C. distal humeral epiphysis

D. thoracic vertebral body

E. carpal navicular bone

D is correct.

The vertebral bodies are characteristic sites for metastatic carcinoma. Metastatic carcinoma is rarely seen in the distal femoral metaphysis, proximal tibial metaphysis, or distal humeral epiphysis. Metastatic carcinoma to the bones of the hands and feet is rare.

17.043 Which of the following types of malignancy has the GREATEST tendency for solitary bone metastasis imitating a primary bone neoplasm?

A. squamous cell pulmonary carcinoma

B. mammary duct cell carcinoma

C. renal cell carcinoma

D. prostatic adenocarcinoma

E. small-cell undifferentiated carcinoma

C is correct.

Renal cell carcinoma is known for solitary metastases from an occult primary. The other primary tumors listed are more frequently associated with multiple metastases.

17.044 Which of the following diseases is MOST likely to be confused with osseous metastatic disease from prostatic adenocarcinoma on the basis of clinical and radiographic examination?

A. fibrous dysplasia

B. aneurysmal bone cyst

C. hyperparathyroidism

D. Paget's disease (osteitis deformans)

E. osteogenesis imperfecta

D is correct.

Paget's disease produces deformed bone with dense osteoblastic lesions similar to metastatic prostatic carcinoma. Fibrous dysplasia produces a mottled area of rarefied bone with indistinct margins. Aneurysmal bone cysts produce a ballooning lytic area. Hyperparathyroidism produces multiple cystic lytic areas. Osteogenesis imperfecta causes thin, brittle bone cortex that is rarefied on radiographs.

17.045 A well-circumscribed round lytic lesion in the metaphyseal cortex of a long bone composed of vascularized osteoblastic tissue producing immature benign-appearing osteoid is BEST characterized as a(n):

A. osteoblastoma

B. osteoid osteoma

C. osteoblastic osteosarcoma

D. osteochondroma

E. chondroblastoma

B is correct.

An osteoid osteoma is a vascularized proliferation of immature osteoid in the cortex of a long bone. Osteoblastomas occur in the medullary space of bones, not the cortex. Osteoblastic osteosarcomas are infiltrative, poorly circumscribed, lesions that involve both the medullary and cortical zones of a long bone. Osteochondromas are bony protuberances covered by cartilage occurring on the surface of a long bone. Chondroblastomas cause lytic areas in the epiphysis, and contain immature chondroid and giant cells.

17.046 The histologic differential diagnosis of a typical osteoblastoma includes all of the following EXCEPT:
  A. chondroblastoma
  B. giant cell tumor
  C. well-differentiated osteosarcoma
  D. osteoid osteoma
  E. osteochondroma

E is correct.
Osteochondromas are composed of mature cancellous bone and cartilage, not osteoid and giant cells as are osteoblastomas. Chondroblastomas have giant cells causing some areas to resemble osteoblastomas. Giant cell tumors have giant cells and may have an occasional osteoid, thereby resembling an osteoblastoma. Well-differentiated osteosarcomas may resemble an osteoblastoma on histology. Osteoid osteomas and osteoblastomas are virtually identical on microscopy.

17.047 The presence of a Codman's angle (or triangle) on X-rays of a bone lesion indicates that the process has gone through which of the following maneuvers?
  A. extended down into the diaphyseal marrow, resulting in tumor bone production
  B. extended down into the diaphyseal marrow, resulting in bone lysis
  C. lifted the periosteum, resulting in reactive bone production
  D. crossed the epiphyseal plate cartilage and entered the epiphysis
  E. crossed the joint cartilage and entered the joint space

C is correct.
Lifting the periosteum causing reactive bone formation causes a Codman's triangle.

17.048 All of the following are true of chondrosarcomas EXCEPT:
  A. are more common in patients over 40 years of age
  B. more commonly occur in long bones
  C. more commonly occur in the axial skeleton
  D. usually not sensitive to chemotherapy

B is correct.
Chondrosarcomas occur most frequently in the axial skeleton.

17.049 The basic defect in osteopetrosis (Albers–Schönberg disease) is the activity of which cell?
  A. osteoblast
  B. osteoclast
  C. histiocyte
  D. macrophage

B is correct.
The basic defect is a hereditary defect in osteoclast activity which results in inadequate bone resorption and, thus, a net increase in bone mass. There is thickening of the cortical bone and narrowing of the medullary cavity.

17.050 Of the following, which is the result of a deficiency in vitamin D?
  A. osteomalacia
  B. osteogenesis inperfecta
  C. osteomyelitis
  D. achondroplasia

A is correct.
Rickets in children and osteomalacia in adults are both the result of a deficiency in vitamin D. The bone is composed of relatively normal amounts of osteoid which is deficient in its mineralization.

17.051 Patients with sickle cell disease are particularly prone to osteomyelitis due to:
  A. *Staphylococcus* species
  B. *Pseudomonas aeruginosa*
  C. *Escherichia coli*
  D. *Salmonella* species

D is correct.

Patient's with sickle cell disease are particularly prone to osteomyelitis which, for reasons as yet unknown, is often caused by *Salmonella* species.

17.052 Patients with hypertrophic osteoarthropathy often have an underlying condition which is usually:
  A. osteosarcoma
  B. lymphoma
  C. bronchogenic carcinoma
  D. achondroplasia

C is correct.

This disorder is characterized by new bone formation at the periosteum at the distal end of the long bones, metacarpal and metatarsal bones, and proximal phalanges. Patients with this condition usually have an underlying disease, usually bronchogenic carcinoma.

17.053 Patients with McCune–Albright syndrome present with focal skin pigmentation (*café au lait* spots) and precocious sexual development in association with:
  A. fibrous dysplasia
  B. fibrous histiocytoma
  C. fibrosarcoma
  D. Paget's disease of bone

A is correct.

In this syndrome, there are focal lesions characterized by the abnormal proliferation of fibrous tissue and immature woven bone in multiple sites (polyostotic fibrous dysplasia).

17.054 Which one of the following conditions is associated with an increased risk of osteosarcoma?
  A. osteopetrosis
  B. Paget's disease of bone
  C. fibrous dysplasia
  D. hypertrophic osteoarthropathy

B is correct.

In patients with severe polyostotic disease, the development of osteosarcoma may be as high as 10%.

17.055 Ewing's sarcoma is commonly associated with:
  A. characteristic translocation involving chromosomes 11 and 22
  B. deletion of the retinoblastoma gene
  C. Philadelphia chromosome
  D. deletion on chromosome 13

A is correct.

Ewing's sarcoma is an uncommon malignancy of bone usually occurring between the ages of 10 and 20 years. It has been associated with a translocation between chromosomes 11 and 22. There is also an association with neuroectodermal tumors.

17.056 Which one of the following statements is TRUE concerning synovial sarcoma?
  A. usually occurs in the proximity of a joint, but does not arise from the synovium
  B. arises from the synovium
  C. usually occurs in patients > 60 years of age
  D. is associated with Paget's disease of bone

A is correct.

These uncommon tumors occur in the proximity of joints, but do not usually involve either the joint or synovium. They are so named because of their histologic resemblance to developing synovium.

17.057 All of the following are true of osteosarcoma EXCEPT:
   A. commonly occurs in axial skeleton
   B. commonly occurs in long bones
   C. commonly occurs between ages 10 and 25 years
   D. associated with a deletion on chromosome 13
   E. may be associated with prior history of irradiation

A is correct.
Osteosarcomas typically occur in the metaphyses of long bones. The most common site is the distal femur.

17.058 All of the following are true of well-differentiated liposarcoma EXCEPT:
   A. occurs in the soft tissue of an extremity
   B. occurs in retroperitoneum
   C. commonly metastasizes to regional lymph nodes
   D. atypical lipoblasts (floret cells) present on histology
   E. may have areas of chronic inflammation and fibrosis on histology

C is correct.
These malignancies usually occur in adults. The well-differentiated types are low-grade lesions that tend to occur in the retroperitoneum or deep soft tissues of an extremity. They rarely, if ever, metastasize, but may recur following excision.

17.059 Osteosarcomas are typically treated with:
   A. radiation only
   B. chemotherapy only
   C. surgical resection only
   D. surgical resection and adjuvant chemotherapy
   E. surgical resection and radiation

D is correct.
Patients with osteosarcomas are routinely treated with preoperative chemotherapy (with or without radiotherapy) followed by surgical resection of the tumor.

17.060 Chondrosarcomas are typically treated with:
   A. radiation only
   B. chemotherapy only
   C. surgical resection only
   D. surgical resection and adjuvant chemotherapy
   E. none of the above

C is correct.
Chondrosarcomas do not respond to chemotherapy and, in most cases, treatment is limited to surgical resection.

17.061 Which one of the following lesions may occasionally give rise to chondrosarcoma?
   A. osteogenesis imperfecta
   B. osteopetrosis
   C. osteomyelitis
   D. osteopenia
   E. osteochondromatosis

E is correct.
Multiple osteochondromas may occur in multiple hereditary exostoses. There is an increased risk for the development of chondrosarcomas in these patients.

17.062 Which one of the following entities has an underlying defect of abnormal collagen synthesis?
   A. osteogenesis imperfecta
   B. osteopetrosis
   C. osteomyelitis
   D. osteopenia
   E. osteochondromatosis

A is correct.
This is a hereditary disorder of collagen synthesis which results in death *in utero* or in abnormalities of the skeleton and other collagen-rich tissues such as the sclera, joints, ligaments, eyes, ears, teeth, and skin.

17.063 Which one of the following conditions is associated with hearing loss, dental abnormalities and blue sclerae?

    A. osteogenesis imperfecta
    B. osteopetrosis
    C. osteomyelitis
    D. osteopenia
    E. osteochondromatosis

A is correct.
Osteogenesis imperfecta is a hereditary disorder of collagen synthesis which results in death *in utero* or in abnormalities of the skeleton and other collagen-rich tissues such as the sclera, joints, ligaments, eyes, ears, teeth, and skin. Characteristic findings are skeletal fragility, blue sclerae, hearing loss, and dental alterations.

17.064 Which one of the following conditions is associated with a net increase in bone mass?

    A. osteogenesis imperfecta
    B. osteopetrosis
    C. osteomyelitis
    D. osteopenia
    E. osteochondromatosis

B is correct.
The basic defect is a hereditary defect in osteoclast activity which results in inadequate bone resorption and, thus, a net increase in bone mass. There is thickening of cortical bone and narrowing of the medullary cavity.

17.065 Which one of the following tumors commonly involves bones of the axial skeleton?

    A. malignant fibrous histiocytoma
    B. osteosarcoma
    C. Ewing's sarcoma
    D. well-differentiated liposarcoma
    E. chondrosarcoma

E is correct.
Chondrosarcomas occur most commonly in the bones of the axial skeleton.

17.066 Which one of the following is a tumor of soft tissue that typically involves an extremity or the retroperitoneum?

    A. malignant fibrous histiocytoma
    B. osteosarcoma
    C. Ewing's sarcoma
    D. well-differentiated liposarcoma
    E. chondrosarcoma

D is correct.
Well-differentiated liposarcomas usually occur in adults. They are low-grade lesions that tend to occur in the retroperitoneum or deep soft tissues of an extremity. They rarely, if ever, metastasize, but may recur following excision.

17.067 The most common etiologic agent of hematogenous osteomyelitis is:

    A. *Pseudomonas aeruginosa*
    B. *Escherichia coli*
    C. *Proteus mirabilis*
    D. *Staphylococcus aureus*
    E. *Salmonella typhimurium*

D is correct.
Pyogenic osteomyelitis is usually caused by bacteria and approximately 80–90% of cases of hematogenous osteomyelitis are caused by *Staphylococcus aureus*.

17.068 The typical location for presentation of synovial sarcoma is:

    A. synovium
    B. soft tissue in close proximity to a joint
    C. retroperitoneum
    D. deep intramuscular soft tissue
    E. mediastinal lymph node

B is correct.
These uncommon tumors occur in the proximity of joints, but do not usually involve either the joint or synovium. They are so named because of their histologic resemblance to developing synovium.

17.069   Which one of the following is TRUE concerning osteosarcomas?
  A. are associated with translocation between chromosomes 11 and 22
  B. commonly arise in bones of the pelvis
  C. are associated with deletion of the q14 locus on chromosome 13
  D. are not sensitive to chemotherapeutic agents
  E. typically arise in the diaphysis of a long bone

C is correct.
Genetic and environmental factors have been strongly implicated as having etiologic roles in the development of osteosarcoma. Patients who develop retinoblastoma have homozygous mutations in the q14 locus on chromosome 13. Patients who survive the retinoblastoma are at an increased risk of developing osteosarcoma.

17.070   Which one of the following conditions carries an increased risk of osteosarcoma?
  A. McCune–Albright syndrome
  B. Albers–Schönberg disease (osteopetrosis)
  C. osteogenesis imperfecta
  D. hypertrophic osteoarthropathy
  E. Paget's disease of bone

E is correct.
There is an increased risk of the development of osteosarcoma in patients with Paget's disease of bone. This risk increases up to 10% in patients with polyostotic disease.

17.071   Fibrous dysplasia is found in which one of the following diseases?
  A. McCune–Albright syndrome
  B. Albers–Schönberg disease (osteopetrosis)
  C. osteogenesis imperfecta
  D. hypertrophic osteoarthropathy
  E. Paget's disease of bone

A is correct.
Fibrous dysplasia is characterized by the abnormal proliferation of fibrous tissue and immature woven bone in a localized area of the skeleton. A polyostotic form may occur in association with *café au lait* spots and endocrinopathy, and is called the McCune–Albright syndrome.

17.072   Anemia and neutropenia are found in which one of the following diseases?
  A. McCune–Albright syndrome
  B. Albers–Schönberg disease (osteopetrosis)
  C. osteogenesis imperfecta
  D. hypertrophic osteoarthropathy
  E. Paget's disease of bone

B is correct.
The basic defect is a hereditary defect in osteoclast activity which results in inadequate bone resorption and, thus, a net increase in bone mass. There is thickening of cortical bone and narrowing of the medullary cavity. The latter obliterates the bone marrow, resulting in anemia and neutropenia.

17.073   Which one of the following conditions is associated with cranial nerve compression?
  A. Paget's disease of bone
  B. fibrous dysplasia
  C. hypertrophic osteoarthropathy
  D. osteopenia
  E. osteitis fibrosa cystica

A is correct.
Clinical presentation varies depending on which bones are involved. Thickening of the calvarium may result in narrowing of the foramina of cranial nerves with signs of cranial nerve damage.

17.074   Which one of the following conditions commonly involves bones of the appendicular skeleton (long bones)?
  A. osteosarcoma
  B. chondrosarcoma
  C. Ewing's sarcoma
  D. osteochondroma
  E. osteitis fibrosa cystica

A is correct.
Osteosarcoma typically occurs in the metaphyses of long bones. The most common site is the distal femur.

17.075   Which one of the following tumors often exhibits a biphasic morphology with epithelioid and spindle cell components?
   A. liposarcoma
   B. malignant fibrous histiocytoma
   C. synovial sarcoma
   D. rhabdomyosarcoma
   E. cystosarcoma

C is correct.
These uncommon tumors occur in the proximity of joints, but do not usually involve either the joint or synovium. They are so named because of their histologic resemblance to developing synovium. The neoplasms often have a biphasic pattern consisting of both epithelioid and spindle cells.

17.076   Which one of the following is a malignant soft tissue tumor of older adults characterized by a storiform pattern of tumor cells with associated giant cells?
   A. liposarcoma
   B. malignant fibrous histiocytoma
   C. synovial sarcoma
   D. rhabdomyosarcoma
   E. cystosarcoma

B is correct.
These tumors are the most common malignant soft tissue tumor of adults. They usually occur as a mass in the deep soft tissues of an extremity. The morphologic pattern is typically a background of spindle-shaped fibroblasts in a storiform pattern mixed with bizarre multinucleate tumor giant cells.

17.077   A newborn infant manifests weakness, poor motor tone, and decreased spontaneous motor activity. The possible diagnoses include all of the following EXCEPT:
   A. congenital fiber-type disproportion
   B. progressive spinal muscular atrophy
   C. Duchenne muscular dystrophy
   D. genetic defect of glycogen metabolism
   E. nemaline (rod) myopathy

C is correct.
Duchenne muscular dystrophy is X-linked. However, newborn boys with this disease are normal at birth and during the very early stages of development.

17.078   Of the patients with the following muscle diseases, which develop clinical weakness at the earliest age?
   A. Duchenne muscular dystrophy
   B. Becker's muscular dystrophy
   C. polymyositis
   D. McArdle's disease
   E. nemaline (rod) myopathy

E is correct.
Nemaline or rod myopathy consists of hypotonia and delayed motor development which usually present at birth or in early infancy. Pathologic findings include the appearance of aggregates of sub-sarcolemmal spindle-shaped particles referred to as 'nemaline rods'.

17.079   Duchenne muscular dystrophy has recently been shown to result from:
   A. an abnormal isoenzyme of fast-twitch (type 2 fiber) muscle myosin ATPase
   B. a defective ion channel in the transverse tubular system
   C. a deficiency of a protease inhibitor intrinsic to muscle
   D. a deficiency of a high-molecular-weight protein associated with the muscle surface membrane
   E. absence of a normal neurotrophic molecule

D is correct.
The HMW protein dystrophin is normally found adjacent to the sarcolemmal membrane. Patients with Duchenne muscular dystrophy are deficient in this protein.

17.080 Immobilization of a muscle for many weeks results in:
  A. uniform atrophy of all muscle fibers
  B. atrophic fibers appearing in groups
  C. selective atrophy of type 2 (fast-twitch, strength) fibers
  D. selective atrophy of fibers on the margins of fascicles
  E. normal histologic appearance on routine H & E-stained sections of muscle

C is correct.
In immobilization, the muscle atrophy which occurs primarily involves the type 2 fibers.

17.081 What is the site of the abnormality in nemaline or rod myopathy?
  A. pigmented nucleus of brain stem
  B. anterior horn of spinal cord
  C. dorsal root ganglion
  D. peripheral nerve
  E. neuromuscular junction
  F. muscle membrane
  G. muscle contractile apparatus

G is correct.
Nemaline or rod myopathy is the result of a developmental abnormality in the architecture of the muscle fiber causing muscle weakness at birth (neonatal hypotonia).

17.082 What is the site of the abnormality in myasthenia gravis?
  A. pigmented nucleus of brain stem
  B. anterior horn of spinal cord
  C. dorsal root ganglion
  D. peripheral nerve
  E. neuromuscular junction
  F. muscle membrane
  G. muscle contractile apparatus

E is correct.
Myasthenia gravis is an autoimmune disease with a decreased number of muscle acetylcholine receptors in the synaptic region secondary to circulating antibodies to these receptors.

17.083 A middle-aged patient with progressive weakness that improves with administration of an acetylcholinesterase-blocking agent MOST likely has which one of the following conditions?
  A. diffuse axonal injury
  B. Down syndrome
  C. Duchenne muscular dystrophy
  D. multiple sclerosis
  E. myasthenia gravis
  F. polymicrogyria
  G. spinal muscular atrophy
  H. subdural hematoma

E is correct.
Myasthenia gravis is an autoimmune disease with a decrease in the number of muscle acetylcholine receptors in the synaptic region secondary to circulating antibodies to these receptors. Acetylcholinesterase-blocking agents allow a build-up of acetylcholine which improves symptoms in these patients.

17.084 A young boy with large calf muscles and difficulty in getting up from the floor is MOST likely to have which one of the following conditions?
- A. diffuse axonal injury
- B. Down syndrome
- C. Duchenne muscular dystrophy
- D. multiple sclerosis
- E. myasthenia gravis
- F. polymicrogyria
- G. spinal muscular atrophy
- H. subdural hematoma

C is correct.
Duchenne muscular dystrophy is an X-linked disorder which becomes clinically evident by the age of 5 years. Patients have a progressive weakness beginning in the pelvic girdle muscles, which requires children to use the upper extremities to stand up from a seated position. Enlargement of the calf muscles or pseudohypertrophy occurs in these patients. Initially, the increased muscle size is due to an increase in the size of muscle fibers but, later, with the development of atrophy, there is an increase of fat in the connective tissue.

17.085 Sex-linked recessive inheritance occurs in which one of the following conditions?
- A. diffuse axonal injury
- B. Down syndrome
- C. Duchenne muscular dystrophy
- D. multiple sclerosis
- E. myasthenia gravis
- F. polymicrogyria
- G. spinal muscular atrophy
- H. subdural hematoma

C is correct.
Duchenne muscular dystrophy is an X-linked disorder which becomes clinically evident by the age of 5 years. Patients have a progressive muscle weakness.

17.086 A humoral-mediated autoimmune response has been implicated in the pathogenesis of:
- A. polymyositis
- B. dermatomyositis
- C. inclusion-body myositis
- D. postinfluenzal myositis
- E. granulomatous myositis

B is correct.
A greater number of B cells and a higher CD4:CD8 ratio suggests that dermatomyositis is a humorally mediated disease.

17.087 Autoimmune blockade of synaptic neurotransmitter release underlies:
- A. Alzheimer's disease
- B. Guillain–Barré syndrome
- C. diffuse axonal injury
- D. myasthenia gravis
- E. Eaton–Lambert syndrome

E is correct.
A myasthenia gravis-like syndrome called Eaton–Lambert syndrome may occur in patients with malignancy. The release of acetylcholine, rather than its action (as in myasthenia gravis), is blocked by an autoantibody.

17.088 Progressive muscle weakness which culminates in death in the second to early in the third decades is characteristic of:
- A. Duchenne muscular dystrophy
- B. Werdnig–Hoffmann disease
- C. inclusion-body myositis
- D. myasthenia gravis
- E. McArdle's disease

A is correct.
Duchenne muscular dystrophy is an X-linked disorder which manifests by around 5 years of age and consists of muscle weakness. There is progression with death occurring by the age of the early 20s.

17.089 Episodic weakness associated with intense exercise in a young adult is characteristic of:
   A. Duchenne muscular dystrophy
   B. Werdnig–Hoffmann disease
   C. inclusion-body myositis
   D. myasthenia gravis
   E. McArdle's disease

E is correct.
McArdle's disease is a genetic deficiency of muscle phosphorylase. It is a rather mild disease which may go unrecognized until later in life. Patients have weakness, stiffness, and pain associated with intense exercise, and a failure of lactate to appear in the blood.

17.090 A 74-year-old woman presents with weakness in her legs. A muscle biopsy shows little histologic change, but a histochemical preparation shows large distinct clusters of both type 1 and type 2 muscle fibers. The MOST likely diagnosis is:
   A. acute inflammatory polyneuropathy
   B. amyotrophic lateral sclerosis
   C. slowly progressive peripheral neuropathy
   D. Friedreich's ataxia
   E. Werdnig–Hoffmann disease

C is correct.
In a slow chronic neuropathy, surviving neurons sprout collateral axons and reinnervate denervated fibers. As the muscle fiber type is determined by the innervating neuron, reinnervated muscle fibers may change fiber type to match the new neuron. This results in loss of the normal 'checkerboard' mixture of type 1 and 2 fibers, and the appearance of groups of muscle fibers of the same fiber type (fiber-type grouping).

17.091 Which one of the following diseases carries the MOST favorable prognosis?
   A. acid maltase deficiency
   B. congenital central core myopathy
   C. Duchenne muscular dystrophy
   D. infantile spinal muscular atrophy
   E. systemic carnitine deficiency

B is correct.
Central core disease is a congenital myopathy consisting of early-onset hypotonia and a nonprogressive muscle weakness.

17.092 A 58-year-old man with small-cell carcinoma of the lung develops a proximal muscle weakness with autonomic dysfunction. The muscle weakness is MOST likely due to:
   A. antitumor antibodies that block acetylcholine release
   B. hypercalcemia interfering with muscle action-potential propagation
   C. peripheral neuropathy resulting from chemotherapy toxicity
   D. tumor involvement of the brachial plexus
   E. radiation-induced demyelination of peripheral nerves

A is correct.
A myasthenia gravis-like syndrome may be seen in some patients with malignancy. It is believed that the release of acetylcholine is blocked by antibodies directed against tumor antigens.

17.093 A 69-year-old man presents with muscle weakness and pain. A muscle biopsy is performed, and reveals intrafasicular lymphocytic infiltrates and scattered fibers with small round eosinophilic or basophilic sarcoplasmic inclusions. The MOST likely diagnosis is:
   A. dermatomyositis
   B. inclusion-body myositis
   C. myasthenia gravis
   D. polymyositis
   E. viral myositis

B is correct.
Inclusion-body myositis is a relatively rare inflammatory myopathy characterized by small eosinophilic or basophilic inclusions in muscle fibers.

SECTION 18: NERVOUS SYSTEM AND EYE

18.001   Demyelination is the principal pathologic process in all of the following diseases EXCEPT:
    A. globoid cell leukodystrophy (Krabbe's disease)
    B. progressive multifocal leukoencephalopathy
    C. multiple sclerosis
    D. periventricular leukomalacia
    E. perivenous encephalomyelitis

D is correct.
Periventricular leukomalacia refers to ischemic infarcts in the periventricular white matter. This may occur in premature newborns.

18.002   Dementia may be a clinical manifestation of all of the following EXCEPT:
    A. Alzheimer's disease
    B. Huntington's disease
    C. idiopathic Parkinsonism
    D. Jakob–Creutzfeldt disease
    E. amyotrophic lateral sclerosis

E is correct.
Amyotrophic lateral sclerosis is a degenerative disorder which results in loss of both lower and upper motor neurons. Patients demonstrate muscle atrophy, fasciculations, and weakness due to the lower motor neuron loss, and hyperreflexia and spasticity secondary to the upper motor neuron loss. Dementia is not a feature of this disease.

18.003   Which one of the following types of neuron is particularly susceptible to ischemia?
    A. hypothalamic neurons
    B. Purkinje cells of the cerebellum
    C. pigmented neurons of the locus ceruleus
    D. anterior horn cells of the spinal cord
    E. dorsal root ganglion neurons

B is correct.
Among the cells most sensitive to ischemia are the Purkinje cells of the cerebellum and the pyramidal neurons of the hippocampus.

18.004   Which one of the following congenital brain abnormalities may be attributed to some insult or event occurring late in development?
    A. Arnold–Chiari malformations
    B. hydranencephaly
    C. holoprosencephaly
    D. agenesis of the corpus callosum
    E. diastematomyelia

B is correct.
Hydranencephaly is an extreme form of prosencephaly in which virtually the entire cerebrum is absent. The head is normally formed, suggesting that the brain formed normally, but was then destroyed by an intrauterine event. These are late destructive lesions occurring after 25 weeks of gestation.

18.005   Which one of the following is not a potential consequence of blunt head trauma?
    A. diffuse axonal damage
    B. Guillain–Barré polyneuritis
    C. fat embolism
    D. 'border-zone' cerebral infarction
    E. territorial cerebral infarction

B is correct.
Guillain–Barré syndrome is characterized by an ascending paralysis. Many cases occur after an acute influenza-like illness. The disease is primarily an inflammatory disorder of the peripheral nerves.

18.006   Which one of the following diseases is NOT thought to be autoimmune in nature?
  A. multiple sclerosis
  B. Guillain–Barré polyneuritis
  C. myasthenia gravis
  D. perivenous encephalomyelitis
  E. periventricular leukomalacia

E is correct.
Periventricular leukomalacia is caused by ischemic infarcts in the periventricular white matter. This disease may occur in premature newborns.

18.007   Which one of the following congenital brain abnormalities does NOT represent a disorder of neuronal cell migration?
  A. agyria
  B. pachygyria
  C. heterotopias
  D. lissencephaly
  E. porencephaly

E is correct.
Porencephaly is a cystic defect in the brain most likely caused by necrosis during development. Disorders of neuronal migration include lissencephaly and polymicrogyria.

18.008   A 64-year-old man is brought to the hospital with severe chest pain radiating to the left arm. ECG and cardiac enzyme studies reveal changes which are interpreted as due to acute myocardial infarction. There is no evidence of a focal neurologic deficit. The patient then enters cardiac arrest and is resuscitated, but remains comatose for 24 h before death ensues. Which one of the following is MOST likely to be seen on either gross or microscopic examination of this patient's brain after autopsy?
  A. a large area of necrosis and petechial hemorrhage in the territory of left middle cerebral artery
  B. herniation of the left uncus
  C. shrunken neurons with eosinophilic cytoplasm and pyknotic nuclei in the hippocampus and in the Purkinje cells of the cerebellum
  D. a large amount of blood in the ventricle
  E. multiple microscopic abscesses in the cerebrum

C is correct.
During the period of cardiac arrest, the patient experienced generalized anoxia. The neurons in the hippocampus and the Purkinje cells of the cerebellum are the cells most sensitive to hypoxia.

18.009 A 46-year-old woman is brought to the emergency room because of a severe headache of sudden onset. No significant past history is given by her family. She is found dazed, but there is no loss of consciousness. No hemiparesis or focal neurologic deficit is found, but there is nuchal rigidity. A lumbar puncture reveals blood in the cerebrospinal fluid. This patient MOST likely has:
   A. a large hemorrhagic infarct in the right middle cerebral artery territory
   B. a large hemorrhage in the thalamus with extension of blood to the ventricle
   C. a cerebral abscess which has extended to the ventricle
   D. epidural hemorrhage
   E. rupture of a berry aneurysm

E is correct.
The sudden onset of the event with no significant past history along with no focal neurologic defects and bloody CSF strongly suggest acute subarachnoid hemorrhage. The most likely cause is a ruptured berry aneurysm.

18.010 Which one of the following statements is TRUE of berry aneurysms?
   A. have same structure as a normal intracranial artery
   B. lack a muscular media, but have an intact internal elastic lamina
   C. lack an internal elastic lamina, but have an intact muscular media
   D. have a thin fibrous wall and lack both a muscular media and internal elastic lamina
   E. lack a consistent histologic pattern

D is correct.
A berry aneurysm is a thin-walled outpouching situated at arterial branch points of the circle of Willis or nearby major vessels. At the neck of the aneurysm, the muscular wall and intimal elastic lamina are either absent or rudimentary.

18.011 The MOST frequent cause of multiple microabscesses in the brain is:
   A. abscess of lung
   B. otitis media
   C. bacterial endocarditis
   D. acute cystitis
   E. acute immunodeficiency syndrome

C is correct.
Multiple abscesses of the brain are most usually secondary to embolic bacterial seeding from infected heart valves.

18.012 Which one of the following is characterized by intracytoplasmic inclusion bodies in neurons?
   A. herpes simplex encephalitis
   B. rabies
   C. progressive multifocal leukoencephalopathy
   D. toxoplasmosis
   E. Jakob–Creutzfeldt disease

B is correct.
The typical histologic finding in rabies is the presence of cytoplasmic round-to-oval eosinophilic inclusions in the neurons. These inclusions are called Negri bodies.

18.013 Which of the following is characterized by rapidly progressive dementia and diffuse atrophy of the brain?
   A. herpes simplex encephalitis
   B. rabies
   C. progressive multifocal leukoencephalopathy
   D. toxoplasmosis
   E. Jakob–Creutzfeldt disease

E is correct.
Jakob–Creutzfeldt disease is a spongiform encephalopathy caused by a prion. The predominating clinical presentation is rapidly progressive dementia.

18.014 Which one of the following has a predilection for temporal lobe involvement?
  A. herpes simplex encephalitis
  B. rabies
  C. progressive multifocal leukoencephalopathy
  D. toxoplasmosis
  E. Jakob–Creutzfeldt disease

A is correct.
Herpes simplex encephalitis is the most common type of sporadic acute encephalitis. Most infections are caused by HSV-1 and predominantly involve the temporal and medial frontal lobes of the brain.

18.015 Which one of the following organisms may infect the fetus by a transplacental route and cause necrotizing calcification in the brain?
  A. herpes simplex virus
  B. rabies virus
  C. *Cryptococcus neoformans*
  D. *Toxoplasma gondii*
  E. *Candida albicans*

D is correct.
Toxoplasma gondii is an intracellular protozoan which may cross the placenta and infect infants *in utero*. The infected infant presents with destructive lesions of the central nervous system, with necrosis and calcifications.

18.016 Which one of the following may be diagnosed by skeletal muscle biopsy?
  A. Alzheimer's disease
  B. Huntington's disease
  C. idiopathic Parkinsonism
  D. Jakob–Creutzfeldt disease
  E. amyotrophic lateral sclerosis

E is correct.
Amyotrophic lateral sclerosis is a degenerative disorder affecting both lower and upper motor neurons. There is marked muscle atrophy, which can be seen on muscle biopsy. The other conditions listed are not associated with specific muscle alterations.

18.017 Which one of the following congenital vascular lesions of the brain is MOST likely to be an incidental finding at autopsy rather than a clinical manifestation?
  A. arteriovenous malformation
  B. venous angioma
  C. capillary telangiectasis
  D. berry aneurysm

C is correct.
Capillary telangiectasias are microscopic foci of dilated thin-walled vessels lying between normal brain parenchyma. They occur most frequently in the pons and are not likely to cause a clinical problem.

18.018 Lewy bodies are found in association with which one of the following diseases?
  A. chronic alcoholism
  B. Alzheimer's disease
  C. idiopathic Parkinsonism
  D. selective atrophy of frontal lobes
  E. Jakob–Creutzfeldt disease

C is correct.
Some of the neurons in the brain of patients with idiopathic Parkinson's disease may contain intracytoplasmic, eosinophilic, round inclusions surrounded by a pale rim. These structures are called Lewy bodies and contain neurofilament antigens.

18.019 Pick bodies are found in association with which one of the following diseases?
  A. chronic alcoholism
  B. Alzheimer's disease
  C. idiopathic Parkinsonism
  D. selective atrophy of frontal lobes
  E. Jakob–Creutzfeldt disease

D is correct.
Pick bodies are cytoplasmic, round-to-oval, filamentous inclusions which stain with special silver stains. They are composed of neurofilaments and endoplasmic reticulum. They are seen in Pick's disease, in which there is prominent atrophy of the frontal and temporal lobes of the brain.

18.020   Atrophy of mammillary bodies is seen in association with which one of the following diseases?
    A. chronic alcoholism
    B. Alzheimer's disease
    C. idiopathic Parkinsonism
    D. selective atrophy of frontal lobes
    E. Jakob–Creutzfeldt disease

A is correct.

In chronic alcoholism, some patients demonstrate confusion, nystagmus, ataxia and extraocular paralysis known as Wernicke–Korsakoff syndrome. The brain in these patients shows atrophy of the mammillary bodies at autopsy.

18.021   The MOST common primary brain tumor in adults is:
    A. astrocytoma
    B. medulloblastoma
    C. neurofibroma
    D. ependymoma
    E. hemangioblastoma

A is correct.

Astrocytomas are gliomas which account for approximately 80% of adult primary brain tumors. They are usually located in the cerebral hemispheres.

18.022   The MOST common tumor of the spinal cord is:
    A. astrocytoma
    B. medulloblastoma
    C. neurofibroma
    D. ependymoma
    E. hemangioblastoma

D is correct.

Ependymomas generally begin near the ependymal lining of the ventricular system. In the first two decades of life, they tend to occur near the fourth ventricle. In mid-life, they most commonly occur in the spinal cord. They are the most common tumor of the spinal cord.

18.023   Which one of the following tumors may be multiple and associated with *café au lait* spots?
    A. astrocytoma
    B. medulloblastoma
    C. neurofibroma
    D. ependymoma
    E. hemangioblastoma

C is correct.

The familial Recklinghausen's disease or neurofibromatosis is characterized by multiple neurofibromas and hyperpigmented skin macules called *café au lait* spots.

18.024   Which one of the following tumors may be associated with erythrocytosis?
    A. astrocytoma
    B. medulloblastoma
    C. neurofibroma
    D. ependymoma
    E. hemangioblastoma

E is correct.

von Hippel–Lindau disease has a predilection to develop capillary hemangioblastomas in the cerebellum, retina, brain stem, and spinal cord. Approximately 10% of patients with hemangioblastomas have polycythemia.

18.025   Which one of the following tumors frequently spreads to the subarachnoid space of the brain and spinal cord?
    A. astrocytoma
    B. medulloblastoma
    C. neurofibroma
    D. ependymoma
    E. hemangioblastoma

B is correct.

Medulloblastomas are neoplasms which occur in the midline of the cerebellum in children. In adults, the lesions tend to occur more laterally. They are rapidly growing tumors with a propensity to invade and spread in the subarachnoid space.

18.026   Which one of the following microscopic abnormalities is typically seen in diffuse axonal injury?
   A. neurofibrillary tangles and neuritic plaques
   B. round, layered, eosinophilic cytoplasmic inclusions in pigmented neurons (Lewy bodies)
   C. small, round, eosinophilic cytoplasmic inclusions (Negri bodies)
   D. large block-like eosinophilic intranuclear inclusions
   E. reactive axonal swellings ('retraction balls')
   F. dissolution of central neuronal Nissl substance
   G. axonal torpedoes in Purkinje cells

E is correct.
Diffuse axonal injury is seen with diffuse-impact blunt head trauma. On microscopy, there is evidence of widespread axonal injury with reactive axonal swellings called 'retraction balls'.

18.027   Which one of the following microscopic abnormalities is typically seen in Parkinson's disease?
   A. neurofibrillary tangles and neuritic plaques
   B. round, layered, eosinophilic cytoplasmic inclusions in pigmented neurons (Lewy bodies)
   C. small, round, eosinophilic cytoplasmic inclusions (Negri bodies)
   D. large block-like eosinophilic intranuclear inclusions
   E. reactive axonal swellings ('retraction balls')
   F. dissolution of central neuronal Nissl substance
   G. axonal torpedoes in Purkinje cells

B is correct.
Some of the neurons in the brain of patients with idiopathic Parkinson's disease may contain intra-cytoplasmic, eosinophilic, round inclusions surrounded by a pale rim. These structures are called Lewy bodies and contain neurofilament antigens.

18.028   Which one of the following microscopic abnormalities is typically seen in Alzheimer's disease?
   A. neurofibrillary tangles and neuritic plaques
   B. round, layered, eosinophilic cytoplasmic inclusions in pigmented neurons (Lewy bodies)
   C. small, round, eosinophilic cytoplasmic inclusions (Negri bodies)
   D. large block-like eosinophilic intranuclear inclusions
   E. reactive axonal swellings ('retraction balls')
   F. dissolution of central neuronal Nissl substance
   G. axonal torpedoes in Purkinje cells

A is correct.
Alzheimer's disease is a cortical degenerative disorder characterized by dementia. Neurofibrillary tangles are seen on histologic examination of the brain of affected patients. The tangles consist of filaments in the cytoplasm of neurons that displace or encircle the nucleus. Neuritic plaques are focal, round, accumulations of dilated neuritic processes surrounding a central amyloid core.

18.029 The neuronal response to axonal injury is typically which one of the following?
- A. neurofibrillary tangles and neuritic plaques
- B. round, layered, eosinophilic cytoplasmic inclusions in pigmented neurons (Lewy bodies)
- C. small, round, eosinophilic cytoplasmic inclusions (Negri bodies)
- D. large block-like eosinophilic intranuclear inclusions
- E. reactive axonal swellings ('retraction balls')
- F. dissolution of central neuronal Nissl substance
- G. axonal torpedoes in Purkinje cells

F is correct.
Following axonal injury, the cell body of a neuron swells. The Nissl substance disappears and the nucleus moves towards the periphery of the cell.

18.030 Which one of the following microscopic abnormalities is typically seen in herpetic encephalitis?
- A. neurofibrillary tangles and neuritic plaques
- B. round, layered, eosinophilic cytoplasmic inclusions in pigmented neurons (Lewy bodies)
- C. small, round, eosinophilic cytoplasmic inclusions (Negri bodies)
- D. large block-like eosinophilic intranuclear inclusions
- E. reactive axonal swellings ('retraction balls')
- F. dissolution of central neuronal Nissl substance
- G. axonal torpedoes in Purkinje cells

D is correct.
Large eosinophilic intranuclear inclusion bodies with a halo (type A intranuclear inclusions) are typically seen in herpesvirus, cytomegalovirus, and measles encephalitis.

18.031 What is the site of the abnormality in amyotrophic lateral sclerosis?
- A. pigmented nucleus of brain stem
- B. anterior horn of spinal cord
- C. dorsal root ganglion
- D. peripheral nerve
- E. neuromuscular junction
- F. muscle membrane
- G. muscle contractile apparatus

B is correct.
Amyotrophic lateral sclerosis is a degenerative disorder resulting in the loss of both lower and upper motor neurons. There is atrophy of the anterior (motor) roots and corticospinal tracts.

18.032 All of the following are typical of global ischemia of the brain caused by cardiac arrest EXCEPT:
- A. watershed infarcts
- B. laminar necrosis
- C. ischemic changes especially on the surface of the brain
- D. necrosis of Purkinje cells of the cerebellum
- E. necrosis of cells in Sommer's sector of the hippocampus

C is correct.
In the cerebral cortex, the neuronal loss produces uneven destruction with preservation of some layers and involvement of others. This pattern is called pseudolaminar necrosis. The pyramidal cells of Sommer's sector of the hippocampus, Purkinje cells of the cerebellum, and pyramidal neurons in the neocortex are the most susceptible to hypoxia.

18.033 All of the following are characteristics of amyotrophic lateral sclerosis EXCEPT:
  A. association with a papovavirus
  B. involvement of motor neurons of the anterior horn
  C. involvement of lateral corticospinal tracts
  D. symmetric hyperreflexia and spasticity
  E. symmetric muscle atrophy and fasciculation

A is correct.
There has been no reported association between amyotrophic lateral sclerosis and papovavirus.

18.034 All of the following are true regarding neoplasms of the central nervous system EXCEPT:
  A. more than half of primary brain tumors arise from glial cells
  B. frequency of CNS tumors is roughly evenly divided between brain and spinal cord
  C. metastases outside the CNS are rare
  D. the most common source of metastases to the brain is bronchogenic carcinoma

B is correct.
The vast majority of CNS neoplasms are found in the brain.

18.035 A 35-year-old woman with mitral stenosis and atrial fibrillation suddenly develops left-sided paralysis. It is diagnosed to be due to a cerebral embolism. Such an embolus MOST commonly impacts in a branch of the:
  A. anterior cerebral artery
  B. basilar artery
  C. vertebral artery
  D. middle cerebral artery
  E. posterior cerebral artery

D is correct.
Emboli to the brain primarily lodge in the distribution of the middle cerebral artery. The incidence is approximately equal in the right and left hemispheres of the brain.

18.036 A 2-year-old child presents with fever, headache, prostration, and nuchal rigidity. The cerebrospinal fluid is cloudy, and microscopic examination reveals innumerable neutrophils. CSF protein is increased and glucose is decreased. The MOST likely etiologic agent is:
  A. *Escherichia coli*
  B. *Hemophilus influenzae*
  C. *Streptococcus pneumoniae*
  D. *Staphylococcus aureus*

B is correct.
Causative organisms in meningitis tend to vary with the age of the patient. In newborns, *E. coli* and group B streptococci are the most common pathogens. In infants and young children, *H. influenzae* is the usual organism involved. In adolescents and young adults, *Neisseria meningitidis* is more likely to be the agent involved and, in older adults, it is *S. pneumoniae* and *Listeria monocytogenes*.

18.037 A 54-year-old man with rapidly progressive dementia has a brain biopsy which shows diffusely distributed vacuoles and gliosis in the gray matter without inflammation. The white matter was unremarkable. The MOST likely diagnosis is:
  A. Alzheimer's disease
  B. multiple sclerosis
  C. progressive multifocal leukoencephalopathy
  D. Jakob–Creutzfeldt disease
  E. subacute sclerosing panencephalitis

D is correct.
Jakob–Creutzfeldt disease produces a characteristic spongiform alteration in the gray matter. The clinical manifestation of this disease is a rapidly progressive dementia. It is believed to be caused by a prion.

18.038   Which one of the following disorders is thought to be associated with measles virus?

    A. kuru

    B. postencephalitic Parkinsonism

    C. progressive multifocal leukoencephalopathy

    D. Jakob–Creutzfeldt disease

    E. subacute sclerosing panencephalitis

E is correct.

Subacute sclerosing panencephalitis is predominantly a disease of children. It is caused by the measles virus reactivated several years after the measles attack or immunization against measles. It presents as an encephalitis with intranuclear inclusions in neurons and glial cells.

18.039   A 50-year-old man develops headaches, vomiting, apathy, convulsions, and papilledema. On radiologic examination, a lesion is found in the left cerebral hemisphere with extension to the opposite hemisphere through the corpus callosum. Biopsy shows pleomorphic hyperchromatic cells in a pseudopalisade arrangement around foci of necrosis. The MOST likely diagnosis is:

    A. astrocytoma

    B. ependymoma

    C. metastatic carcinoma

    D. glioblastoma multiforme

    E. medulloblastoma

D is correct.

Astrocytomas usually present with seizures, headaches, and focal neurologic symptoms. Glioblastoma multiforme is a high-grade tumor with foci of necrosis and hemorrhage. Anaplastic tumor cells line the edges of the necrotic zones, giving the appearance of pseudopalisading.

18.040   A 7-year-old child develops headaches, vomiting, and a staggering gait. A cerebellar neoplasm is diagnosed. The neoplasm is MOST likely a(n):

    A. ependymoma

    B. glioblastoma multiforme

    C. medulloblastoma

    D. neuroblastoma

    E. oligodendroglioma

C is correct.

Medulloblastomas are cerebellar tumors occurring predominantly in children. These tumors have a propensity to seed into the subarachnoid space. The tumor is highly malignant, but radiosensitive.

18.041   A tumor located in the cerebellopontine angle and attached to the vestibular branch of the eighth cranial nerve is MOST likely to be which one of the following neoplasms?

    A. astrocytoma

    B. ependymoma

    C. meningioma

    D. schwannoma

D is correct.

Schwannomas are benign tumors which arise from Schwann cells. In the cranial cavity, the most common location for these tumors is the cerebellopontine angle in association with cranial nerve VIII. These tumors are sometimes called 'acoustic neuromas'.

18.042   Which one of the following is the MOST common tumor of the spinal canal contents in adults?

    A. astrocytoma

    B. ependymoma

    C. metastatic carcinoma

    D. schwannoma

D is correct.

The schwannoma is a well-demarcated encapsulated neoplasm and is the most common spinal tumor in adults. It usually involves the posterior nerve roots.

18.043 Brain stem hemorrhage is MOST frequently associated with which one of the following?
  A. herniation of cingulate gyrus
  B. herniation of uncus
  C. herniation of tonsils of cerebellum
  D. herniation of frontal lobe through a surgical defect in the skull

B is correct.
Downward displacement of the brain stem results in tearing of the penetrating arteries and veins, and hemorrhage in the midbrain and pons. Uncal herniation is most likely to be associated with this.

18.044 Depigmentation of the substantia nigra and locus ceruleus is typically seen in which one of the following diseases?
  A. Alzheimer's disease
  B. Huntington's disease
  C. idiopathic Parkinson's disease
  D. myasthenia gravis
  E. Wernicke–Korsakoff syndrome

C is correct.
Idiopathic Parkinson's disease is characterized by loss of facial expression, slow voluntary movements, altered gait, and a tremor. The typical pathologic finding in these patients at autopsy is pallor or decreased pigmentation of the substantia nigra and locus ceruleus.

18.045 Atrophy of the caudate nucleus is a typical finding in which one of the following diseases?
  A. Alzheimer's disease
  B. Huntington's disease
  C. idiopathic Parkinson's disease
  D. myasthenia gravis
  E. Wernicke–Korsakoff syndrome

B is correct.
Huntington's disease appears in patients between ages 20 and 50 years. It is characterized by uncontrolled movements and progressive dementia. At autopsy, the brain of these patients shows marked atrophy of the caudate nucleus. The putamen and globus pallidus may also show signs of atrophy.

18.046 Atrophy of mammillary bodies is typically seen in which one of the following diseases?
  A. Alzheimer's disease
  B. Huntington's disease
  C. idiopathic Parkinson's disease
  D. myasthenia gravis
  E. Wernicke–Korsakoff syndrome

E is correct.
In chronic alcoholism, some patients demonstrate confusion, nystagmus, ataxia, and extraocular paralysis; this is known as the Wernicke–Korsakoff syndrome. At autopsy, the brain in these patients shows atrophy of the mammillary bodies.

18.047 Focal collections of swollen nerve cell processes with a central amyloid core are typically seen in which one of the following diseases?
  A. Alzheimer's disease
  B. Huntington's disease
  C. idiopathic Parkinson's disease
  D. myasthenia gravis
  E. Wernicke–Korsakoff syndrome

A is correct.
In Alzheimer's disease, a typical finding is the presence of neuritic plaques, which are focal spherical accumulations of silver-staining neuritic processes surrounding a central amyloid core.

18.048 Macrophage-mediated destruction of oligo-dendrocyte-derived myelin is typically seen in which one of the following conditions?
  A. diffuse axonal injury
  B. Down syndrome
  C. Duchenne muscular dystrophy
  D. multiple sclerosis
  E. myasthenia gravis
  F. polymicrogyria
  G. spinal muscular atrophy
  H. subdural hematoma

D is correct.
Multiple sclerosis is a demyelinating disorder with cellular immunity against myelin components.

18.049 A persistent vegetative state following an apparently uncomplicated closed head trauma is MOST likely associated with which one of the following conditions?
  A. diffuse axonal injury
  B. Down syndrome
  C. Duchenne muscular dystrophy
  D. multiple sclerosis
  E. myasthenia gravis
  F. polymicrogyria
  G. spinal muscular atrophy
  H. subdural hematoma

A is correct.
Diffuse axonal injury is seen with diffuse-impact blunt head trauma. Even without grossly obvious brain damage, these patients remain comatose and vegetative. On microscopy, there is evidence of widespread axonal injury.

18.050 Damage to bridging veins is MOST likely to be seen in which one of the following conditions?
  A. diffuse axonal injury
  B. Down syndrome
  C. Duchenne muscular dystrophy
  D. multiple sclerosis
  E. myasthenia gravis
  F. polymicrogyria
  G. spinal muscular atrophy
  H. subdural hematoma

H is correct.
Bridging veins run from the cerebral hemispheres through the subarachnoid and subdural spaces. These vessels are susceptible to tearing in the subdural space and are the source of bleeding in subdural hematomas.

18.051 Which one of the following changes is MOST typically seen in the neuron following axonal transection?
  A. acute neuronal necrosis
  B. block-like eosinophilic intranuclear inclusions in neurons
  C. central chromatolysis
  D. nemaline (rod body) myopathy
  E. numerous small, round, eosinophilic structures in white matter
  F. fiber-type grouping
  G. round eosinophilic, layered, cytoplasmic inclusions in neurons
  H. Wallerian degeneration

C is correct.
After an axon is cut, changes occur in the neuronal cell body consisting of rounding of the cell, peripheral nuclear displacement, and loss of Nissl substance (chromatolysis), especially near the center of the cell.

18.052   Which one of the following alterations appears as an eosinophilia of the neuronal cytoplasm and nuclear pyknosis?
A. acute neuronal necrosis
B. block-like eosinophilic intranuclear inclusions in neurons
C. central chromatolysis
D. nemaline (rod body) myopathy
E. numerous small, round, eosinophilic structures in white matter
F. fiber-type grouping
G. round eosinophilic, layered, cytoplasmic inclusions in neurons
H. Wallerian degeneration

A is correct.
In acute neuronal necrosis such as may occur in anoxia, there is shrinkage of the neuronal body, loss of Nissl substance, eosinophilia of the cytoplasm, and nuclear pyknosis.

18.053 Macrophage-like actions by Schwann cells are responsible for which one of the following alterations?
A. acute neuronal necrosis
B. block-like eosinophilic intranuclear inclusions in neurons
C. central chromatolysis
D. nemaline (rod body) myopathy
E. numerous small, round, eosinophilic structures in white matter
F. fiber-type grouping
G. round eosinophilic, layered, cytoplasmic inclusions in neurons
H. Wallerian degeneration

H is correct.
After transection of an axon, the distal portion undergoes Wallerian degeneration. This is characterized by the Schwann cells breaking down myelin and engulfing the fragmented axons.

18.054   Herpesvirus infection is associated with which one of the following alterations?
A. acute neuronal necrosis
B. block-like eosinophilic intranuclear inclusions in neurons
C. central chromatolysis
D. nemaline (rod body) myopathy
E. numerous small, round, eosinophilic structures in white matter
F. fiber-type grouping
G. round eosinophilic, layered, cytoplasmic inclusions in neurons
H. Wallerian degeneration

B is correct.
In herpes simplex virus encephalitis, the neurons as well as the glial cells contain eosinophilic intranuclear inclusions called 'Cowdry bodies'.

18.055 Dopaminergic neurons of the substantia nigra demonstrate which one of the following alterations in idiopathic Parkinson's disease?

    A. acute neuronal necrosis
    B. block-like eosinophilic intranuclear inclusions in neurons
    C. central chromatolysis
    D. nemaline (rod body) myopathy
    E. numerous small, round, eosinophilic structures in white matter
    F. fiber-type grouping
    G. round eosinophilic, layered, cytoplasmic inclusions in neurons
    H. Wallerian degeneration

G is correct.

In Parkinson's disease, the substantia nigra shows loss of pigmentation along with the accumulation of intracytoplasmic eosinophilic, round, layered inclusions in the dopaminergic neurons. These inclusions are called Lewy bodies.

18.056 Which one of the following alterations is the MOST typical histologic finding 12–24 h after infarction?

    A. acute neuronal necrosis
    B. block-like eosinophilic intranuclear inclusions in neurons
    C. central chromatolysis
    D. nemaline (rod body) myopathy
    E. numerous small, round, eosinophilic structures in white matter
    F. fiber-type grouping
    G. round eosinophilic, layered, cytoplasmic inclusions in neurons
    H. Wallerian degeneration

A is correct.

The typical reaction after an infarction is acute neuronal necrosis. There is shrinkage of the neuronal body, loss of Nissl substance, eosinophilia of the cytoplasm, and nuclear pyknosis.

18.057 An elderly patient with tremor is MOST likely to have which one of the following alterations?

    A. acute neuronal necrosis
    B. block-like eosinophilic intranuclear inclusions in neurons
    C. central chromatolysis
    D. nemaline (rod body) myopathy
    E. numerous small, round, eosinophilic structures in white matter
    F. fiber-type grouping
    G. round eosinophilic, layered, cytoplasmic inclusions in neurons
    H. Wallerian degeneration

G is correct.

In Parkinson's disease, the substantia nigra shows loss of pigmentation along with the accumulation of intracytoplasmic eosinophilic, round, layered inclusions in the dopaminergic neurons. These inclusions are called Lewy bodies.

18.058 Parkinson's disease may be associated with all of the following EXCEPT:
A. loss of neurons of substantia nigra
B. gliosis of substantia nigra
C. inflammatory cell infiltrate in substantia nigra
D. eosinophilic nuclear inclusions in neurons of substantia nigra
E. clinical dementia

C is correct.
There is no inflammatory infiltrate in the brain in Parkinson's disease.

18.059 Chronic ethanol abuse may cause all of the following EXCEPT:
A. degeneration of lateral corticospinal tracts
B. degeneration of vermis of cerebellum
C. atrophy of mammillary bodies
D. loss of myelin in pons
E. peripheral neuropathy

A is correct.
Degeneration of the lateral corticospinal tracts has not been observed secondary to alcoholism.

18.060 Middle-aged patients with Down syndrome virtually always develop:
A. atrophy of dendritic arborizations
B. occlusive hydrocephalus
C. neuritic plaques and neurofibrillary tangles
D. Wallerian degeneration
E. posterior column spinal cord degeneration

C is correct.
There is a marked tendency to Alzheimer-type changes such as neurofibrillary tangles and neuritic plaques in the brain of patients with Down syndrome. These changes may occur as early as age 30 years.

18.061 Integrity of the dura is important in a head trauma patient because:
A. the dura is a relatively effective barrier to infection
B. intracranial hematoma formation is less likely with the dura intact
C. opening the dura relieves intracranial pressure build-up
D. damage to the superior sagittal sinus can cause venous infarction
E. an intact dura rules out cranial fracture

A is correct.
The dura may serve as a barrier to infection. When it is not intact, infectious agents may more easily gain access to the brain.

18.062 Perivenous encephalomyelitis is thought to be the result of:
A. an autoimmune attack on CNS myelin
B. exposure to canine distemper virus
C. inappropriate astrocytic expression of major histocompatibility antigens
D. a neurotoxin elaborated by an anaerobic bacillus
E. a systemic vasculopathy

A is correct.
Perivenous encephalomyelitis is a rare disease that follows an acute course leading to either death or recovery. The basic lesion is a perivenous demyelination with a border of lymphocytes and macrophages. The disease is thought to be due to autoimmune events triggered by exogenous antigens.

18.063 Cingulate gyrus herniation may occur in a patient with:
  A. global cerebral anoxia with brain swelling
  B. hydrocephalus
  C. a subdural hematoma
  D. a cerebellar astrocytoma
  E. rachischisis

C is correct.
Cingulate gyrus herniation may occur with a unilateral lesion. The ipsilateral cerebral hemisphere is pushed to the contralateral side. The cingulate gyrus is pushed under the falx to the contralateral side.

18.064 The onset of symptoms is sudden in each of the following clinical situations EXCEPT:
  A. cerebral thrombosis
  B. cerebral embolism
  C. subarachnoid hemorrhage
  D. cerebral intraventricular hemorrhage

A is correct.
Cerebral thrombosis is clinically slowly progressive within a span of hours to days. Cerebral embolism and all intracranial hemorrhages are usually of abrupt onset.

18.065 Uncal herniation of the brain is LEAST likely to cause which one of the following conditions?
  A. posterior cerebral artery compression
  B. third cranial nerve compression
  C. infarction of anterior cerebral artery territory
  D. Duret hemorrhages in the tegmentum

C is correct.
Due to the anatomic arrangement, anterior cerebral artery compression is not likely to occur with uncal herniation.

18.066 Calcifications are commonly seen in which one of the following tumors?
  A. astrocytoma
  B. medulloblastoma
  C. neurofibroma
  D. ependymoma
  E. hemangioblastoma
  F. oligodendroglioma
  G. metastatic carcinoma

F is correct.
Oligodendrogliomas account for approximately 5–15% of gliomas. These neoplasms are well-circumscribed gelatinous masses, and often contain cysts, focal hemorrhages, and calcifications.

18.067 Perivenous encephalomyelitis is a rare complication of:
  A. antifungal chemotherapy
  B. childhood measles infection
  C. combined radiotherapy and methotrexate chemotherapy
  D. immunosuppression (for transplants, AIDS, etc.)
  E. various systemic viral infections

E is correct.
Perivenous encephalomyelitis is a rare disease that follows an acute course leading to either death or recovery. The basic lesion is a perivenous demyelination with a border of lymphocytes and macrophages. It is thought to be due to autoimmune events triggered by exogenous antigens. The disease may follow viral illnesses or vaccination against smallpox, typhoid/paratyphoid, and rabies.

The following case history relates to questions 18.068 and 18.069. A 50-year-old man arrives at the hospital following a motor-vehicle accident. Initially, he is awake and coherent, but his mental status declines markedly over the next several hours.

18.068   The diagnostic test MOST likely to yield a diagnosis for this patient is:
   A. careful neurological examination
   B. lumbar puncture
   C. imaging of brain (CT scan and/or MRI)
   D. cerebral arteriogram
   E. none of the above because the likely lesion is only demonstrable on microscopy

C is correct.
In a patient with head injury, initial alertness followed by rapid deterioration of mental status is probably due to epidural hemorrhage. Brain imaging is most likely to allow an accurate diagnosis.

18.069   The MOST appropriate immediate therapeutic intervention is:
   A. administration of agents designed to reverse brain swelling
   B. administration of anticoagulant therapy
   C. administration of broad-spectrum antibiotics
   D. emergency surgery
   E. whole body hypothermia

D is correct.
In a patient with head injury, initial alertness followed by rapid deterioration of mental status is probably due to epidural hemorrhage. This is a neurosurgical emergency requiring prompt surgical intervention.

18.070   Which one of the following microscopic findings suggests an infectious process?
   A. Hirano bodies
   B. Lewy bodies
   C. Marinesco bodies
   D. Negri bodies
   E. Pick bodies

D is correct.
The typical histologic finding in the viral illness rabies is the presence of cytoplasmic round-to-oval eosinophilic inclusions in neurons. These inclusions are called Negri bodies.

18.071   Which one of the following microscopic findings is diagnostic in the case of a 70-year-old man who died with tremor and rigidity, but with an intact intellect?
   A. Hirano bodies
   B. Lewy bodies
   C. Marinesco bodies
   D. Negri bodies
   E. Pick bodies

B is correct.
Idiopathic Parkinson's disease is characterized by loss of facial expression, slow voluntary movements, an altered gait, and a tremor. Many patients show no loss of intellect. Some of the neurons in the brain of these patients may contain intracytoplasmic, eosinophilic, round inclusions surrounded by a pale rim. These structures are called Lewy bodies.

18.072   The complex of cerebellar vermis herniation through the foramen magnum, displacement of the lower brain stem into the spinal canal, and lumbosacral meningomyelocele is known as:
   A. Arnold–Chiari malformation
   B. Friedreich's ataxia
   C. Guillain–Barré syndrome
   D. olivopontocerebellar syndrome
   E. Werdnig–Hoffmann malformation

A is correct.
In the Arnold–Chiari malformation, there is a small posterior fossa and a malformation of the midline cerebellum, with protrusion of the vermis through the foramen magnum, hydrocephalus, and lumbar myelomeningocele. There is often caudal displacement of the medulla, malformation of the tectum, and aqueductal stenosis.

18.073 Which one of the following entities is the MOST common?

    A. Dandy–Walker malformation
    B. neuronal heterotopias
    C. polymicrogyria
    D. schizencephaly
    E. spina bifida occulta

E is correct.

Failure of closure or reopening of the caudal portions of the neural tube results in spina bifida. It may be asymptomatic (spina bifida occulta) and may occur in up to 5% of 'normal' subjects.

18.074 Which one of the following is MOST likely to cause a watershed (border-zone) infarct between the middle cerebral and anterior cerebral arterial territories?

    A. embolic occlusion of middle cerebral artery
    B. a fall on the back of the head
    C. atherosclerotic occlusion of anterior cerebral artery
    D. leukemia
    E. myocardial infarction

E is correct.

A decreased circulation in the entire brain (global ischemia) may produce wedge-shaped zones of coagulation necrosis in the most distal areas of arterial supply. The border zone between the anterior and middle cerebral artery is at greatest risk. Myocardial infarction is the only condition listed that may cause global ischemia secondary to cardiogenic shock.

18.075 Hemorrhagic infarct in the brain involving the middle cerebral artery territory is MOST likely to be caused by:

    A. embolic occlusion of the artery
    B. rupture of a Charcot–Bouchard microaneurysm
    C. atherosclerotic occlusion of the artery
    D. hitting the side of the head on a hard wall
    E. a sequela of temporal lobe (uncus) herniation

A is correct.

Cerebral infarction may be due to thrombosis within a vessel supplying blood to the brain or due to embolization of a thrombus from a distant site. Thrombosis *in situ* is more usual in the extra-cerebral carotid system whereas embolism is the more common cause of occlusion in the intracranial vessels.

18.076 Carbon-monoxide poisoning usually produces which type of anoxia to the brain?

    A. anoxic
    B. anemic
    C. histotoxic
    D. ischemic

B is correct.

Anemic anoxia refers to anoxia secondary to a reduced oxygen content in hemoglobin. Carbon-monoxide poisoning is an example of this.

18.077 The microscopic finding of a spongy appearance in the gray matter of the brain suggests an infection by which one of the following agents?

    A. *Cryptococcus*
    B. prion
    C. herpes simplex virus
    D. *Aspergillus*
    E. *Phycomycetes (Mucor)*

B is correct.

Jakob–Creutzfeldt disease produces a characteristic spongiform alteration in the gray matter. The clinical manifestation of the disease is a rapidly progressive dementia. It is believed to be caused by a prion (proteinaceous infectious particle).

18.078 Which one of the following agents is MOST likely to cause infection of the brain in patients with diabetes mellitus?
  A. *Cryptococcus*
  B. prion
  C. herpes simplex virus
  D. *Aspergillus*
  E. *Phycomycetes* (*Mucor*)

E is correct.
Mucormycosis involving the brain may be a sequela of diabetic ketoacidosis. The organism spreads directly from the nasal sinuses to the brain. It is a rapidly progressive, fatal disease.

18.079 Amyotrophic lateral sclerosis is marked by degeneration and loss of all of the following EXCEPT:
  A. anterior horn cells of the spinal cord
  B. the lateral pyramidal pathway of the spinal cord
  C. motor nuclei of the brain stem
  D. upper motor neurons of the cerebral cortex
  E. neurons of the substantia nigra

E is correct.
Loss of neurons in the substantia nigra is a characteristic of idiopathic Parkinson's disease, but not amyotrophic lateral sclerosis.

18.080 All of the following apply to Parkinson's disease EXCEPT:
  A. tremors at rest and muscular rigidity
  B. involvement of dopaminergic neurons
  C. primary involvement of substantia nigra and locus ceruleus
  D. secondary involvement of parietal cortex
  E. eosinophilic cytoplasmic inclusions in pigmented neurons

D is correct.
The parietal cortex is not involved in Parkinson's disease.

18.081 The MOST common cause of meningitis in neonates is:
  A. *Escherichia coli*
  B. *Hemophilus influenzae*
  C. *Neisseria meningitidis*
  D. *Mycobacterium tuberculosis*
  E. viridans streptococci

A is correct.
Causative organisms in meningitis tend to vary with the age of the patient. In newborns, *E. coli* and group B streptococci are the most common pathogenic organisms.

The following case history relates to questions 18.082 and 18.083. A 20-year-old woman develops lower extremity muscle weakness and numbness following viral influenza. The weakness progresses to involve the upper extremities and cranial nerves. She then requires hospitalization and intubation.

18.082 A diagnostic biopsy of the peripheral nerve is performed. This biopsy is MOST likely to show:
   A. active primary myelin degeneration
   B. amyloid deposition within nerve fascicles
   C. axonal degeneration in a 'dying-back' pattern
   D. intrafascicular vasculitis
   E. numerous redundant, periaxonal, Schwann cells ('onion-bulb' formation)

A is correct.
Acute inflammatory demyelinating polyradiculoneuropathy (Guillain–Barré syndrome) is the most likely diagnosis in this patient. Immune-mediated segmental demyelination is thought to be the primary lesion.

18.083 The probability of survival in this patient is:
   A. nil (<1%)
   B. poor (<33%)
   C. more or less even (33–66%)
   D. good (>67%)
   E. excellent (>99%)

D is correct.
Acute inflammatory demyelinating polyradiculoneuropathy (Guillain–Barré syndrome) is the most likely diagnosis in this patient. Around 5% of patients die with this disease.

18.084 A 70-year-old man with no history of neurological problems or deficiencies dies because of atherosclerotic heart disease. At autopsy, a defect is found in his brain. The neuropathologist states that the defect was congenital, lifelong, and attributable to defective organogenesis *in utero*. What lesion is MOST likely to be found?
   A. agenesis of the corpus callosum
   B. neuronal heterotopias
   C. olfactory aplasia
   D. porencephaly
   E. spina bifida occulta

A is correct.
Agenesis of the corpus callosum is a fairly common malformation. It may be associated with normal intelligence and found incidentally at autopsy.

18.085 Which one of the following genetic alterations confers an increased risk for Alzheimer's disease?
   A. chromosome 17 translocations
   B. defective superoxide dismutase
   C. trinucleotide repeats on chromosome 4
   D. triplication of chromosome 21
   E. truncation of a plasma membrane-associated protein

D is correct.
In Down syndrome, there is a marked predilection for premature Alzheimer-type changes. These changes may be seen as early as age 30 years.

18.086 The MOST common pathophysiological pattern in peripheral neuropathy is:
   A. autoimmune polyneuritis
   B. distal axonopathy ('dying-back')
   C. primary segmental demyelination
   D. proximal axonal swellings due to impaired neurofilament transport
   E. transsynaptic degeneration

B is correct.
This is a very common form of peripheral nerve disease. Histologically, the distal axon undergoes atrophy, with subsequent demyelination.

18.087 'Flame-shaped' masses of neurofilaments within neuronal cell bodies and proximal dendrites are a characteristic feature of:
   A. Alzheimer's disease
   B. motor neuron disease
   C. olivopontocerebellar atrophy
   D. Parkinson's disease
   E. Pick's disease

A is correct.
In Alzheimer's disease, typically there are bundles of filaments which form inclusions in the cytoplasm of the neuron. These neurofibrillary tangles tend to be flame-like in shape.

18.088 Intracerebral hemorrhage primarily involving the putamen is MOST likely to be secondary to which one of the following?
   A. hemorrhagic diathesis
   B. ruptured berry aneurysm
   C. amyloid angiopathy
   D. hypertension

D is correct.
Hypertensive intracerebral hemorrhage has a predilection for the deep gray structures within the cerebral hemispheres. Around 50% originate in the putamen.

18.089 Which one of the following neoplasms is MOST frequently located in the fourth ventricle?
   A. astrocytoma
   B. glioblastoma multiforme
   C. ependymoma
   D. medulloblastoma
   E. meningioma

C is correct.
Ependymomas are derived from the ependymal cells which line the ventricles. A common location for these tumors is the fourth ventricle.

18.090 A cystic tumor of the cerebellum in a 10-year-old child is MOST likely to be which one of the following neoplasms?
   A. astrocytoma
   B. glioblastoma multiforme
   C. ependymoma
   D. medulloblastoma
   E. meningioma

A is correct.
A group of astrocytomas called pilocytic astrocytomas typically occur in children or young adults. They usually have a cystic morphology, occur in the cerebellum, and demonstrate benign behavior.

18.091 Which one of the following neoplasms is located exclusively in the cerebellum?
   A. astrocytoma
   B. glioblastoma multiforme
   C. ependymoma
   D. medulloblastoma
   E. meningioma

D is correct.
Medulloblastomas are midline tumors which usually occur in children and always in the cerebellum. The tumor is very malignant, but radiosensitive.

18.092 Which one of the following neoplasms is MOST likely to appear as a butterfly-like lesion involving both cerebral hemispheres?
   A. astrocytoma
   B. glioblastoma multiforme
   C. ependymoma
   D. medulloblastoma
   E. meningioma

B is correct.
Glioblastoma multiforme is the name given to a highly malignant astrocytoma which often spreads to replace the cerebral hemisphere and extends into the opposite hemisphere. This pattern is sometimes referred to as 'butterfly-like'.

18.093 Which one of the following neoplasms may be associated with hyperostosis of the contiguous bone of the skull?

    A. astrocytoma
    B. glioblastoma multiforme
    C. ependymoma
    D. medulloblastoma
    E. meningioma

E is correct.

Meningiomas are basically benign tumors which arise from meningothelial cells of the arachnoid. They are usually associated with the dura. Certain varieties of meningioma may be associated with hyperostotic reactive changes in the overlying bone of the skull.

18.094 A 25-year-old male contact-lens wearer comes to you with a complaint of redness, irritation, minimal serous discharge, and decreased vision in his right eye. He claims to care for his contact lenses appropriately with sterile solutions. On slit-lamp examination, you see a branching central ulcer in the right eye which stains brightly with fluorescein. The blink response to mechanical stimulation of the cornea is absent in contrast to a normal response in the left eye. Your presumptive diagnosis is:

    A. *Pseudomonas* keratitis
    B. herpes simplex keratitis
    C. *Acanthamoeba* keratitis
    D. *Chlamydia* keratitis
    E. *Candida* keratitis

B is correct.

A branching (dendritic) ulcer with decreased corneal sensation (hypesthesia) is typical of herpes simplex infection of the cornea. *Acanthamoeba* keratitis presents classically as a ring-shaped ulcer, pseudomonal keratitis as a suppurative ulcer, and candidal keratitis as a geographic ulcer with satellite lesions. Chlamydial keratitis typically produces a conjunctivitis.

18.095 A 3-year-old boy is brought to you by his parents, who have noticed that his left eye looks 'funny' and 'wanders'. On external examination, you see that the left eye turns in towards the nose. The pupil in that eye looks white in contrast to the normal black appearance in the right eye. A red reflex is seen on ophthalmoscopy in the right eye, but not in the left. You order a CT scan, which shows calcifications within the left eye. Your presumptive diagnosis is:

    A. proliferative diabetic retinopathy
    B. retinopathy of prematurity
    C. retinitis pigmentosa
    D. retinoblastoma
    E. age-related macular degeneration

D is correct.

The clinical findings (leukocoria and strabismus) and age (<5 years) of the patient are typical of retinoblastoma. Calcifications are often present within the tumor. Proliferative diabetic retinopathy and age-related macular degeneration occur in an older population. Retinitis pigmentosa is not associated with a white pupil. Retinopathy of prematurity may give these clinical findings, but lacks calcification on CT.

18.096 A 65-year-old woman complains of redness, tearing, pain, decreased vision, and seeing halos around lights in the left eye. The onset of her condition was sudden, after going to the movies on the previous evening. She denies feeling anything get into her eye. On external examination, her left eye has circumlimbal injection (redness) which does not blanch with topical epinephrine. The cornea is cloudy and thickened. A red reflex is present on ophthalmoscopy, but retinal details are hazy. You measure her intraocular pressure, which is 54 mmHg in the left eye and 18 mmHg in the right. Your presumptive diagnosis is:

A. acute closed-angle glaucoma
B. chronic closed-angle glaucoma
C. acute open-angle glaucoma
D. chronic open-angle glaucoma
E. congenital glaucoma

A is correct.

Open-angle glaucoma usually develops insidiously with few, if any, symptoms. Closed-angle glaucoma, in contrast, typically has a definable onset, often when the pupil is mid-dilated for prolonged periods of time such as in the dim illumination of a movie theater. The acute rise in intraocular pressure causes redness, pain, injection, and corneal edema. Repeated attacks may cause chronic changes in the aqueous outflow tract and persistent elevated pressure that is unrelieved by the usual treatment for closed-angle glaucoma.

18.097 A 59-year-old lawyer brings glass slides of his enucleated left eye to you for diagnosis and consultation. He has been told that the eye contains a melanoma. You see a monomorphic proliferation of elongated cells, with no distinct cytoplasmic borders, forming broad bundles or bands in the posterior choroid. The cell nuclei are also elongated, and contain dispersed chromatin and longitudinal grooves. No nucleoli or mitotic figures are present, nor is there invasion into the retina or sclera. You:

A. concur with the reported diagnosis and inform him that the histologic findings portend an excellent (92% survival) outcome
B. concur with the reported diagnosis and inform him that the histologic findings portend a good (85% survival) outcome
C. concur with the reported diagnosis and inform him that the histologic findings portend a fair (40% survival) outcome
D. concur with the reported diagnosis and inform him that the histologic findings portend a poor (28% survival) outcome
E. disagree with the reported diagnosis and inform him that he has metastatic disease with a dismal prognosis

A is correct.

The histologic features described are classified as a spindle cell melanoma, and may be further subclassified as spindle A-type (elongated nuclei with longitudinal grooves). This histologic subtype is associated with the best 15-year survival rate, approximately 92%. In contrast, spindle B-type melanoma cell nuclei have small, but identifiable, nucleoli rather than longitudinal grooves. Mixed spindle and epithelioid cell, and pure epithelioid cell melanomas have much worse survival rates. Metastatic melanoma in the choroid occurs, but is usually more pleomorphic and epithelioid in morphology.

18.098   A 70-year-old farmer comes to you with the main complaint of gradually decreasing vision without pain in his right eye. On external examination, you notice vascularized growths, one on each eye, at the nasal limbus, encroaching onto the cornea of the right eye into the visual axis (line of sight). Both growths have a triangular appearance with the base towards the cornea and the apex towards the medial canthus and nose. You decide to excise the growth on the right eye. You expect the clinicopathologic diagnosis from the pathologist to be:

    A. pinguecula
    B. pterygium
    C. pyogenic granuloma
    D. limbal dermoid
    E. squamous cell carcinoma

B is correct.
Although pinguecula and pterygium histologically are similar, pinguecula are confined to the perilimbal conjunctiva and do not encroach upon the cornea. Limbal dermoid is present early in life. The remaining choices may involve the cornea, but do not have a triangular ('winglike') appearance as seen in a pterygium.

18.099   The MOST common primary site for metastatic intraocular neoplasms in women is:

    A. lung
    B. endometrium
    C. ovary
    D. gastrointestinal tract
    E. breast

E is correct.
Breast and lung carcinomas are the two most commonly associated with intraocular metastases. A primary neoplasm in the lung is more likely in men.

18.100   You receive an eye from the eye bank for routine pathologic examination and, on histologic evaluation, observe diffuse retinal thinning with absence of ganglion cells, thinning of the nerve fiber layer, and deep cupping of the optic disc; the remainder of the eye is histologically unremarkable. Your histopathologic diagnosis is:

    A. phthisis bulbi
    B. retinal detachment
    C. cataract
    D. papilledema
    E. open-angle glaucoma

E is correct.
Open-angle glaucoma, if uncontrolled, leads to ischemia of the innermost layers of the retina, for example, in the ganglion cells and their axons which form the nerve fiber layer, and exit the eye at the optic disc. Atrophy of the axons causes loss of substance in the optic disc, resulting in the deep cupping.

18.101   You receive a glass-mounted corneal scraping from a patient and, on Papanicolaou staining, you can see polygonal cells with pale orange-pink cytoplasm and occasional multinucleated cells; the nuclei have a 'ground-glass' appearance and intranuclear inclusions. Your cytopathologic diagnosis is:

    A. corneal intraepithelial neoplasia
    B. squamous cell carcinoma
    C. pterygium
    D. herpes simplex keratitis
    E. melanoma

D is correct.
The cells described are corneal epithelial cells infected by herpes simplex virus. The cytologic findings are typical of herpes and identical to those seen in gynecologic (Papanicolaou smear) and dermatologic (Tzanck preparation) scrapings of herpetic vesicobullous lesions. No dysplastic or malignant nuclear characteristics are described, which may be seen in the remaining choices.

18.102 All of the following diseases may be associated with retinal or subretinal neovascularization EXCEPT:
- A. age-related macular degeneration
- B. diabetic retinopathy
- C. retinopathy of prematurity
- D. hypertensive retinopathy

D is correct.
Proliferation of new blood vessels (neovascularization) may be a complication of diabetes, retinopathy of prematurity, and macular degeneration. Hypertension typically causes hemorrhages, cottonwool spots, exudates, and optic disc edema if severe, but no neovascularization.

18.103 According to the Callender classification, the histologic type of uveal melanoma, in decreasing order of incidence, is:
- A. mixed, spindle B, spindle A, epithelioid
- B. spindle B, spindle A, epithelioid, mixed
- C. epithelioid, mixed, spindle B, spindle A
- D. spindle A, spindle B, mixed, epithelioid

A is correct.
Mixed spindle and epithelioid cell melanoma is the most common histologic type, occurring in around 40% of cases; epithelioid is the least common ($< 5\%$)

18.104 A 75-year-old woman comes to the emergency room complaining of sudden complete loss of vision in the left eye. On direct ophthalmoscopy of the left eye, you see a cloudy gray retina devoid of hemorrhages with a cherry-red spot. The right eye is unremarkable. Your diagnosis is:
- A. central retinal vein occlusion
- B. central retinal artery occlusion
- C. age-related macular degeneration, disciform type
- D. age-related macular degeneration, atrophic type
- E. macular dystrophy

B is correct.
Central retinal artery occlusion causes a sudden complete loss of vision. The retina becomes edematous, and the cherry-red spot is due to increased visibility of the underlying choroid at the point where the retina is normally thinnest: the fovea. Central retinal vein occlusion causes massive retinal hemorrhaging ('strawberry sundae') with diminished, but not absent, vision. Macular diseases may cause loss of central vision, but with retention of peripheral vision.

18.105 A 75-year-old woman comes to the emergency room complaining of sudden loss of central vision in the left eye. On direct ophthalmoscopy, you see a large subretinal hemorrhage in the macula of the left eye. The right eye shows multiple small yellow dots in the macula with no other abnormalities. Your diagnosis of the left eye is:
- A. central retinal vein occlusion
- B. central retinal artery occlusion
- C. age-related macular degeneration (ARMD) disciform type
- D. age-related macular degeneration (ARMD), atrophic type
- E. macular dystrophy

C is correct.
A sudden decrease in central visual acuity in an elderly patient due to bleeding in the macular/foveal subretinal space indicates a choroidal/subretinal neovascular membrane, the 'wet' or disciform type of ARMD. The opposite eye shows funduscopic evidence of the 'dry' form of ARMD. Macular dystrophy presents earlier in life with a gradual decrease in visual acuity and, typically, has a more symmetric funduscopic appearance. Artery and vein occlusions, which often occur in the elderly, do not have the funduscopic appearance of isolated macular/foveal subretinal hemorrhage. Central retinal artery occlusions cause a complete loss of the entire visual field, not just the central field; and central retinal vein occlusions cause severe diminution of the entire visual field.

18.106 A 75-year-old woman comes to the emergency room complaining of sudden loss of central vision in the left eye. On direct ophthalmoscopy, you cannot visualize the retina due to a vitreous hemorrhage. In the right eye, you see multiple intra-retinal small round hemorrhages and discrete small yellowish-white deposits, and cystic spaces in the macula. There appear to be more vessels on the optic disc than usual. You surmise that the vitreous hemorrhage in the left eye is due to:
    A. trauma
    B. retinopathy of prematurity
    C. age-related macular degeneration
    D. proliferative diabetic retinopathy
    E. hypertensive retinopathy

D is correct.

The funduscopic appearance of the right eye is typical of proliferative diabetic retinopathy (neo-vascularization of the optic disc), with associated background changes of dot/blot hemorrhages, exudates, and cystoid macular edema. Vitreous hemorrhage is a common complication of proliferative diabetic retinopathy, and is not usually seen in ARMD or hypertensive retinopathy. Whereas vitreous hemorrhage may be a complication of trauma or retinopathy of prematurity, the findings in the fellow eye are not consistent with those etiologies.

18.107 A 75-year-old woman comes to the emergency room complaining of sudden loss of superior vision in the left eye following cataract surgery 3 months earlier. On direct ophthalmoscopy, you visualize the superior retina without adding plus or minus lenses, but must add six diopters of power (+6D) to focus the inferior retina. The right eye is post-cataract surgery and artificial lens implantation 1 year previously, with good results. Ophthalmoscopy of the right eye is unremarkable. You call in the ophthalmologist and expect that he is MOST likely to find retinal detachment due to:
    A. peripheral retinal tears occurring after the intraocular surgery
    B. an underlying choroidal melanoma
    C. traction from proliferative diabetic retinopathy
    D. high myopia
    E. an underlying metastatic tumor

A is correct.

Patients undergoing cataract surgery are at an increased risk of developing retinal detachment, which typically occurs in the first 1–2 years following surgery as a result of detachment of the vitreous, causing tears in the retina. As the detached retina is displaced anteriorly (towards the cornea), more refractive power is necessary to focus on the detached portion. Although subretinal tumors, either primary or metastatic, may cause retinal detachment, their frequency is much less than detachments following cataract surgery. No funduscopic features of myopia or diabetes are present to suggest those etiologies.

18.108 Cataract is an opacification of the:
    A. cornea
    B. aqueous humor
    C. pupil
    D. lens
    E. vitreous humor

D is correct.
Cataracts are opacities within or opacification of the lens.

18.109 The histologic cell type of uveal melanoma portending the BEST chance of long-term survival is:

A. epithelioid
B. spindle A
C. mixed epithelioid and spindle
D. spindle B
E. necrotic

B is correct.
According to the Callender classification (spindle A, spindle B, epithelioid, and mixed) of uveal melanomas, tumors composed of the spindle A cell type have a >90% 15-year survival rate; spindle B melanomas are slightly worse at around 80–85%. The epithelioid cell type, and mixtures of spindle and epithelioid cell types, have 30–40% 15-year survival rates, as do necrotic unclassifiable tumors.

18.110 Which one of the following ophthalmoscopic findings categorizes a diabetic patient as having proliferative retinopathy?

A. microaneurysms
B. macular edema
C. neovascularization
D. arteriolar–venular shunts
E. cotton-wool spots

C is correct.
The *sine qua non* for the diagnosis of proliferative diabetic retinopathy is the presence of neovascularization of the retina either at the optic disc or elsewhere. The other abnormalities listed may be seen in earlier stages of diabetic retinopathy (background or preproliferative diabetic retinopathy).

18.111 Characteristics of the retinoblastoma gene include:

A. normal gene product functions as a tumor promoter
B. located on chromosome 14 (14q13 locus)
C. mutation of both alleles is necessary for the development of retinoblastoma
D. close proximity to the gene for aniridia

C is correct.
The retinoblastoma gene on chromosome 13q14 is a tumor suppressor gene and codes for a protein which regulates the cell cycle. Mutations of both alleles of chromosome 13 allow unchecked cell division and, therefore, tumor formation. The defective gene locus in aniridia is on chromosome 11p (11p13).

18.112 The MOST common type of glaucoma is:
A. congenital glaucoma
B. open-angle glaucoma
C. chronic angle-closure glaucoma
D. acute angle-closure glaucoma

B is correct.
Chronic open-angle glaucoma affects >2% of the population >40 years of age. Angle-closure glaucoma and congenital forms of glaucoma are much less common.

18.113 Of the following corneal dystrophies, the one which has an autosomal-recessive inheritance pattern is:
A. Fuchs' dystrophy
B. granular dystrophy
C. lattice dystrophy
D. macular dystrophy

D is correct.
Granular and lattice dystrophies of the cornea have an autosomal-dominant inheritance, and Fuchs' dystrophy has no recognized pattern of inheritance. Macular dystrophy is an autosomal-recessive disorder.

SECTION 19: PEDIATRIC DISEASES

19.001 Short- or long-term complications of oxygen therapy in respiratory distress syndrome in the neonate may include all of the following EXCEPT:
   A. necrotizing enterocolitis
   B. bronchopulmonary dysplasia
   C. intraventricular hemorrhage
   D. erythroblastosis fetalis
   E. patent ductus arteriosus

D is correct.
Premature neonates requiring oxygen therapy are at risk of developing not only retinopathy of prematurity, but also necrotizing enterocolitis, intraventricular hemorrhage, persistent patent ductus arteriosus, and bronchopulmonary dysplasia. Erythroblastosis fetalis is not a complication of oxygen therapy, but rather a maternal–fetal blood group incompatibility.

19.002 Malignant neoplasms occurring principally in the infant/childhood years include all of the following EXCEPT:
   A. retinoblastoma
   B. Wilms' tumor
   C. hepatoblastoma
   D. medulloblastoma
   E. hemangioma

E is correct.
Hemangioma is a common benign tumor of infancy which typically regresses spontaneously. All of the other tumors listed are malignant pediatric tumors.

19.003 A mother brings her 10-year-old son to you, complaining of his chronic productive cough and foul-smelling floating bowel movements, symptoms which have persisted for several years. You note on examination that he is small for his age and you hear decreased breath sounds in the left lung field, but find no other specific abnormalities on physical examination. Additional studies that you suspect will be abnormal in this case include all of the following EXCEPT:
   A. chest X-ray
   B. CT scan of the abdomen/retroperitoneum
   C. sputum culture
   D. fecal culture
   E. sweat chloride test

D is correct.
Signs and symptoms of cystic fibrosis usually appear in childhood, and reflect the organs either primarily or secondarily damaged by mucus impaction: lungs; pancreas; intestines; and liver. Bronchiectasis and secondary bronchopneumonia are common complications of bronchial mucus plugging. Pancreatic exocrine atrophy leads to malabsorption; fecal cultures are usually not rewarding. Elevated sweat chloride is diagnostic of the disease.

19.004 You have just delivered a 7.5-lb baby boy, estimated gestational age 38 weeks, to a 31-year-old mother of two; at 5 min after birth, you observe that the neonate is pink with blue extremities, crying heartily, showing a heart rate of 140 beats/min, moving all extremities actively, and grimacing to a catheter placed in the nostril. You estimate that this neonate will have:
  A. 100% survival during the first month of life
  B. 80% survival during the first month of life
  C. 60% survival during the first month of life
  D. 40% survival during the first month of life
  E. 20% survival during the first month of life

A is correct.
The Apgar score at 5 min in this scenario is 8, which is associated with a nearly 100% survival rate by age 1 month.

19.005 Sudden infant death syndrome (SIDS) MOST commonly occurs during which age range?
  A. 0–6 months
  B. 6–12 months
  C. 12–18 months
  D. 18–24 months
  E. 24–30 months

A is correct.
SIDS is most common in the first half of the first year of life, and should be diagnosed with extreme caution, if at all, after the first year.

19.006 MOST birth defects are due to:
  A. intrauterine infection
  B. genetic abnormalities
  C. birth trauma
  D. maternal metabolic disease
  E. unknown causes

E is correct.
Most birth defects are probably multifactorial, involving a variety of genetic and environmental factors.

19.007 A 6-foot 4-inch, 150-lb, myopic, 14-year-old boy comes to you for a physical examination for football tryouts. He has no physical complaints. You find on external examination that he has kyphoscoliosis (abnormal curvature of the spine) and pectus excavatum (depression of the sternum). You suspect that he has Marfan's syndrome. The MOST important part of your physical examination, in terms of the patient's long-term well-being, is:
  A. auscultation of the lungs
  B. auscultation of the heart
  C. ophthalmoscopy
  D. palpation of the abdomen
  E. neurologic testing

B is correct.
Patients with Marfan's syndrome may have aneurysms of the aorta, which may rupture suddenly and cause death. Cardiac auscultation and imaging studies are therefore important in these patients.

19.008 Incomplete formation of a lumen in a normally hollow organ is called:
  A. agenesis
  B. aplasia
  C. atresia
  D. hypoplasia
  E. dysplasia

C is correct.
Incomplete luminal formation in a normally hollow organ is termed atresia.

19.009   The abnormal organization of cells into tissues is called:
   A. agenesis
   B. aplasia
   C. atresia
   D. hypoplasia
   E. dysplasia

E is correct.
In the developmental sense, dysplasia refers to abnormal organization of cells within a tissue or organ.

19.010   Complications of oxygen therapy for respiratory distress syndrome include all of the following EXCEPT:
   A. patent ductus arteriosus
   B. kernicterus
   C. bronchopulmonary dysplasia
   D. necrotizing enterocolitis
   E. intraventricular hemorrhage

B is correct.
Kernicterus, or bile-staining of the basal ganglia of the brain, is a complication of erythroblastosis fetalis, not of oxygen therapy in the premature neonate.

19.011   The virus responsible for the congenital infection resulting in the tetrad of deafness, cataracts, mental retardation, and cardiovascular defects is:
   A. cytomegalovirus
   B. herpes simplex virus
   C. varicella–zoster virus
   D. rubella virus
   E. human immunodeficiency virus

D is correct.
A variety of viral agents may cause intrauterine fetal infections, but rubella, particularly during the first trimester, causes the associated findings of deafness, mental retardation, cataracts, and cardiovascular malformations.

19.012   The MOST common cause of death in children after the age of 1 year is:
   A. malignancy
   B. congenital anomalies
   C. pneumonia
   D. accident
   E. homicide

D is correct.
Whereas congenital/perinatal processes are the most common causes of death in the neonate/infant, accidents are by far the most common cause of death in the pediatric population after the first year of life.

19.013   An overgrowth of mature tissue normally present within an organ or body site is a(n):
   A. teratoma
   B. hamartoma
   C. hygroma
   D. adenoma
   E. choristoma

B is correct.
A hamartoma is a tumor due to the proliferation of histologically mature tissue normally present at that site (for example, chondroid hamartoma of the lung). A choristoma consists of tissue not normally present at that site (for example, a dermoid cyst within the orbit). A hygroma is a benign neoplasm of lymphatic tissue; a teratoma, which may be mature or immature, contains elements of all three germ layers. An adenoma results from proliferation of glandular tissue.

19.014   The major determinant of survival in the preterm neonate is the maturity of which one of the following organs?
   A. brain
   B. lungs
   C. kidneys
   D. liver

B is correct.
Pulmonary maturity and function is the single most important determinant in survival of the immature neonate. All other organ systems, being perhaps marginal, are adequate for survival.

19.015   Hemolytic disease of the fetus/newborn due to maternal–fetal ABO incompatibility is MOST commonly a result of which specific mismatch?
   A. fetus type B, mother type AB
   B. fetus type O, mother type A
   C. fetus type AB, mother type B
   D. fetus type A, mother type O

D is correct.
Hemolytic disease of the fetus/newborn, when due to maternal–fetal ABO mismatch, is most commonly seen when the mother is type O and has circulating IgG anti-A antibodies. These may cross the placenta and bind to the fetal erythrocytes, causing their premature destruction.

19.016 Cystic fibrosis is associated with which one of the following genetic abnormalities?
   A. 13q14 deletion/mutation
   B. 11p13 deletion/mutation
   C. trisomy 21
   D. trisomy 13
   E. 7q deletion/mutation

E is correct.
The gene defect causing cystic fibrosis has been mapped to chromosome 7q31–32; most cases are deletions of a three base-pair sequence which normally codes for phenylalanine at position 508 of the amino-acid sequence of the transmembrane conductance regulator protein.

19.017   Retinoblastoma is associated with which one of the following genetic abnormalities?
   A. 13q14 deletion/mutation
   B. 11p13 deletion/mutation
   C. trisomy 21
   D. trisomy 13
   E. 7q deletion/mutation

A is correct.
The retinoblastoma gene has been localized to the q14 locus of chromosome 13; mutations or deletions within this gene cause an abnormal gene product which fails to regulate cell DNA cycling, leading to uncontrolled proliferation.

19.018 Wilms' tumor is associated with which one of the following genetic alterations?
   A. 13q14 deletion/mutation
   B. 11p13 deletion/mutation
   C. trisomy 21
   D. trisomy 13
   E. 7q deletion/mutation

B is correct.
Wilms' tumor is often associated with deletions or mutations of chromosome 11p; the majority are at locus p13 and, as with retinoblastoma, are believed to be a defect in a tumor supressor gene.

19.019 You are present at the premature birth of a female neonate born to a G4, P2, Ab1 woman known to abuse alcohol. At 5 min, you observe that the neonate is completely limp and blue, has a weak irregular heartbeat with a rate of 50 beats / min, has no spontaneous respirations, and does not respond to a catheter placed in the nostril. Resuscitation measures were instituted at birth and are ongoing. You can predict that the chances of this neonate surviving for 1 month are:

    A. 0%

    B. 20%

    C. 50%

    D. 80%

    E. 100%

B is correct.

The Apgar score for this neonate is 1 at 5 min; such a score is associated with an 80% mortality during the first month of life.

19.020 A parent brings her 2-year-old daughter to you for evaluation of mental developmental delay. On physical examination, you notice that the child has eyes with extremely large pupils that do not constrict with light and, in fact, appear black without a visible iris. You palpate a large right-sided abdominal mass. Karyotypic analysis identifies a deletion in the short arm of chromosome 11 (11p-). If the mass is removed and examined histologically, the MOST important prognostic histologic parameter is the:

    A. presence of rosettes

    B. presence of nuclear anaplasia

    C. presence of necrosis

    D. presence of invasion

    E. presence of lymphocytic host response

B is correct.

This child exhibits signs of the WAGR syndrome (Wilms' tumor, aniridia, genitourinary abnormalities and mental retardation) due to deletions / mutations on chromosome 11p13. A poor prognosis in Wilms' tumor, when based on histologic parameters, correlates with the presence of nuclear anaplasia.

19.021 You are called to the home of a single 19-year-old mother, who is G4, P3, Ab1, and known to abuse tobacco and illicit drugs. She reports finding her 4-month-old son face down and not breathing 15 min after having placed him in the crib (awake) for his afternoon nap. A previous sibling died at age 6 months reportedly as a result of SIDS (sudden infant death syndrome). You are suspicious in this case because:

    A. SIDS usually occurs after 6 months of age

    B. SIDS has been associated with a supine sleeping position

    C. there are no known maternal risk factors for SIDS

    D. SIDS does not tend to occur in siblings

    E. SIDS deaths occur following a period of sleep and usually during the night

E is correct.

Risk for the occurrence of SIDS increases with certain maternal factors (youth, low socioeconomic status, cigarette / drug abuse), familial factors (prior siblings dying of SIDS), and infant factors (prone sleeping position, age < 6 months). SIDS deaths usually occur at night or after a period of sleep, and the diagnosis should be regarded with suspicion where the infant was awake immediately prior to death.

19.022   Congenital deformations in comparison to congenital malformations:

    A. occur earlier in gestation
    B. recur more often in subsequent gestations
    C. are more common
    D. are more severe

C is correct.
Congenital deformations typically occur later in pregnancy, after organogenesis has taken place. The deformations are not usually severe or life-threatening, and do not increase the risk of occurrence in subsequent pregnancies. The frequency of deformations is greater than that of malformations.

19.023   A nursing mother, a migrant worker from Mexico, brings her only child, a 2-month-old girl, to you because of persistent vomiting and diarrhea after feeding. You note that the infant is at the 5th percentile for weight and 15th percentile for height compared with normal infants of that age, although the mother reports that the child was of normal size and weight at birth. You note that the child has leukocoria ('white pupils') bilaterally. Analysis of a urine specimen confirms your clinical diagnosis. You recommend:

    A. dietary restriction of phenylalanine
    B. dietary restriction of galactose
    C. dietary restriction of tyrosine
    D. dietary restriction of fructose

B is correct.
Failure to thrive may be due to enzyme deficiencies associated with all of the metabolic disorders listed, but the presence of cataracts is most consistent with the diagnosis of galactosemia.

19.024   The organs significantly and functionally affected by cystic fibrosis, either directly or indirectly, include all of the following EXCEPT:

    A. lungs
    B. liver
    C. pancreas
    D. intestines
    E. skin

E is correct.
Although cystic fibrosis may be detected because of elevated chloride levels in sweat, the skin is not functionally impaired in cystic fibrosis. All other organs listed may be affected by mucus inspissation and its complications.

19.025   An example of a specific type of congenital malformation due to dystopia is:

    A. esophageal stricture
    B. spina bifida
    C. syndactyly
    D. microcephaly
    E. cryptorchidism

E is correct.
Dystopia refers to the retention of an organ at the site of its location during development, such as the testis within the inguinal canal.

19.026   Accidents are the leading cause of death in the age range:

    A. birth to < 1 year
    B. birth to age 4 years
    C. ages 1–4 years
    D. ages 1–14 years
    E. ages 5–14 years

D is correct.
Although congenital and perinatal problems account for most deaths in the first year of life, accidents are the leading cause of death in the subsequent years of childhood (ages 1–14 years).

19.027 The MOST common intrauterine infection of the fetus is:
  A. herpes simplex virus
  B. varicella–zoster virus
  C. cytomegalovirus
  D. rubella virus
  E. human immunodeficiency virus

C is correct.
All of the viruses listed may cause intrauterine infections, but cytomegalovirus is the most commonly identified viral agent.

19.028 The major long-term complication of perinatal hypoxia in a live-born term neonate is:
  A. neurological deficit
  B. patent ductus arteriosus
  C. bronchopulmonary dysplasia
  D. necrotizing enterocolitis
  E. caput succedaneum

A is correct.
The major long-term complication in patients surviving hypoxia in the perinatal period is neurologic, such as cerebral palsy. Patent ductus arteriosus, bronchopulmonary dysplasia, and necrotizing enterocolitis are complications associated with oxygen therapy for respiratory distress syndrome. Caput succedaneum is not usually associated with long-term complications.

19.029 So-called 'small, round, blue, cell tumors' of childhood include all of the following EXCEPT:
  A. neuroblastoma
  B. retinoblastoma
  C. lymphangioma
  D. Wilms' tumor
  E. lymphoma

C is correct.
Of the neoplasms listed, lymphangioma is the only one not characterized histologically by the presence of closely packed small cells with scant cytoplasm, imparting a blue appearance to the tissue when mounted on a glass slide. Lymphangioma demonstrates an infiltrating pattern of dilated vascular spaces containing lymph fluid.

19.030 A very low-birth-weight neonate is, by definition, one whose weight is:
  A. $< 500\,g$
  B. $< 1000\,g$
  C. $< 1500\,g$
  D. $< 2000\,g$
  E. $< 2500\,g$

C is correct.
A low birth-weight is defined as $< 2500\,g$, and a very low birth-weight is $< 1500\,g$.

19.031 What is the lowest ratio of antenatal lecithin to sphingomyelin considered sufficient to minimize the risk of postnatal respiratory distress syndrome?
  A. 0.0 : 1.0
  B. 0.5 : 1.0
  C. 1.0 : 1.0
  D. 1.5 : 1.0
  E. 2.0 : 1.0

E is correct.
When the ratio of lecithin to sphingomyelin reaches or exceeds 2 : 1, the lungs are considered sufficiently mature, rendering the risk of respiratory distress syndrome minimal.

19.032   The risk for developing sudden infant death syndrome (SIDS) in a neonate/infant may be reduced by:
    A. the mother being a teenager
    B. being premature at birth
    C. having a sibling with SIDS
    D. sleeping in a supine position
    E. being <6 months of age

D is correct.
The risk for SIDS increases with maternal factors (young age, low socioeconomic status, drug abuse), familial factors (SIDS in a sibling), and infant factors (age <6 months, premature at birth, prone sleeping position).

19.033   Symmetric (proportionate) intrauterine growth retardation (type I IUGR) is characteristic of which group of etiologic factors?
    A. fetal
    B. maternal
    C. placental
    D. paternal

A is correct.
When the growth retardation preferentially spares the brain, the retardation is termed 'asymmetric' or 'disproportionate', and indicates that maternal or placental factors are responsible for the retardation. When fetal factors are involved, the retardation is usually symmetric (the brain is not spared and is growth-retarded proportional to the remainder of the body).

19.034   Significant hemolytic disease in the newborn due to maternal–fetal ABO mismatch occurs MOST often in mothers with maternal blood type:
    A. AB
    B. A
    C. B
    D. O

D is correct.
Mothers with blood type O may have naturally occurring, circulating IgG anti-A antibodies that cross the placenta and coat the erythrocytes of type A fetuses, causing hemolytic disease. Other maternal–fetal ABO mismatches are much less commonly the cause of significant hemolytic disease.